Obesity Treatment

Establishing Goals, Improving Outcomes, and Reviewing the Research Agenda

NATO ASI Series

Advanced Science Institutes Series

A series presenting the results of activities sponsored by the NATO Science Committee, which aims at the dissemination of advanced scientific and technological knowledge, with a view to strengthening links between scientific communities.

The series is published by an international board of publishers in conjunction with the NATO Scientific Affairs Division

A	Life Sciences	Plenum Publishing Corporation
B	Physics	New York and London
C	Mathematical and Physical Sciences	Kluwer Academic Publishers Dordrecht, Boston, and London
D	Behavioral and Social Sciences	
E	Applied Sciences	
F	Computer and Systems Sciences	Springer-Verlag
G	Ecological Sciences	Berlin, Heidelberg, New York, London,
H	Cell Biology	Paris, Tokyo, Hong Kong, and Barcelona
I	Global Environmental Change	

PARTNERSHIP SUB-SERIES

1. Disarmament Technologies	Kluwer Academic Publishers
2. Environment	Springer-Verlag
3. High Technology	Kluwer Academic Publishers
4. Science and Technology Policy	Kluwer Academic Publishers
5. Computer Networking	Kluwer Academic Publishers

The Partnership Sub-Series incorporates activities undertaken in collaboration with NATO's Cooperation Partners, the countries of the CIS and Central and Eastern Europe, in Priority Areas of concern to those countries.

Recent Volumes in this Series:

Series A: Life Sciences

Obesity Treatment

Establishing Goals, Improving Outcomes, and Reviewing the Research Agenda

Edited by

David B. Allison and
F. Xavier Pi-Sunyer

Obesity Research Center
Saint Luke's/Roosevelt Hospital
Columbia University College of Physicians and Surgeons
New York, New York

Plenum Press
New York and London
Published in cooperation with NATO Scientific Affairs Division

Proceedings of a NATO Advanced Research Workshop on
Obesity Treatment,
held June 2–5, 1993,
in New York, New York

NATO-PCO-DATA BASE

The electronic index to the NATO ASI Series provides full bibliographical references (with keywords and/or abstracts) to about 50,000 contributions from international scientists published in all sections of the NATO ASI Series. Access to the NATO-PCO-DATA BASE is possible in two ways:

—via online FILE 128 (NATO-PCO-DATA BASE) hosted by ESRIN, Via Galileo Galilei, I-00044 Frascati, Italy

—via CD-ROM "NATO Science and Technology Disk" with user-friendly retrieval software in English, French, and German (©WTV GmbH and DATAWARE Technologies, Inc. 1989). The CD-ROM also contains the AGARD Aerospace Database.

The CD-ROM can be ordered through any member of the Board of Publishers or through NATO-PCO, Overijse, Belgium.

Library of Congress Cataloging-in-Publication Data

```
Obesity treatment : establishing goals, improving outcomes, and
   reviewing the research agenda / edited by David B. Allison and F.
   Xavier Pi-Sunyer.
       p.    cm. -- (Nato ASI SERIES. Series A, Life sciences ; 278)
     "Proceedings of a NATO Advanced Research Workshop on Obesity
   Treatment, held June 2-5, 1993, in New York, New York"--T.p. verso.
     "Published in cooperation with NATO Scientific Affairs Division."
   Includes bibliographical references and index.
     ISBN 0-306-45115-8
     1. Obesity--Congresses.   I. Allison, David B.   II. Pi-Sunyer, F.
   Xavier.   III. North Atlantic Treaty Organization.   Scientific
   Affairs Division.   IV. NATO Advanced Research Workshop on Obesity
   Treatment (1993 : New York, N.Y.)   V. Series.
     [DNLM: 1. Obesity--therapy--congresses.   WD 210 O126 1995]
   RC628.033  1995
   616.3'98--dc20
   DNLM/DLC
   for Library of Congress                                95-35961
                                                             CIP
```

ISBN 0-306-45115-8

© 1995 Plenum Press, New York
A Division of Plenum Publishing Corporation
233 Spring Street, New York, N. Y. 10013

10 9 8 7 6 5 4 3 2 1

Printed in the United States of America

ORGANIZING COMMITTEE

David B. Allison, Ph.D. and F. Xavier Pi-Sunyer, M.D.
New York Obesity Research Center
St. Luke's/Roosevelt Hospital
Columbia University College of Physicians and Surgeons

Jules Hirsch, M.D.
New York Obesity Research Center
Rockefeller Universtiy

Per Bjorntörp, M.D., Ph.D.
University of Gothenberg

Albert J. Stunkard, M.D.
University of Pennsylvania

Claude Bouchard, Ph.D.
Laval University

SPONSORS

The North Atlantic Treaty Organization (NATO)
The National Institutes of Diabetes, Digestive, and Kidney Diseases (NIDDK)
The National Heart, Lung, and Blood Institute (NHLBI)
The National Institute of Child Health and Development (NICHD)

CONTRIBUTORS

American Psychological Association
Best Foods
Boots Pharmaceuticals, Inc.
Campbell Soup Company
Eli Lilly and Company
Food Education Society of England
Health Management Resources
Hoffman-LaRoche, Inc.
Jenny Craig, Inc.
Lederle Laboratories - American Cyanamide
M&M Mars
Mead Johnson Nutritional Group
MetPath, Inc.
NutraSweet Company
Pepsi-Cola Company
Pritikin Systems, Inc.
Ross Laboratories - New Directions
Sandoz Nutrition Corporation
Servier Amérique
Weight Watchers International

PREFACE

Treatment outcome has certainly improved since Stunkard and McLaren-Hume (1959) reviewed the literature and found that less than 25% of obese patients lost 20 pounds or more and less than 5% lost 40 pounds or more. However, one of the few points on which almost all obesity researchers agree is that to date, our results are quite modest and we are generally unsuccessful in promoting effective weight maintenance among obese persons. As the title of a more recent article, "Improving long-term weight loss: *Pushing the limits of treatment*," (Brownell & Jeffrey, 1987, [emphasis added]) suggests, many believe that we have pushed our current treatment paradigms to the limit.

It was with this background in mind that we organized the meeting from which these proceedings issue. The purpose of the three day international meeting was to evaluate the current knowledge base and conceptual paradigms of obesity treatment and to suggest directions for future research and clinical practice. Rather than simply for research reporting, the meeting was primarily for research generation. All speakers were established scientists in the field who were asked to summarize our state of knowledge in a given area rather than present the results of their latest research. Great efforts were taken to ensure that panel discussions occupied a central portion of the conference, and that the questions *"What else do we need to know?"* and *"How do we find it out?"* were consistently addressed. To that end, in addition to the group of obesity experts, several methodologists were also invited. These methodologists not only gave preplanned talks on the third day of the meeting, but were present throughout to offer commentary on information presented by the substantive researchers and issues raised in panel discussions.

The meeting was intended to be somewhat "extra-paradigmatic." We hoped to step back from established conceptions of treatment research and explore alternative conceptions and strategies. As such, the program did not include talks which elaborated on the application of established techniques or minor variants thereof to achieve weight loss. Rather, broader addresses which focused on issues for which there are fewer clear answers were solicited. Consequently, participants were chosen who could integrate diverse and complex research findings and offer some perspective on "the big picture." Participants were also selected who hold diverse opinions and expertise. For example, we were mindful to include investigators who represent both the "mainstream" and the "outskirts" of the obesity research community. We aimed to promote an atmosphere where divergent ideas would be freely expressed but critically examined, and anticipated that this would lead to conceptions of obesity treatment that would take us outside the confines of our current paradigms.

A second objective of the meeting was to produce these published proceedings in the hopes that such a publication could have a major impact on the field by summarizing our current state of knowledge and, more importantly, clarifying the future research agenda. It is hoped that this document will spark new and innovative research among a wide audience of investigators and ultimately lead to better outcomes for obese persons. Only time will tell how well we have met these objectives.

David B. Allison, Ph.D.   F. Xavier Pi-Sunyer, M.D., M.P.H.

REFERENCES

Brownell, K. D., & Jeffrey, R. W. (1987). Improving long-term weight loss: Pushing the limits of treatment. Behavior Therapy, 18, 353-374.

Stunkard, A. J., & McLaren - Hume, M. (1959). The results of treatment for obesity. Archives of Internal Medicine, 103, 79-85.

CONTENTS

IN SEARCH OF OPTIMAL WEIGHTS FOR U.S. MEN AND WOMEN

Theodore B. VanItallie and Edward A. Lew

Department of Medicine
Columbia University College of Physicians and Surgeons
St. Luke's/Roosevelt Hospital
New York, NY 10025

INTRODUCTION

An "optimal" body weight has to be optimal for a particular purpose, otherwise the concept has little meaning. Although one can visualize situations in which substantially larger fat stores (and hence increased weight) would be biologically beneficial, this discussion will be limited to consideration of surveys of adiposity status in relation to morbidity and mortality outcomes in members of the U.S. population who were ostensibly healthy at study inception. The term "adiposity" is used here in recognition of the fact that weight for height is only one of an array of physical attributes related to adiposity that have been (and continue to be) used as indices of adiposity in epidemiological studies. Such attributes include body mass index (BMI), skinfold thicknesses measured at various sites, total body fat content (adjusted for stature), percent fat, pattern of regional fat distribution as inferred from such indices as the waist-hip circumference ratio (WHR), and visceral fat content in relation subcutaneous or total body fat content (VanItallie & Lew, 1992 and 1993; Sjostrom, 1993).

During the last three decades, the relationship between relative weight and morbidity and mortality risk has been examined in a number of epidemiological investigations of different segments of diverse populations drawn mostly from the middle class but sometimes limited to persons in particular occupations or persons with distinct life styles, and screened in different ways to exclude those in impaired health and smokers. The disparities among findings in different studies shed light on the ranges of mortality associated with the risks of adiposity under various circumstances.

Unfortunately, the disparate findings of some of the surveys generated a certain amount of confusion. However, when various sources of bias in the surveys were identified, it was possible to develop improved criteria to assess their design and validity. Samples of such sources of bias are shown in Table 1.

For the present analysis, we have drawn on results of four major epidemiological studies, conducted on U.S. residents, that for the most part obviated the biases listed in Table 1. They are: (1) the American Cancer Society Study; (2) the Framingham Heart Study; (3) the

Table 1. Sources of Bias in Prospective Studies of the Association between One or More Adiposity Indicators and Morbidity and Mortality Risk.

* <u>Failure to control for cigarette smoking</u>
    (Results in an artifactually high morbidity and mortality in lean subjects, with consequent underestimation of mortality risk among the "overweight".)

* <u>Failure to exclude subjects in impaired health at start of study</u>
    (May result in an artifactually high morbidity and mortality in lean subjects and distortion of the overall findings.)

* <u>Study population with special characteristics</u>
    (Use of a cohort in which there is an over-representation of people whose occupation or socioeconomic status [for example] inherently biases the relationship of relative weight or fatness to subsequent health and longevity. For example, longshoremen and policemen are in occupations that tend to screen out those in impaired health ["healthy worker effect"] both before and during a prospective investigation.)

* <u>Cohort size too small</u>
    (With a relatively small cohort [as in the Framingham Heart Study] longer follow-up periods are required to permit emergence of a strong association between overweight and mortality.)

* <u>Insufficiently long follow-up period</u>
    (The adverse effects of overweight/obesity on health and longevity may be delayed, sometimes for 10 to 16 years or longer.)

* <u>Inappropriate control of intermediate risk factors</u>
    (If the goal of the study is to determine the effect of adiposity on mortality, it is inappropriate to control for factors like hypertension or hyperglycemia-hyperinsulinemia that are associated with obesity or represent a later phase of the underlying metabolic disorder.)

* <u>Misclassification biases arising from the heterogeneity of the adiposity syndrome and the surrogate measure of adiposity used as the independent variable</u>
    (One subgroup of the obese population may be at substantially higher risk than another subgroup [e.g. those with visceral obesity vs those with femoral-gluteal obesity]. When the subgroups are not properly distinguished, the overall risk of the subgroups combined will be diluted.)

---

[a]Adapted from Simopoulos & VanItallie, 1984; Manson et al., 1987; VanItallie & Lew, 1990; Sjöström, 1993.

Nurses' Health Study; and (4) the Seventh Day Adventist Study. Characteristics of these studies are summarized in Table 2. Data from these investigations were examined to identify the BMI ranges (and the values for other markers related to adiposity) associated with the lowest morbidity and mortality risk.

AMERICAN CANCER SOCIETY (ACS) STUDY

All-Cause Mortality

Among the nonsmoking subjects followed in the ACS Study (Lew & Garfinkel, 1979;

Table 2. Characteristics of Four Major Prospective Epidemiological Studies Conducted in the United States

Study		Authors	Number of Subjects	Duration of Study	Smoking Taken Into Account	Adiposity Index	Outcomes Investigated
American Cancer Society Study		Lew & Garfinkel (1979)	336,442 Men[a] 410,060 Women[a]	13 yr	Yes	Relative Weight	All-cause and disease-specific mortality
Framingham Heart Study	(1)	Hubert et al. (1983)	2,252 Men 2,818 Women	26 yr	No	Metropolitan Relative Weight (1959)	Cardiovascular disease morbidity
	(2)	Garrison et al. (1983)	2,252 Men[a] 2,818 Women[a]	26 yr	Yes	Metropolitan Relative Weight (1959)	All-cause mortality
	(3)	Harris et al. (1988)	597 Men 1,126 Women	1–23 yr (mean, 9.5)	Yes	Body Mass Index (kg/m^2)	All-cause mortality in nonsmoking older persons
(Framingham Offspring Study)	(4)	Garrison & Kannel (1993)	1,193 Men 1,254 Women (all nonsmokers)	Not applicable	Yes	Subscapular Skinfold/ Body Mass Index	Cardiovascular disease risk factors
Nurses Health Study	(1)	Manson et al. (1990)	115,886 Women[a]	8 yr	Yes	Body Mass Index	Coronary heart disease morbidity and mortality
	(2)	Colditz et al. (1990)	113,861 Women	8 yr	Not applicable	Body Mass Index	Incidence of non-insulin dependent diabetes
	(3)	Stampfer et al. (1992)	90,302 Women	8 yr	Not applicable	Body Mass Index	Risk of symptomatic gallstones
Seventh Day Adventist Study[b]		Lindsted et al. (1991)	8,828 Men (all nonsmoking and nondrinking)	26 yr	Yes	Body Mass Index	All-cause and disease-specific mortality

[a] These numbers are the totals for subjects in ostensibly good health. Of these, 34,436 were nonsmoking men and 375,381 were nonsmoking women. The optimal BMI ranges were developed from the experience among the nonsmoking men and women who were in ostensibly good health at the study's inception.

[b] Because of their distinctive lifestyle, Seventh-Day Adventists constitute a highly selected population with a significantly lower mortality than the general population.

3

Table 3. Mortality Ratios from Diabetes, Coronary Heart Disease (CHD), and Cancer by Body Mass Index (BMI) in Smoking and Nonsmoking Women Combined Aged 50-59 Years.

BMI (kg/m^2)[a]	Mortality ratios (%)[b]		
	Diabetes	CHD	Cancer
20.0 to 22.5	64	82	92
22.5 to 27.5	100	100	100
27.5 to 30.0	228	145	114
30.0 to 32.5	435	164	116
32.5 to 35.0	712	216	112
≥35	1,232	311	182

[a]Based on weights in indoor clothing without shoes.
[b]In relation to death rates among those 90 to 109% of average weight. Death rates among women of average weight exceeded those among women with below-average ("optimal") weights.

(Lew & Garfinkel, 1979)

Lew, 1985), the lowest all-cause mortality ratios (MRs) were observed in men aged 30-59 years whose BMIs ranged from 20.5-23.0 kg/m^2 and in women aged 30-59 years whose BMIs ranged from 19.0-21.5 kg/m^2. The lowest MRs of men aged 60-89 years occurred in those whose BMIs ranged from 19.0-22.5 kg/m^2. Among women aged 60-89 years, the lowest MRs were observed in those with BMIs ranging from 19.0-22.0 kg/m^2

Disease-Specific Mortality

Coronary heart disease (CHD). Among ACS Study men of all ages who had never smoked, CHD MR was lowest in those whose weights were 80-89% of average (BMIs of about 19.5-22.0 kg/m^2). Among women of all ages who had never smoked, CHD MR was lowest in those whose weights were < 80% through 89% of average (BMIs of 19.0-21.0 kg/m^2).

In the ACS Study, men aged 30-59 considered all together, regardless of smoking habits, experienced the lowest MRs from CHD in the BMI range 20.2-22.0 kg/m^2. Among corresponding women aged 30-59, the lowest MRs from CHD were in the BMI range 19.0-21.0 kg/m^2.

Diabetes mellitus. In the same cohort in which smoking habits were disregarded, the lowest MRs from diabetes among men aged 50-79 years occurred in those whose BMIs ranged from 20.0-22.0 kg/m^2. Among women aged 50-79 years, those with the lowest MRs from diabetes had BMIs of 19.0-21.0 kg/m^2.

The association of an increasing BMI with rising MRs from diabetes, CHD and cancer in ACS Study women (smoking and nonsmoking) aged 50-59 years is shown in Table 3.

FRAMINGHAM HEART STUDY

The Framingham Heart Study (FHS) population has been examined and followed biennially since 1949. Hence, the FHS is now in its 44th year. The FHS also has generated a collateral investigation known as the Framingham Offspring Study.

In a 26-year follow-up of the participants in the FHS, Hubert et al. (1983) reexamined the relationship between the degree of obesity and the incidence of cardiovascular disease, using Metropolitan Relative Weight (MRW) as the obesity index. MRW was defined as percentage of "desirable weight" (the ratio of actual weight to desirable weight x 100). Because of the much longer period of follow-up in this study, the effects of overweight were more fully reflected. Desirable weight for each sex was derived from the Metropolitan Life Insurance Company tables published in 1959 by taking the midpoint of the desirable weight range for medium build at a specified height. When these midpoints are translated into BMIs, the value for men is 22 kg/m^2; that for women is 21 kg/m^2.

On entry into the FHS, the disease-free cohort (smokers and nonsmokers were not distinguished) were already considerably overweight. On average, men were 18.9% and women 0.5% above desirable weight. Hubert et al. divided the subjects into three MRW categories, (1) < 110% [a BMI less than 4.2 kg/m^2 for men and less than 23.1 kg for women]; (2) 110-29% [for men, 24.2-28.4 kg/m^2; for women, 23.1-27.1 kg/m^2], 3) 130%+ [for men, about 28.6+ kg/m^2; for women about 27.3+ kg/m^2]. The authors found that the incidence of CHD increased with increasing MRW, the gradient of the risk being steeper in men and women under the age of 50. However, there was an even stronger gradient of risk for sudden death with increasing MRW in each age group for both men and women. Thus, it was clearly demonstrated that when cardiovascular disease (CVD), CHD, and sudden death were the dependent variables, the weight category associated with the most favorable outcomes was a MRW of < 110% (corresponding to BMIs lower than 24.2 and 23.1 for men and women respectively). MRWs in the 110-129% category and higher are associated with a significantly increased risk of CVD, CHD, and sudden death.

Logistic regression analyses indicated that weight gain in the Framingham cohort was positively and significantly related to risk of CVD over 26 years in both sexes. Weight gain into middle and older ages was independently associated with an increased risk of CVD. Weight loss was associated with a decreased risk of CVD. Thus, to cite Hubert et al., "Not only was there a powerful relationship of MRW to disease risk in Framingham, but also, the change in MRW after the young adult years made an independent contribution to the prediction of CVD."

Several additional items of interest emerged in the report of Hubert et al. First, in the highest weight class of the Framingham cohort (MRW > 130%), only 8% of the men and 18% of the women were free of CVD risk factors. Second, in Framingham men, a strong and significant association between MRW and CHD incidence did not emerge until the 8-year follow-up, after which the strength of the relationship remained fairly constant.

In another 26-year follow-up of the FHS participants, Garrison et al. (1983) considered the relationship between relative weight and 26-year mortality among smokers and nonsmokers. When a multiple logistic regression analysis was applied to those subjects with an MRW above 100%, a positive and statistically significant relationship was demonstrated between MRW and mortality, after adjustment for cigarette smoking and age. Of the three age-groups of nonsmoking men studied (age at entry 30-39, 40-49, 50-62 years), only one failed to show minimum mortality in the 100-109% MRW class. Thus, nonsmokers aged 30-39 years showed minimum mortality in the 100-119% MRW range (BMI = 22.0-26.0 kg/m^2). Garrison et al. concluded from their data that "... the concept of "desirable weight', as defined by the Metropolitan Life Insurance Co. in 1959, is validated by the Framingham Heart Study."

The oldest age group studied by Garrison et al. in their analyses of relative weight and long-term mortality in Framingham smokers and nonsmokers consisted of men aged 50-62 years. In a subsequent examination of body mass index and mortality among nonsmoking older persons, Harris et al. (1988) looked at the relationship of weight at age 65 years and subsequent mortality in a population of 1723 nonsmokers who were followed-up from one to 23 years (mean, 9.5 years) during the FHS. These investigators found that among men aged 65 years, the BMI range associated with the lowest subsequent mortality was 23.0-25.2 kg/m^2. For women aged 65 years, the optimal BMI range was 24.1-26.1 kg/m^2.

In this population, the principal causes of death were CVD (49.8% of male and 48.5% of female deaths) and cancer (26.3% of male and 24.9% of female deaths). Among men, the MRs were 130% for those with BMIs ranging from 25.3-28.4 kg/m^2 and 170% for those with BMIs > 28.5 kg/m^2. Among women, MRs were 140% for those with BMIs of 26.2-28.6 kg/m^2 and 200% for those with BMIs > 28.7 kg/m^2.

Duration of overweight contributed to mortality risk in this elderly population. Those who were heavy at both ages 55 and 65 years were at significantly higher risk than those who were heavy only at age 65 years. It was also found that those losing 10% of BMI from ages 55 to 65 were at increased risk of death (MR=200%) regardless of the level of BMI at age 65 years.

Harris et al. concluded their report by recommending that, in future research on an elderly population "...with high rates of chronic illness and disability, it would be useful to examine the relationship of weight with outcomes such as functional status, health care use, and prevalence of illness."

In harmony with this recommendation, Garrison and Kannel (1993) have recently reported the results of their efforts to develop adiposity standards "consistent with optimum cardiovascular health without the lengthy follow-up required for mortality studies." The population on which their report was based consisted of 2447 nonsmoking men and women aged 20- 59 years, drawn from the Framingham Offspring Study (FOS). However, only the data from men and women aged 20-39 years were used to determine "healthy weight" estimates for men and women separately. This determination was accomplished by using the right subscapular skinfold (RSS) thickness as the independent variable, with the dependent variables being eight generally recognized CVD risk factors. Right subscapular skinfold thickness values from the younger subset were divided into deciles and a "summary threshold of adiposity" (STA) was determined as being the highest decile of RSS thickness at which CVD risk factors showed the minimum value. After the health-optimal STAs (corresponding to RSS thicknesses of < 12 mm for men and < 15 mm for women) were established in the group of younger subjects, they were used to define the subgroup of the entire sample (aged 20-59 years) that consisted of men and women who had RSS thickness values below the STA and who could therefore be considered to have a healthy adiposity status. Using data from this subgroup, the authors estimated a "healthy weight" table.

When men and women with RSS at or above the STA were excluded, 469 men and women (19% of the original sample of 2447) remained who were considered to have healthy adiposity status (HAS). In the group who exhibited HAS, the mean BMI for the men was 22.5 kg/m^2; that for the women was 21.0 kg/m^2. The approach used by Garrison and Kannel to select the STA gave equal weight to each CVD risk factor. The principal reason for using this method of weighing arose from awareness by these authors that, in terms of changes in CVD risk factors, the responses of obese individuals to the same degree and duration of adiposity can be quite variable.

According to the authors' calculations, there is a very high probability (above 90%) that an unhealthy adiposity is present in men and women with a BMI greater than 24.5 kg/m^2. The probability is high (about 50%) that unhealthy adiposity exists in men and women with a BMI greater than 22.0 kg/m^2.

In the discussion of their findings, Garrison and Kannel point out "As only one measure of central adiposity, subscapular skinfolds may not detect potentially important regional adiposity, and more detailed studies of fat distribution and quantification would be likely to yield more precise estimates of unhealthy adiposity thresholds at various depots."

THE NURSES' HEALTH STUDY (NHS)

The NHS, now in its seventeenth year, has provided valuable information about the effect of overweight on risk of CHD, clinical diabetes and symptomatic gallstones.

Coronary Heart Disease

During 8 years of follow-up of the NHS cohort, Manson et al. (1990) identified 605 first coronary events, including 306 nonfatal myocardial infarctions, 83 deaths due to CHD and 216 cases of confirmed angina pectoris. The 115,886 middle-aged women in the cohort were divided by self-reported weight into BMI quintiles (<21, 21-<23, 23-<25, 25-<29, and > 29 kg/m^2). The mean ages (+SD) of the subjects (yr) in each quintile were: <21 (40.1+7.1); 21-<23 (41.7+7.1); 22-<25 (43.1+7.1); 25-<29 (43.8+7.0); > 29 kg/m^2 (43.8+6.7).

For increasing levels of current BMI, the relative risks of nonfatal myocardial infarction and fatal and nonfatal CHD combined, adjusted for age and cigarette smoking, in the five BMI groups were 100, 130, 130, 180, and 330%. The authors reported that the current BMI was a more important determinant of coronary risk than that at age 18. Also, weight gain during the intervening years increased the risk of CHD in middle-aged women.

These data, adjusted for age and smoking, indicate that the leanest women (with BMIs corresponding to less than 95% of 1983 MRW [Metropolitan Life Insurance Company, 1984]) had the lowest rates of CHD; CHD risks among women of average weight were 30 percent higher than those of the lean women. CHD rate increased by 80% in mildly to moderately overweight women (BMI 25 to 29 kg/m^2) and by 230% in the women whose BMIs were > 29 kg/m^2.

As the authors pointed out, the highest BMI category (> 29 kg/m^2) corresponds to a weight 30% or more above the 1983 MRW. Approximately 25% of US women 35 to 64 years of age fall into this category. An additional 20% of middle-aged US women fall into the second highest BMI category (25 to 29 kg/m^2). Seventy percent of the CHD observed in the women whose BMIs were 29 kg/m^2 or higher and 40% of the CHD in the entire cohort was attributable to their overweight.

Because of its relatively short (8-year) follow-up, the excess morbidity and mortality from CHD associated with overweight was probably underestimated in the NHS, especially as women with diagnosed CHD and stroke were excluded from entry into the study.

Diabetes Mellitus

Colditz et al. (1990) have reported on the role of overweight as a risk factor for clinical diabetes in the NHS cohort. During 8 years of follow-up of the NHS cohort, 873 infinite cases of noninsulin dependent diabetes mellitus (NIDDM) occurred among women initially free of diagnosed diabetes. The ages of the subjects ranged from 30 to 65 years. The age-adjusted relative risks of NIDDM at various BMI levels are shown in Table 4.

The data indicate that the relative risk of diabetes is elevated for women with BMIs > 22 kg/m^2 and is especially pronounced for women with a BMI greater than 25 kg/m^2. Thus, in the BMI range of 25 to 27 kg/m^2, women had more than a fivefold increase in diabetes risk within the NHS cohort; 90.4 percent of diabetes diagnoses were attributable to a BMI higher than 22 kg/m^2. Compared to women whose weight was stable after age 18 years, women who gained weight after that age exhibited an increased risk of developing NIDDM. The more the weight gain the greater was the risk. Women who gained more than 3 kg had a substantially higher risk of diabetes than those gaining less than 3 kg.

Compared to weight-stable women, those who gained 10 to 20 kg after age 18 had a relative risk of developing diabetes of 460% (adjusting for age and for BMI at age 18). As

Table 4. Body Mass Index and Risk of Non-Insulin -Dependent Diabetes in Middle-Aged American Women.1,2

Body mass index (kg/m^2)	Age-adjusted relative risk
< 22	1.0
22 - 22.9	2.2
23 - 23.9	3.6
25 - 26.9	5.5
27 - 28.9	10.1
31 - 32.9	29.6
≥ 35	60.9

[a] Based on a cohort of 113,861 women 30-55 years of age at the beginning of the study and followed for 8 years thereafter.

[b] Adapted from Colditz et al., 1990.

Colditz et al. emphasize, "To the extent that body mass index is an imperfect measure of adiposity, even the strong association between body mass index and diabetes that we observed may represent an underestimate of the true relation between adiposity and diabetes." Another likely cause of underestimation of this relation was the relatively short follow-up period.

Gallstones

In 1989, Maclure et al. reported on a four-year prospective study of 88,837 members of the NHS cohort (age range 34 to 59) in which the relationship between BMI status and risk of symptomatic gallstones was assessed. Overall, these authors observed a roughly linear relation between relative weight and risk of gallstones. Women whose BMIs were less than 20 kg/m^2 had the lowest risk of gallstones; among those whose BMIs four years earlier had been 24-25 kg/m^2, the age-adjusted relative risk was 170%. Among women whose BMIs were 32 kg/m^2 or greater four years earlier, the age-adjusted relative risk of symptomatic gallstones was 600%.

In this cohort, the risk of having gallstones during the follow-up period (1980 to 1984) was doubled among women who gained 5 to 9 kg between the age of 18 years and 1976. The risk tripled among women who gained 10 kg or more. On the basis of their findings, the authors concluded that "...even a slight excess of weight may be an important determinant of the increased risk of gallstones in middle-aged women."

SEVENTH DAY ADVENTIST STUDY

In the Seventh Day Adventist (SDA) Study, Lindsted et al. (1991) examined the relationship between BMI and 26-year mortality among 8828 nonsmoking, nondrinking SDA men. The cohort included 439 men with BMIs below 20 kg/m^2. Lindsted and associates divided the SDA cohort into BMI quintiles, as follows: I < 22.3; II 22.4-24.2; III 24.3-25.7; IV 25.8-27.5; V > 27.5 kg/m^2. Among men aged 50-89 years, those in quintile I exhibited the lowest adjusted relative risk for all-cause mortality, CHD mortality, cancer mortality and cerebrovascular disease mortality (Table 5). These relationships remained after the authors controlled for demographic characteristics, smoking history, activity level, dietary pattern, coffee consumption and medical illness. Nor was there any increase in the mortality experience of the "very lean" (those with BMIs below 20 kg/m^2) compared with the "lean" (BMI 20-22 kg/m^2).

Table 5. All-Cause and Coronary Heart Disease Mortality in the Seventh Day Adventist Study.[1,2]

	Hazard ratios (from univariate survival analysis) comparing BMI quintiles I-IV to V				
	BMI quintiles				
Age (yr)	≤ 22.3	22.4-24.2	24.3-25.7	25.8-27.5	≥ 27.5
All-cause mortality					
50-59	0.5	0.8	0.8	1.1	1.0
60-69	0.5	0.5	0.7	0.7	1.0
70-79	0.6	0.6	0.7	0.7	1.0
80-89	0.7	0.9	0.9	0.9	1.0
90-99	1.1	1.0	1.0	0.9	1.0
Coronary heart disease mortality					
50-59	0.4	0.5	1.2	1.0	1.0
60-69	0.3	0.5	0.6	0.6	1.0
70-79	0.5	0.4	0.6	0.6	1.0
80-89	0.6	0.8	0.9	0.8	1.0
90-99	1.3	1.0	1.1	1.1	1.0

[a] Based on a 26-year follow-up of 8,828 nonsmoking and nondrinking Seventh Day Adventist men

[b] Adapted from Lindsted et al., 1991

The participants in the study were predominantly married Caucasians. Their mean BMI was 25 kg/m^2. It is noteworthy that during the 26-year follow-up, mean age at death was highest (80.5 years) in the lowest BMI quintile and lowest (75.8 years) in the highest quintile. The authors point out that the subjects in the highest BMI category showed the least adherence to a fruit and vegetable dietary pattern as well as the greatest history of past smoking (31.6% vs 23.6% in quintile I). Although the results for quintile V of the multivariate analyses were similar to those of the univariate analyses, "control for confounding in the Cox model (in the words of the authors) may have been incomplete."

The protective effects of a BMI < 22 kg/m^2 against CHD mortality decreased with increasing age; however, the effect remained until the tenth decade of life. In their commentary on this crossover, the authors suggest that "If mortality is postponed and a maximal lifespan exists, deaths must occur in a narrower interval preceding the (end of the) lifespan." This effect is sometimes referred to as "compression of mortality."

In interpreting the findings of Lindsted et al. it is important to keep in mind that SDA men are a very select group drawn from the general population. Thus, their abstinence from smoking and alcohol, their (preponderantly) vegetarian diet, their relatively disciplined life style, and their generally higher educational attainment (a relatively high proportion of SDA men are college educated) represent factors known to be associated with a decreased mortality risk.

DISCUSSION

Mortality- and Morbidity-Optimal BMI Ranges

Information about the BMI ranges associated with (1) lowest all-cause mortality; (2)

Table 6. Body Mass Indices (BMIs) Associated with Lowest All-Cause Mortality in Men and Women at Various Ages

Study	Authors	Number of Subjects	Duration of follow-up (yr)	Age (yr)	Optimal BMI range (kg/m²)
			Men		
American Cancer Society	Lew & Garfinkel (1979)	336,442	13	30 - 59 [a] 60 - 89 [a]	20.5 - 23.0 [c] 19.0 - 22.5 [c]
Framingham Heart Study	Garrison et al. (1983)	2,252	26	30 - 39 [a] 40 - 49 [a] 50 - 62 [a]	22.0 - 26.0 22.0 - 24.0 22.0 - 24.0
Framingham Heart Study	Harris et al. (1988)	597 [b]	1 - 23 (mean 9.5)	65	23.0 - 25.2
Seventh Day Adventist	Lindsted el al. (1991)	8,828 [b]	26	50 - 89	≤ 22.3
			Women		
American Cancer Society	Lew & Garfinkel (1979)	410,060	13	30 - 59 [a] 60 - 89 [a]	19.0 - 21.5 [c] 19.0 - 22.0 [c]
Framingham Heart Study	Harris et al. (1988)	1,126 [b]	1 - 23 (mean 9.5)	65	24.1 - 26.1

[a] nonsmoking study subjects were drawn from overall numbers of men and women who participated (see Table 2, footnote 2)
[b] all nonsmokers
[c] adjusted for weight of street clothing (2.27 kg for men and 1.36 kg for women)

Table 7. Body Mass Indices Associated with Lowest Coronary Heart Disease Mortality in Men and Women at Various Ages

Study	Authors	Number of Subjects	Duration of follow-up (yr)	Age (yr)	Optimal BMI range (kg/m²)
			Men		
American Cancer Society	Lew & Garfinkel (1979)	336,442	13	all ages [a] 30 - 59 [b]	19.5 - 22.0 20.0 - 22.0
Seventh Day Adventist	Lindsted el al. (1991)	8,828 [c]	26	50 - 89	≤ 22.3
			Women		
American Cancer Society	Lew & Garfinkel (1979)	410,060	13	all ages [a] 30 - 59 [b]	19.0 - 21.0 19.0 - 21.0

[a] Nonsmoking subjects were drawn from overall numbers of men and women who participated
[b] Smoking disregarded
[c] Entire cohort consisted of nonsmokers

lowest CHD mortality; (3) lowest incidence of CVD, CHD, and sudden death; and (4) lowest morbidity from CHD, clinical diabetes, and symptomatic gallstones is summarized in Tables 6-9. Table 10 shows the right subscapular skinfold (RSS) thicknesses and BMI values associated with the lowest concurrent levels of CVD risk factors. Tables 11 and 12 assemble the same overall information separately for men and women by age categories. As a practical matter, the lowest mortality and morbidity experience generally occurs in a significant segment of the

Table 8. Body Mass Indices Associated with Lowest 26-Year Incidence of Cardiovascular Disease, Coronary Heart Disease and Sudden Death (smoking not taken into account).

Study	Authors	Number of Subjects	Age (yr)	Optimal BMI range (kg/m^2)
Framingham Heart Study	Hubert et al. (1983)	2,252 (men)	all ages	< 24.2
		2,818 (women)	all ages	< 23.1

Table 9. Body Mass Indices Associated with Lowest Selected Morbidity in a Middle-Aged Female Population (Nurses' Health Study Cohort).

Nature of illness	Study	Number of Subjects	Duration of follow-up (yr)	Optimal BMI range (kg/m^2)
Coronary heart disease	Manson et al. (1990)	115,886 [a,b]	8	< 21
Clinical non-insulin-dependent diabetes	Colditz et al. (1990)	113,861 [b]	8	< 22
Symptomatic gallstones	Maclure et al. (1989)	88,837 [c]	8	< 20

[a] Data adjusted for age and cigarette smoking
[b] Age range at start of study, 30-55 years
[c] Age range at start of study 34-59 years

Table 10. Right Subscapular Skinfold (RSS) Thicknesses and Body Mass Indices Associated with Lowest Concurrent Levels of Cardiovascular Disease Risk Factors.

Study	Authors	Number of Subjects	Age (yr)	Optimal RSS thickness (mm)	Optimal BMI range (kg/m^2)
Framingham Heart Study (Framingham Offspring Study)	Garrison & Kannel (1993)	1,193 (men [a])	20-59	< 12	≤ 22.5
		1,254 (women [a])	20-59	< 15	≤ 21.0

[a] All nonsmoking

studied population. (For example, in the ACS Study optimal mortality experience occurred in approximately 15% of the population under examination.)

These data, in aggregate, suggest that for otherwise healthy U.S. men of all ages, a BMI range that is optimal for both morbidity and mortality could be < 22.5 kg/m^2. For U.S. women the optimal range could be < 21 kg/m^2. The fact that the findings of widely disparate studies of BMI ranges associated with the lowest morbidity and mortality are so similar lends support to the validity of these proposed optimal ranges.

Table 11. Data for Men

All-cause mortality

Age range (yr)	Study	Optimal BMI range (kg/m^2)
30 - 69	Garrison et al. (1983)	22.0 - 26.0
30 - 59	Lew & Garfinkel (1979)	20.5 - 23.0
40 - 49	Garrison et al. (1983)	22.0 - 24.0
50 - 62	Garrison et al. (1983)	22.0 - 24.0
50 - 89	Lindsted et al. (1991)	< 22.3
60 - 89	Lew & Garfinkel (1979)	19.0 - 22.5
65	Harris et al. (1988)	23.0 - 25.2

Coronary heart disease mortality

All ages	Lew & Garfinkel (1979)	19.5 - 22.0
30 - 59 *	Lew & Garfinkel (1979)	20.0 - 22.0
50 - 89	Lindsted et al. (1991)	≤ 22.3

Cardiovascular disease, coronary heart disease, sudden death

All ages *	Hubert et al. (1983)	< 24.2

Lowest concurrent levels of cardiovascular disease risk factors

20 - 59	Garrison et al. (1993)	≤ 22.5

*Smoking not taken into account.

Table 12. Data for Women

All-cause mortality

Age range (yr)	Study	Optimal BMI range (kg/m^2)
30 - 59	Lew & Garfinkel (1979)	19.0 - 21.5
60 - 89		19.0 - 22.0
65	Harris et al. (1988)	24.1 - 26.1

Coronary heart disease mortality

All ages	Lew & Garfinkel (1979)	19.0 - 21.0

Cardiovascular disease, coronary heart disease, sudden death

All ages	Hubert et at. (1983)	< 23.1

Coronary heart disease morbidity

30 - 55	Manson et al. (1990)	< 21.0

Noninsulin-dependent diabetes morbidity

30 - 55 *	Colditz et al. (1990)	< 22.0

Risk of symptomatic gallstones

34 - 59 *	Maclure et al. (1989)	< 20.0

Lowest concurrent levels of cardiovascular disease risk factors

20 - 59	Garrison & Kannel (1993)	≤ 21.0

* Smoking not taken into account.

Limitations of the BMI as a Surrogate for Adiposity

As has been pointed out many times, the BMI (kg/m^2) is an imperfect surrogate for adiposity. The values from which BMIs are derived (height and weight) are frequently inaccurate, either because height and weight are not measured properly or because they are self-reported. Moreover, as people age they lose height (particularly women); hence, on a per person basis, the BMI in an elderly individual may be spuriously increased. In very large surveys like the ACS Study (Lew & Garfinkel, 979), BMIs were not calculated for each participant but based on height and weight averages of subgroups. Thus, the precision of a specific BMI value is frequently illusory-- such values are often simply approximations.

It should also be noted that, as people age, the body's fat-free mass decreases while its content of fat increases (Cohn, 1993). Such changes take place even if the BMI remains the same. Thus, older individuals may be fatter than would be suggested by the BMI (Micozzi & Harris, 1990). The alteration in body composition that occurs with advancing age may help explain the finding that, in the elderly, abdominal obesity, as inferred from the WHR, can be a better predictor than the BMI of morbidity and mortality risk (Folsom et al., 1993; Rimm et al., 1993).

Hazards of Weight Gain During Adult Life

The findings of the four investigations provide little basis for liberalizing weight standards for people as they get older. Indeed, there is convincing evidence that any substantial weight gain during adult life is an independent risk factor for NIDDM, CVD and CHD. For example, in a 26-year follow-up of Framingham men, it was found that an increase of 20% above 1959 MRW (to a BMI of 26.4 kg/m^2) was associated with a 29% increase in the relative risk of developing CVD. In the NHS, an increase in weight of 10 to 20 kg after age 18 increased the relative risk of nonfatal and fatal CHD (combined) to 170%. In the same population, an increase in weight of 10 to 20 kg increased the relative risk of NIDDM to 460%. The relative risk of having symptomatic gallstones tripled among women who gained 10 kg or more after age 18.

In the Health Professionals Follow-up Study, E. Rimm et al (1993) have found that weight gain in adulthood is a risk factor for CHD in men. Their study involved a three-year follow-up of 29,122 men aged 40 to 75 years in 1986, with no previous CVD. Their analysis showed that the multivariate relative risk rose from 123% associated with gains of weight ranging from 3-6 kg, to 207% for gains of 19+ kg.

Taken in concert, these observations indicate that weight gain after linear growth has ceased can be harmful to health. They also show that the relative risk of developing CVD, CHD and NIDDM rises monotonically as the amount of weight gained increases.

Should Weight Standards Be Liberalized for People as They Age?

In 1985, Andres et al. reported on their analysis for "age effects" of data taken from the Build Study 1979 (Society of Actuaries and Association of Life Insurance Medical Directors, 1980). They constructed parabolic curves expressing the relationship between MRs and BMIs for each of ten age-sex groups and computed the BMI nadirs of the various curves. Thus, for each age-sex group, they determined the range of BMIs associated with less than expected mortality. They found that "for both men and women there was a powerful effect of age on the body mass index associated with minimal mortality." Based on their calculations, they decided that, for men and women aged 50-69 years, a BMI range of 25.2 to 27.3 kg/m^2 was optimal, compared with an optimal range of 19.5 to 23.4 kg/m^2 for men and women aged 20-39 years. From this analysis and the findings of 23 other population studies (most of which may have suffered from some of the flaws listed in Table 1), Andres et al. concluded that weight standards should be adjusted for age. They acknowledged, however, that "more studies are required, especially in persons over age 70; the data are too sparse to make any recommendations with confidence to elderly persons."

The recommendation that weight standards be age-adjusted was, in fact, adopted in the "revised suggested weights for heights" published in 1990 by the US Department of Agriculture (USDA) and the Department of Health and Human Services (DHHS).

Although the 1990 US government "weight guidelines" have been roundly criticized (Willett et al., 1991), the notion of adjusting weight standards for age is still accepted by many health professionals. Therefore, further discussion is needed about the problems generated by age-specific weight-for-height or BMI tables such as those recommended by Andres et al. (1985) and USDA-DHHS (1990).

As one example, the calculations of Andres et al. (1985) seem to suggest that as people age, some degree of weight gain is not only not harmful but actually desirable. Thus, for a woman 70 inches tall, the tables devised by Andres et al. (1985) provide for an increase in weight from a range of 122-162 pounds at age 25 to 167-207 pounds at age 65. The implication that such a weight gain is safe and even desirable is totally at odds with other evidence reviewed herein indicating that weight gains of this magnitude (35-45 pounds) during adult life significantly increase morbidity and mortality risk.

Apart from the reported dangers to health associated with appreciable weight gain after cessation of linear growth, is the substantial evidence from the studies listed in Table 2 and reviewed herein that, for nonsmoking men and women, a BMI close to 21.5 kg/m^2 maintained throughout adult life is associated with the lowest mortality risk and the lowest risk of developing such obesity-associated illnesses as CHD, hypertension, NIDDM and gallbladder disease.

The disturbing discrepancy between the findings of Andres et al. (1985) on the one hand, and observations of the ACS study, the FHS, the NHS, and the SDA Study on the other hand, makes it appropriate to examine more closely some of the pitfalls inherent in using sources like the Build Study 1979 to support the position that weight standards should be liberalized as people age. Some of the pertinent limitations of this study are detailed below.

Difficulties in Selecting Populations for Determining the Effects of Overweight On Mortality at the Older Ages

In endeavoring to determine the effects of overweight on mortality at the older ages, it is necessary to face up to the fact that a very high proportion of obese persons at those ages suffer as well from other (often obesity-related) impairments that materially increase mortality; for instance, hypertension, electrocardiographic abnormalities, myocardial hypertrophy, hypercholesterolemia, and NIDDM. Thus, in the FHS, some 74% of the male subjects aged 55-62 years and 83% of the female subjects at entry (1950) exhibited these and other health problems. The older the subject and the greater the degree of overweight, the higher the prevalence of adverse findings (Lew, unpublished data).

Lew and Wilber (1982) analyzed the 26-year follow-up data from the FHS in terms of the mortality experience for (1) subjects in ostensibly good health at entry; (2) subjects in impaired health at entry; and (3) effects of variations in relative weight on mortality in the presence of health impairments, based on criteria for standard life insurance. They found that, for persons in impaired health, the MRs (for all ages and both sexes combined) were well above the anticipated normal values over the entire relative weight range; the minimum relative mortality (128%) was recorded among those 5-15% overweight. In contrast, the corresponding MRs for ostensibly healthy subjects were all well below the anticipated normal values, with the lowest MR (68%) among those 5-15% underweight.

Of particular interest was the observation (Lew, published data) that, among Framingham men aged 55-62 at entry (in 1950), about 25% of those 15-25% underweight were free of health impairments as compared with only 5% of those 35% or more overweight. If the customary criteria of insurability had been applied to the middle-aged Framingham population, it is obvious that a high proportion of the overweight men would have been rejected for life insurance coverage at standard rates. However, the small fraction of older overweight men who were free of health impairments and therefore insurable would have been a highly selected group and more comparable to the nonoverweight as regards mortality risk.

The Framingham experience may serve as an informative backdrop to the investigations of mortality in relation to relative weight among insured lives. Such investigations have been automatically directed at persons in "good health" since the subjects had to meet the customary standards of insurability. These standards are more exacting at the older ages than those dictated by the concept of "acceptable health" in medicine. The insurance experience produced distinctly lower mortality at the older ages because it reflected the selection of persons in good health regardless of weight status. Had the prevailing standards of acceptable health at the older ages commonly used by physicians been applied, many more persons would have been accepted for insurance and the experience would have shown higher mortality.

As mentioned earlier, Andres et al. (1985) proposed broader and more liberal ranges of mortality-optimal BMIs based on data from the Build Study 1979, which dealt with the mortality experience among persons insured 1954-72. Andres and associates interpreted the findings of the Build Study 1979 as indicating that, for men aged 60-69, the BMI associated with lowest mortality was 26.6 kg/m^2, a value of 24% higher than the BMI (21.4 kg/m^2) associated with minimal mortality at ages 20-29. Among women aged 60-69, optimal BMI was 27.3 kg/m^2, 40% higher than the optimal BMI (19.5 kg/m^2) at ages 20-29.

These authors may not have been aware that during the period covered by the Build Study 1979, men and (particularly) women aged 60 and older applied for life insurance only infrequently and were very carefully screened before the insurance was issued. This strict selection was reflected in the relatively high declination rates on applications for insurance at the older ages. As a result, the Build Study 1979 showed little extra mortality among slightly and moderately overweight policy holders at ages 60 and older.

In contrast, the American Cancer Society's Study (Lew and Garfinkel, 1979) came up with distinctly elevated mortality among corresponding overweight individuals aged 60-69. For men in this age range who were 20-29% overweight, the MR was 123%. For women aged 60-69 years and 20-29% overweight, it was 137%.

The compilers of the 1983 Metropolitan height and weight tables ended them at age 59 because they appreciated the problematic nature of the mortality experience at ages 60 and older.

Excess Death Rate vs Mortality Ratio at the Older Ages

Examination of MRs among nonsmoking ACS Study subjects whose weights exceeded the average for members of their age by 0% or more discloses that the magnitude of these ratios decreased with each decade of advancing age (Figure 1). This decline in MR (a finding reported in many surveys) might suggest to some that the risk of being overweight diminishes with aging. Those who make such an interpretation should bear in mind that, as the death rate rises with advancing age (Fig 2), even a small elevation in relative mortality (e.g. an MR of 125%), produces increasingly larger numbers of extra deaths per 1000, so that the excess death rate (EDR) becomes the more significant measure of extra mortality at the older ages. Thus, as indicated in Table 13, an MR of 250% (for example) could increase a 45-year old white man's risk of dying from 3.7 to 9.3 per 1000, an increase in risk of dying of 5.6 per 1000. An MR of 125% would increase a 75-year old white man's risk of dying by 13.4 per 1000.

As shown in Fig 3, the seriousness of a "high" MR in a young adult may be overestimated if one fails to consider the low mortality rates that obtain at that age level. By the same token, the significance of a "lower" MR may be underestimated in an older person

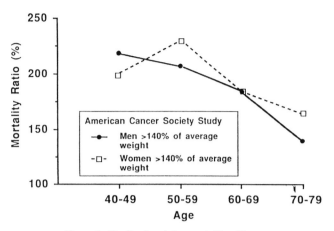

Figure 1. Decline in relative mortality with age.

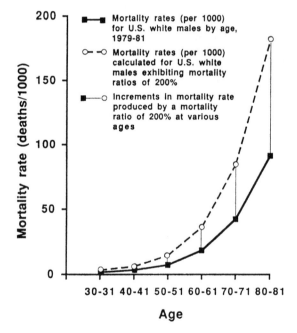

Figure 2. Effect of the rising mortality rate associated with aging on magnitude of the increments in mortality rate produced at various ages by a mortality ratio of 200%. (From VanItallie & Lew, 1993, with permission).

whose normal mortality rate is already high.

Some may be tempted to regard an MR of, say, 150% as being trivial and not worthy of much concern. This point of view is certainly inappropriate from the public health perspective. Thus, if a degree of overweight that gives rise to an MR of 50% occurs in one million people whose average age is 40, out 1300 extra deaths will result. It should also be kept in mind that MRs that may not seem particularly worrisome in early adult life become increasingly ominous as people get older and the absolute probability of dying increases in accelerating fashion.

Table 13. Extra Deaths Per 1000 Resulting from Different Mortality Ratios (MRs) at Various Ages. (Based on U. S. 1989 mortality statistics for white males).

Age (yr)	Death rate (per 1000)	Extra deaths per 1000 at specified MRs (%)					
		125	150	200	250	300	350
20	1.4	0.35	0.70	1.4	2.1	2.8	3.5
25	1.6	0.40	0.80	1.6	2.4	3.2	4.0
30	1.7	0.43	0.85	1.7	2.6	3.4	4.3
35	2.1	0.53	1.05	2.1	3.2	4.2	4.7
40	2.6	0.65	1.30	2.6	3.9	5.2	6.5
45	3.7	0.93	1.85	3.7	5.6	7.4	9.3
50	5.6	1.40	2.80	5.6	8.4	11.2	14.0
55	9.3	2.35	4.70	9.3	14.1	15.6	23.5
60	15.2	3.80	7.60	15.2	22.8	30.4	38.0
65	22.8	5.70	11.40	22.8	34.2	45.6	57.0
70	34.8	8.70	17.40	34.8	52.2	64.6	87.0
75	53.7	13.40	26.90	53.7	80.6	107.4	134.0
80	82.8	20.70	41.40	82.8	124.2	165.6	207.0
85	125.6	31.40	62.80	125.6	188.0	251.2	
90	181.0	45.30	90.50	181.0	272.0		
95	252.0	63.00	126.00	252.0			
100	320.0	80.00	160.00	320.0			

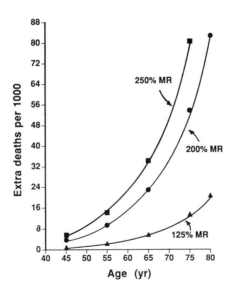

Figure 3. Effect of age on extra deaths per 1000 at different mortality ratios.

Longevity is Not the Most Appropriate Dependent Variable

Although death is an unequivocal end point, it is becoming evident that from a health policy standpoint, it is preferable to use morbidity or some index of disability as the dependent

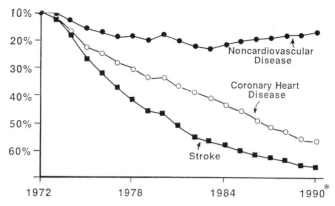

Figure 4. Percent decline in age-adjusted mortality rates since 1972. (Source: Data calculated by the National Heart, Lung, and Blood Institute).
*Provisional data for 1990.

variable in studies that attempt to relate adiposity to health outcome.

There are a number of reasons why this is so. First, far more information is available now about morbidity outcomes than was obtainable in the past (Grundy, 1987). The concept of "active life expectancy" is beginning to take hold, as opposed to life expectancy per se (Manton and Stallard, 1991). Second, with respect to certain important diseases, there has developed in recent years an increasing divergence of morbidity from mortality incidence. Notable examples are the remarkable drops in age-adjusted mortality rates from CHD and stroke that have occurred in the U.S. since 1972. During the last two decades, the mortality rate from the principal cause of death, CHD, has creased about 50%; that from stroke has fallen by 57% (Fig 4). There is evidence, however, that CHD morbidity rates have not declined in pace with the reduction in mortality rates (Agostino et al., 1989). In their description of trends in CHD mortality, morbidity, and risk factor levels, as disclosed by the Minnesota Heart Survey, Burke et al (1989) have reported that, between 1968 and 1986, age-adjusted CHD mortality rates declined dramatically in Twin Cities residents. Among those aged 30 to 74 years CHD mortality declined by 52% in men and 58% in women. But the same study also showed that attack rates based on hospitalized definite myocardial infarction did not change from 1970 to 1985. (Incidentally, it is of interest to note that, between 1973 and 1987, BMIs increased by 1 unit and 1.7 units in Twin Cities men and women respectively.)

Increases in hospital discharges for MI were recorded between the late 1970s through 1986 by the National Hospital charge Survey (National Center for Health Statistics, 1987). But, as Burke et al. point out, in 1985, "... there was a greater financial incentive in 1985 than in 1980 for hospitals to identify and document every acute MI and unstable angina case." According to Burke et al, other reasons for the increase in acute CHD discharge diagnoses could be a higher survival rate in the 1980s of out-of-hospital cardiac arrests, increased use of coronary artery bypass surgery and angioplasty in patients without acute symptoms as well as the greater attention paid to post-procedural EKG changes and increases in enzyme levels.

Whatever the case, the marked decline in CHD mortality since 1972 (unaccompanied by any concurrent decrease in prevalence of obesity [Guthrie et al., 1986]) cannot fail to have weakened somewhat the association between adiposity and life expectancy. In contrast, the association between adiposity and CHD morbidity is likely to have remained strong. After all, people who recover from MIs still suffer from CHD morbidity.

Apart from the implications of the decline in CHD mortality, there are many other reasons why health surveys concerned with the adverse effects of adiposity should increasingly focus on morbidity (e.g. diabetes) and functional disability rather than on years of life expectancy. This change in emphasis recognizes that concern about extending the duration of life has to be matched with concern about the proportion of the later years that can be lived in an active, nonimpaired state. If morbidity outcomes and various measures of functional status are used increasingly as the dependent variables in epidemiological investigations like those discussed in the present analysis, it seems likely that standards for the various surrogates of adiposity status (be they BMI, WHR, visceral fat content or subscapular skinfold thickness) will become more rather than less stringent.

REFERENCES

Agostino, R. B., Kannel, W. B., Belanger, A. J., & Sytkowski, P. A. (1989). Trends in CHD and risk factors at age 55-64 in the Framingham Study. International Journal of Epidemiology, 18(suppl 1), S67-S72.

Andres, R., Elahi, D., Tobin, J. D., Muller, D. C., & Brant, L. (1985). Impact of age on weight goals. Annals of International Medicine, 103 (6 pt 2), 1030-1033.

Burke, G. L., Sprafka, J. M., Folsom, A. R., Luepker, R. V., Norsted, S. W., & Blackburn, H. (1989). Trends in CHD mortality, morbidity and risk factor levels from 1960 to 1986: The Minnesota Heart Survey. International Journal of Epidemiology, 18(suppl 1), S73-S81.

Cohn, S. H. (1993). Neutron activation in obesity research. In: Recent Developments in Body Composition Analysis: Methods and Application, J. G. Kral & T. B. VanIttalie, eds. Smith-Gordon, London, (p 35-42).

Colditz, G. A., Willett, W. C., Stampfer, M. J., Manson, J. E., Hennekens, C. H., Arky, R. A., & Speizer, F. E. (1990). Weight as a risk factor for clinical diabetes in women. American Journal of Epidemiology, 132, 501-513.

Folsom, A. R., Kaye, S. A., Sellers, T. A., et al. (1993). Body fat distribution and 5-year risk of death in older women. JAMA, 269, 483-487.

Garrison, R. J., Feinleib, M., Castelli, W. P., & MacNamara, P. (1983). Cigarette smoking as a confounder of the relationship between relative weight and long-term mortality. JAMA, 249, 2199-2203.

Garrison, R., J., & Kannel, W. B. (1993). A new approach to estimating healthy body weights. International Journal of Obesity, 17.

Grudy, E. (1987). Future patterns of morbidity in old age. In Advanced Geriatric Medicine. F. I. Laird and J. Grimley Evans, eds. John Wright, Bristol (pp. 53-72).

Guthrie, H. A., Habicht, J-P, Johnson, S. R., & VanItallie, T. B. (1986). Nutrition Monitoring in the United States: A Progress Report from the Joint Nutrition Monitoring Evaluation Committee. DHHS Publication No. (PHS) 86-1255. Hyattsville, MD (pp 54 and 61).

Harris, T., Cook, E. F., Garrison, R., Higgins, M., Kannel, W., & Goldman, L. (1988). Body mass index and mortality among nonsmoking older persons. The Framingham Heart Study. JAMA, 259, 1520-1524.

Hubert, H. B., Feinleib, M., McNamara, & Castelli, W. P. (1983). Obesity as an independent risk factor for cardiovascular disease: A 26-year follow-up of participants in the Framingham Heart Study. Circulation, 67, 968-977.

Lew, E. A., & Garfinkel, L. (1979). Variations in mortality by weight among 750,000 men and women. Journal of Chronic Diseases, 32, 563-576.

Lew, E. A. (1985). Mortality and weight: Insured lives and the American Cancer Society Studies. Annals of Internal Medicine, 103(6 pt 2), 1024-1029.

Lew, E. A., & Wilber, J. (1982). Supplementary observations on 1979 Build and Blood Pressure Studies. Rec Soc Actuaries, 8(4), 1157-1180.

Lindsted, K., Tonstad, S., & Kuzma, J. W. (1991). Body mass index and patterns of mortality among Seventh-day Adventist men. International Journal of Obesity, 15, 397-406.

Maclure, K. M., Hayes, K. C., Colditz, G. A., Stampfer, M. J., Speizer, F. E. & Willett, W. C. (1989). Weight, diet, and the risk of symptomatic gallstones in middle-aged women. New England Journal of Medicine, 321, 563-569.

Manson, J. E., Stampfer, M. J., Hennekens, C. H., & Willett, W. C. (1987). Body weight and longevity: A reassessment. JAMA, 257, 353-358.

Manson, J. E., Colditz, G. A., Stampfer, M. J., Willett, W. C., Rosner, B., Momson, R. R., Speizer, F. E., & Hennekens, C. H. (1990). A prospective study of obesity and risk of coronary heart disease in women. New England Journal of Medicine, 372, 882-889.

Manton, K. G., & Stallard, E. (1991). Cross-sectional estimates of active life expectancy for the U.S. elderly and oldest-old populations. Journal of Gerontology, 46, S170-S182.

Metropolitan Life Insurance Company. (1959). New weight standards for men and women. Statistician Bulletin, 40, 1-4.

Metropolitan Life Insurance Company. (1984). 1983 Metropolitan height and weight tables. Statistician Bulletin,, 64,2-9.

Micozzi. M. S., & Harris, T. H. (1990). Age variations in the relation of body mass indices to estimates of body fat and muscle mass. American Journal of Physical Anthropology, 81, 375-379.

National Center for Health Statistics. (1987). Advance Data 1986. Summary: National Hospital Discharge Survey, 145, 1-15.

Rimm, E. B., Stampfer, H. J., Ascherio, E. G., Colditz, G. A., & Willett, W. C. Height, obesity , and fat distribution as independent predictors of coronary heart disease (CHD).

Simopoulos, A. P., & VanItallie, T. B. (1984). Body weight, health, and longevity. Annals of Internal Medicine, 100, 285-295.

Sjostrom, L. (1993). Impacts of body weight, body composition, and adipose distribution on morbidity and mortality. In: Obesity: Theory and Therapy. Second edition, A. J. Stunkard, and T. A. Wadden, eds. Raven Press, New York, (pp. 13-41).

Society of Actuaries and Association of Life Insurance Medical Directors of America. (1980). Build Study, 1979. Philadelphia: Recording and Statistical Corporation.

Stampfer, M. J., Maclure, M., Colditz, G. A., Manson, J. E., & Willett, W. C. (1992). Risk of gallstones in women with severe obesity. American Journal of Clinical Nutrition, 55, 652-658.

U. S. Department of Agriculture, U. S. Department of Health and Human Services. (1990). Nutrition and Your Health: Dietary Guidelines for Americans. Third edition. Washington. D. C.: U. S. Government Printing Office.

VanItallie. T. B., & Lew, E. A. (1990). Overweight and underweight. In: Mortality Trends by Age and Time Elapsed, E. A. Lew and J. Gajewski, eds. Praeger. New York, (pp. 13.1-13.22).

VanItallie. T. B., & Lew, E. A. (1992). Assessment of morbidity and mortality risk in the overweight patient. In : Treatment of the Seriously Obese Patient. T. A. Wadden and T. B. VanItallie, eds. The Guilford Press, New York, (pp. 3-32).

VanItallie. T. B., & Lew E. A. (1993). Estimation of the effect of obesity on health and longevity. A perspective for the physician. In: Obesity: Theory and Therapy, Second edition. A. J. Stunkard, T. A. Wadden, eds. Raven Press, New York, (pp. 219-230).

Willett, W. C., Stampfer, M., Manson, J., & VanItallie, T. B. (1991). New weight guidelines for Americans: Justified or Injudicious? American Journal of Clinical Nutrition. 53, 1102-1103.

WHAT IS THE WEIGHT REQUIRED FOR SUBSTANTIAL HEALTH GAINS?

Steven B. Heymsfield

Obesity Research Center
Department of Medicine
St. Luke's-Roosevelt Hospital Center
Columbia University College of Physicians and Surgeons
New York, New York 10025

INTRODUCTION

The formal title of this presentation is "What is the weight required for substantial health gains?" The original impetus for this topic was the observation that small amounts of weight loss in obese subjects tended to produce large changes in health risks (Kanders, & Blackburn, 1992). In addition to addressing this issue, I will present a more general review of the critical issues in interpreting the relations between weight loss and changes in health outcome.

The major assumptions upon which obesity treatment is founded are:

• obesity is associated with increased health risks, and
• weight reduction in obese subjects will reduce these health risks.

Many weight loss studies, including treatment with behavior modification and surgery, conclusively show that weight loss indeed does improve some of the pathophysiological changes associated with obesity (Kanders & Blackburn, 1992; Goldstein, 1992). What, however, are some of the important issues in interpreting these results?

Before embarking on this review, I want to emphasize two key requirements that must be met in order to fulfill the generally accepted but not fully validated mandate to treat obesity: the ability to produce a sustained *long-term* loss in body weight; and to demonstrate improved morbidity and mortality following weight loss treatment. Accomplishing these two aims would give health care practitioners a clear mandate to aggressively treat obesity. By analogy, treatment of hypertension was limited until effective blood pressure lowering medications were introduced in the 1950's. Successive refinements in these medications over three decades have allowed us to normalize blood pressure indefinitely in hypertensive patients. Armed with these therapies, investigators in the 1960's and 1970's showed that treatment of hypertension significantly reduces the risk of stroke and coronary artery disease (Kaplan, 1993; JAMA, 1992). Our own field lacks such definitive outcome studies and for this reason obesity treatment is not yet embraced as central to health care management. A requisite for our field before moving forward is to develop long-term effective weight loss and weight maintenance therapies.

Obesity Treatment, Edited by D.B. Allison
and F.X. Pi-Sunyer, Plenum Press, New York, 1995

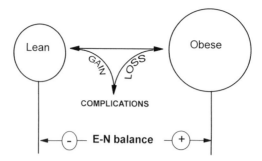

Figure 1. Relations between energy-nitrogen balance, weight change, and complications of obesity. Positive energy-nitrogen balance leads to weight gain and negative balance to weight loss. Gaining or losing weight may result in clinical complications, morbidity, and mortality.

OBESITY, WEIGHT CHANGE, AND OUTCOME

The first issue I wish to explore concerns the relations that exist between weight change and obesity-related complications. The term "complications" is a general one that refers to a range of pathophysiological disturbance beginning with an obesity-related physiologic or biochemical abnormality and progressing to disease and ultimately death.

Obesity is the result of long-term positive energy and nitrogen balance. On the pathway to developing obesity there evolves pathophysiologic complications which are followed later by increased morbidity and mortality. For specific conditions, what is the nature of the functions that relate the outcome variable to BMI? That is, does the complication risk rise linearly, exponentially, and so on? As shown in Figure 1, not all of the complication risk is associated with weight gain. For some obesity-related complications the risk actually rises during weight loss. An important question is whether or not these transient increases in risk outweigh the presumed long-term benefits of weight loss.

The potential relation between a hypothetical outcome and BMI is shown in Figure 2. The figure shows three different possible situations. In the first, patient A has the condition prior to developing obesity and the condition persists unchanged with weight gain. Likewise, with weight loss the outcome variable would show no measurable improvement. In patient B the outcome measure becomes progressively worse in a linear fashion with weight gain. With weight loss this subject would experience proportional improvements in prognosis. The third patient (C) has no abnormality in the lean state, but the outcome measure risk rises exponentially with weight gain. A sharp increase in risk occurs with obesity onset, and likewise a relatively small weight loss results in a marked improvement in the outcome measure.

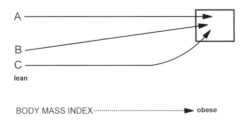

Figure 2. Obesity Complications versus Body Mass Index: Three hypothetical obese subjects who have differing responses of a risk-related physiological functions as they gain or lose weight.

An example of these three situations is the patient with high blood pressure. Some patients are hypertensive when thin, and these patients obviously would have high blood pressure when obese. Another situation is the patient who is normotensive when thin. With progressive weight gain in most patients there tends to be an increase in systolic blood pressure, and this would lead to classification of some patients as hypertensive (Figure 2, patient B). Lastly, a third type of patient might exist who is also normotensive when lean, and then experiences a very sharp rise in blood pressure with weight gain. This patient might have conditions in which physiologic changes of obesity, as seen in patient B, somehow interact with a genetic predisposition to markedly increase blood pressure.

These examples emphasize an important need: to establish the relation between each obesity risk and BMI and to determine how these risks change with weight loss. These relations need to be established across different genders, ages and ethnic groups. An important point deriving from the previous examples is that individuals may respond differently than predicted from group means. We need methods of predicting these individual responses. (See Elashoff; McArdle & Allison; and Rindskopf, this volume).

WEIGHT LOSS AND CHOICE OF OUTCOME MEASURE

The next issue relates to health outcome. There are three stages in the evolution of obesity-related complications: physiologic abnormality, morbidity and disease, and death. The simplest level to study is an obesity-related physiologic abnormality such as glucose intolerance or high blood pressure. Most weight control research is carried out at this level. Morbidity is more complex because most diseases are multifactorial and obesity is usually only a minor contributor to disease risk. For example, atherosclerosis is a complex process and even more complex at the clinical level such as with coronary heart disease. Experiments that examine morbidity are much more complex and costly to carry out than physiologic endpoint studies. Mortality studies are even more complex than morbidity studies. In the long run, our field must demonstrate that people are healthier and live longer if they either do not become obese or, if once obese, they lose weight and then maintain their weight loss. More quality studies are needed at all three levels, but in the long run we need to demonstrate improved morbidity and mortality related to our treatments. In carrying out such studies, an obvious first step is to study subjects at highest risk. For example, obese diabetic or hypertensive patients would be good initial study populations because they are likely to benefit most from long-term weight loss.

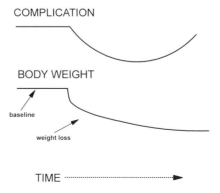

Figure 3. Influence of time on obesity-related complication or physiologic abnormality. The upper panel shows a physiologic endpoint that transiently improves with weight loss but returns to an abnormal level with long-term weight loss.

WEIGHT LOSS DURATION AND OUTCOME

One often overlooked concern is duration of weight loss. A consistent finding is that short term weight loss is associated with marked improvements in most health outcome indices. Defining short-term is difficult, but usually represents between three and six months of weight loss. More importantly, I include here ongoing weight loss as compared to weight stability or weight maintenance. In contrast, some health outcome indices, which are normalized during short-term weight loss, return to their baseline level over the long-term (Figure 3).

This occurs despite sustained weight loss. An example is serum levels of cholesterol, which decrease with short-term weight loss and rise back to their initial levels with long-term weight reduction. Thus, examining the relation between health outcome indices and weight loss requires a clear distinction between short and long-term effects.

MEASUREMENT ISSUES

Are there important methodological considerations in examining the relations between outcome measures and BMI? Weight loss studies involve measurement considerations. The first concern is referred to as "regression-to-the-mean". All physiological measurements normally vary, and those subjects with a high initial level tend to have a lower follow-up level and vise versa. Patients in many weight loss studies are segregated into groups according to their initial level of the health outcome variable. The phenomenon of regression to the mean alone would predict that those subjects with a high initial level (e.g., blood pressure) will have a significant reduction in the health outcome measure at follow-up (i.e., with weight loss). Properly designed studies ideally compensate for regression -to-the-mean by including several baseline measurements/visits and control groups of patients that are equally high on the risk factor at baseline but receive no treatment.

A second concern involves measurement bias. This is particularly true for blood pressure. Digit preference and observer bias requires use of a random zero blood pressure syphgmomanometer to quantify systolic and diastolic blood pressure changes. Although this equipment is rarely used in obesity/weight loss studies, it is standard equipment in blood pressure medication studies. Another problem with blood pressure measurements is use of improper size cuffs in obese patients. A small blood pressure cuff tends to overestimate blood pressure in obese patients. These concerns often confound interpretation of weight reduction studies.

CONFOUNDING EFFECTS OF WEIGHT LOSS AND DIET CHANGE

The next concern related to health outcome studies is two-fold: the independent effects of diet change and weight loss; and the specific nature of health outcome measure under study. First, weight loss is associated with both a change in amount and composition of foods, and with a decrease in adipose tissue. Each can have independent effects on the health outcome measure, and this is usually not considered in weight loss studies. For example, weight loss diets are often low in salt (i.e., NaCl) and reduction in salt intake has an independent effect on blood pressure change in obese.

TRANSIENT RISK CHANGES WITH WEIGHT LOSS

Although the purpose of weight reduction is to improve an obese patient's health status,

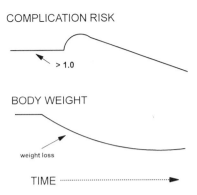

COMPLICATION RISK

> 1.0

BODY WEIGHT

weight loss

TIME

Figure 4. Risk of obesity-related complication with weight loss. The risk of some endpoints, such as cholelithiasis, may increase transiently with weight loss.

some risks may actually transiently increase with weight loss. An example is shown in Figure 4 of what is currently theorized for the effects of weight loss on gallstones.

There appears to be an increase in bile lithogenicity with short-term weight loss and this finding is paralleled by a rise in the incidence in gallstones and acute cholecystitis. Most investigators, however, suggest that once this lithogenic phase passes that post-obese subjects will no longer be at increased risk of gallstone formation (Heshka, Heymsfield, Nunez, Fittante, Legaspi, & Pi-Sunyer, submitted for publication). Some obesity-related outcomes may thus transiently worsen with weight loss but improve over the long term.

SUMMARY

Obesity is a preventable disorder and ideally prevention would negate the adverse health outcomes related to excess adipose tissue. Unfortunately efforts at obesity prevention are still in an early stage and the practitioner must therefore treat established obesity. The underlying hypothesis of this treatment is that obesity is associated with adverse health outcomes and that voluntary weight loss reduces a subject's morbidity and improves their life span. While most investigators agree that weight reduction therapy is beneficial, the following points related to treatment studies need to be considered:

♦ Obesity-related complications may vary in their relation to BMI. That is, some may be linearly related to BMI and others may be exponentially related to BMI. There may also be gender, ethnic, and age differences in how various complications are related to BMI. Future studies need to examine these relations and to consider the other study-design related factors described in this report.

♦ Complications of obesity occur at three stages: physiological, clinical illness or morbidity, and mortality. Weight loss studies are easiest to carry out that examine physiological changes. Studies that examine mortality are far more complex and require long time periods. Most research at present is focused on reversal of physiologic abnormalities associated with obesity. Long-term effective weight loss therapies are needed and advances in treatment should be accompanied by more meaningful outcome studies such as those that examine morbidity and mortality.

♦ Several considerations are important in evaluating studies that examine the effects of weight loss on physiologic endpoints, morbidity, and mortality. These include: duration of weight loss (i.e., short vs. long term); and technical factors such as regression to the mean and measurement bias.

♦ Some adverse health risks may be transiently increased with weight loss. The relative reduction in complication risk in some cases may be greatest for those at highest risk. Studies designed to examine the effects of weight loss on morbidity and mortality would profit from beginning with subject groups at high initial risk.

ACKNOWLEDGEMENTS

Supported by National Institutes of Health Grant PO1-DK42618

REFERENCES

Goldstein, D. J. (1992). Beneficial health effects of modest weight loss. International Journal of Obesity; 1, 397-415.

Heshka, S., Heymsfield, S. B., Nunez, C., Fittante, A. M., Legaspi, B. V., Pi-Sunyer, F. X. (1992). Obesity and Cholelithiasis: Risk of Gallstone Development on a Prescribed 1200 kcal/d Diet. Submitted for publication.

Kanders, B.S., Blackburn, G.L. Reducing primary risk factors by therapeutic weight loss. In T.A. Wadden & T.B. VanItallie

(Eds.), Treatment of the seriously obese patient, (pp. 213-230). New York: Guilford Press.

Kaplan, N.M. (1993). Nonpharmacologic treatment of hypertension. Current Opinion in Nephrology and Hypertension, 1,85-90.

The Trials of Hypertension Prevention Collaborative Research Group. (1992). The effects of nonpharmacologic interventions on blood pressure of persons with high normal levels. JAMA , 26, 1213-1220.

DEFINING SOCIALLY AND PSYCHOLOGICALLY DESIRABLE BODY WEIGHTS AND THE PSYCHOLOGICAL CONSEQUENCES OF WEIGHT LOSS AND REGAIN

David M. Garner

Department of Psychiatry
Michigan State University
East Lansing, MI 48824

INTRODUCTION

Obesity is viewed as a common condition in the United States with an estimated prevalence of as high as 24% for men and 27% for women (Kuczmarski, 1992). The enormity of public concern about obesity is reflected by the estimated $55 billion to be spent annually in the United States by 1995 for weight loss products and services (Marketdata Enterprises, 1989). While the diet industry still commands enormous profits and professionally led weight control programs are the standard treatment offered to those presenting with obesity, there has been a growing wave of public discontentment with both commercial and professional programs over the past several years. This has been partially fueled by highly publicized Congressional and FTC hearings charging the commercial dieting industry with misleading and fraudulent advertising.

There has been seeming unity in the scientific community in condemning deceptive advertising. However, scientists remain sharply divided on the fundamental question of whether traditional behavioral and dietary treatments should be the standard offered to obese individuals. The traditional approach has been sharply challenged recently by reports suggesting that for the vast majority of people: 1) dieting is ineffective in producing <u>lasting</u> and <u>clinically significant</u> amounts of weight loss, 2) dieting is no match for the genetic and biological factors that resist permanent weight loss once obesity has occurred, 3) dieting may aggravate health risk factors associated with obesity, and 4) dieting can lead to serious side-effects such as binge-eating and depression (cf. Bennett, 1987; Garner, 1993; Garner & Wooley, 1991; Hall & Stewart, 1989; Rothblum, 1989; Wooley & Garner, 1991).

These challenges have prompted a counter-charge that: "the public good will not be served if overweight individuals "come to believe that (a) diets do not work, (b) dieting is more dangerous than staying heavy, and (c) excess weight is a trivial risk factor" (p. 508, Brownell & Wadden, 1992). How can the professional, let alone the consuming public, make sense of these contradictory messages from professionals and what should be the standard used in

Obesity Treatment, Edited by D.B. Allison
and F.X. Pi-Sunyer, Plenum Press, New York, 1995

judging the available evidence? The discussion needs to focus on what is known about three interrelated areas of research: 1) the effectiveness of dieting, 2) the risks associated with dieting, and 3) the risks associated with being obese. The analyses of these issues have implications for defining socially and psychologically desirable (or realistically attainable) body weights as well as in evaluating the psychological consequences of weight loss and regain?

THE EFFECTIVENESS OF DIETING

It is of interest that the debate still rages on the effectiveness of dietary and behavioral treatment. Perhaps it is partly a problem of semantics. It is without question that most diets "work" in the short-term although the clinical significance of the weight loss may be questioned for many treatments (cf. Garner & Wooley, 1991). However, there can be little doubt most treatments fail to reverse the obese state, and long-term follow-up studies indicate that 90% to 95% of those who lose weight will regain it within several years (Bennie, 1977; Bjorvell & Rossner, 1985; Graham, Taylor, Hovell, & Siegel, 1983; Jordan, Canavan, & Steer, 1985; Kramer, Jeffery, Foster & Snell, 1989; Murphy et al., 1985; Stalonas, Perri, & Kerzner, 1984; Stunkard & Penick, 1979). This pattern of findings led Brownell (1982) to conclude, over a decade ago, if "cure from obesity is defined as reduction to ideal weight and maintenance of that weight for 5 years, a person is more likely to recover from most forms of cancer than from obesity."

In recent years, there has been a greater emphasis on more aggressive, multicomponent interventions that incorporate exercise, social influence, longer treatment duration, and continued therapeutic contact after the end of formal treatment (Perri & Nezu, 1993; Wadden, 1993). The assumption is that obesity is a "chronic disease" and that it needs continuous treatment over many years. While more comprehensive programs have produced greater weight losses and improved maintenance during the first 18 months after treatment (Perri, McAllister, Gange, Jordan, McAdoo, & Nezu, 1988), the results are still unimpressive when the follow-up is extended over several years (Perri, Nezu, Patti, & McCann, 1989). Very low calorie diets (VLCDs) have been proposed as one solution to the clinically insignificant weight losses achieved in most behavioral programs. Again, initial optimism with VLCDs combined with behavior therapy has been dampened by a sobering series of long-term follow-up studies indicating that the pattern with the VLCD is the same as with other dietary treatments. It is only the rate of weight regain, not the fact of weight regain, that appears open to debate (Andersen, Stokholm, Backer, & Quaade, 1988; Hovell et al., 1988; Wadden, Stunkard, & Liebschutz, 1988).

How are these data to be translated into recommendations for clinical practice? In a review of the current status of the treatment of obesity, Wadden (1993) has responded to recent criticisms of the utility and ethics of current treatments by stating that:

> *"the option of no treatment deserves serious consideration, particularly in the case of older individuals with lower body obesity who are free of health complications. It is an option, however, that cannot be universally endorsed until there are definitive research data"* (p. 211).

While it is encouraging to see that some of the concerns raised about traditional treatment have had an impact, for the debate to become more focused, there needs to be further clarification regarding the nature of the disagreement. First, those who have offered criticism of traditional treatment have generally not suggested that the obese should receive "no treatment." Rather it has been recommended that current evidence should compel greater effort in exploring alternative methods for improving life-style, health risk factors, body image, and the self-esteem of the obese without requiring significant amounts of weight loss (Garner & Wooley, 1991).

Second, the so called anti-diet movement (in my opinion more appropriately termed "the alternative to restrictive dieting approach") has been cast in a somewhat radical light when, in fact, it is based on very conservative principles that govern decision-making in other areas of science and medicine. It is based on the principle that safety and efficacy should be demonstrated before there is wide endorsement of a particular intervention. It is also grounded by the corollary that when there is compelling evidence that a treatment is either unsafe of ineffective, it should not be recommended. At the very least, the public should be fully informed regarding information available on safety and efficacy, and this should be clearly displayed or described for all commercially available products or programs. This conservative standard is applied to the pharmaceutical and cosmetic industries under Title 21 of the Code of Federal Regulations, (CFR, revised, 1993) which requires that "a drug approved for marketing may be labeled, promoted, and advertised by the manufacturer only for those uses for which the drug's safety and effectiveness have been established" (CFR, 201.100, (d)(1), 1993). Moreover, the Federal Code requires that "indications, effects, ... and any relevant warnings, hazards, contraindications, side effects, and precautions must be in the same in language and emphasis" as the approved labeling for the drug (CFR, 201.100, (d)(1), 1993). While some might argue that the effectiveness and safety standards imposed on the drug industry are too rigorous for the obesity field, the highly suggestive data on ineffectiveness and risks associated with dietary and behavioral treatment, should lead to legitimate questioning of their continued widespread use (although this may not preclude experimental use). These standards are particularly relevant given the risks of exploitation by the diet industry following the longstanding exposure of women to the powerful cultural forces to diet (Garner, Garfinkel, Schwartz & Thompson, 1980).

Third, while our understanding of the biology of weight regulation and genetics is incomplete, there are convincing data from these fields to account for the failure of traditional behavioral and dietary treatments. Research on neuroregulatory, hormonal and other physiological mechanisms that play a role in micronutrient selection, appetite, energy metabolism and weight regulation argue for a shift from a strict behavioral paradigm for weight loss to a behavioral paradigm directed toward improving health status, irrespective of weight.

THE RISKS ASSOCIATED WITH DIETING AND WEIGHT LOSS

At this time, it is remains unknown whether dieting is more dangerous than remaining heavy. This argument seems to rest on the assumption that, for most obese people, "staying heavy" is voluntary, and that dieting is viable for reversing the obese state. There are formidable methodological obstacles associated with assessing the risks of dieting versus the risks of obesity, not the least of which is finding a sample for whom treatment has led to long-term maintenance of weight loss.

Given the long history of commercial and research diet programs, it is incredible that there has been so little published data on the risks and the side-effects associated with dieting. As indicated above, the most conservative approach, and one consistent with the ethical and legal standards applied to other health-care products, is for the "burden of proof" to rest on those advocating the safety of weight loss traditional treatment rather than on those not advocating these interventions.

It is well documented that weight loss can lead to initial psychological improvement in those who are upset about their weight (Wadden & Stunkard, 1993). Although perhaps less extensively studied, there is good evidence that the virtually inevitable weight regain is followed by marked psychological distress (Wadden and Stunkard, 1993). In a thoughtful study,

Wadden, Stunkard and Smoller (1986) found that the assessment methods used were important in determining the impact of dieting on obese women participating in a weight loss program. Although women experienced improvement in mood assessment both at the beginning and end of treatment, more than 50% showed a worsening mood during one or more weeks (Wadden et al., 1986). Moreover, assessment by open-ended interview and retrospective reports revealed adverse side effects that were not apparent from standardized self-report measures. In a subsequent study, Wadden, Stunkard and Liebschutz, (1993) found that obese participants describe the weight regain after treatment as having negative effects on: 1) satisfaction with appearance, 2) self-esteem, 3) self-confidence, 4) general level of happiness, 5) physical health, 6) recreational activities, 7) job performance, 8) social activities, 9) outlook for the future and 10) relationship with partner, among other areas. Certainly these findings are important and need to be followed by improved methods for assessing the potential emotional pain associated with the failure experience of weight regain (Wooley & Garner, 1991).

Other reviews have summarized the literature indicating that restrictive dieting and weight suppression can produce emotional disturbance such as anxiety, depression, irritability, anger, social withdrawal and personality changes (cf. Garner, et al., 1985; Keys et al., 1950; Pirke & Ploog, 1987; Wadden & Stunkard, 1993; Wadden, Stunkard & Smoller, 1986). It is well known that restrictive dieting and weight suppression can lead to clinically significant binge-eating (Garner et al., 1985; Polivy & Herman, 1985), and that the treatment of binge-eating generally involves eliminating strict dietary restraint. Thus, there is an inherent conflict between the weight-loss paradigm, and the paradigm for the treatment of binge eating, a symptom increasingly observed in obese individuals seeking treatment (Marcus & Wing, 1987).

The physical risks associated with dieting are not well understood, in part, because this issue has only recently become the focus of intense research interest. However, considering the evidence suggesting that there may be physical and psychological risks associated with dieting and weight loss (including weight regain), three recommendations would seem both conservative and beyond reasonable debate at this point in time. First, the minimal standards for research and for clinical interventions should involve careful documentation of any untoward effects of dieting, weight-loss and weight regain. Secondly, there should be a standard method of reporting both physical and psychological side-effects, such as the adverse event report, currently required for pharmaceuticals. Finally, there should be continued research on the effects of weight loss and weight cycling on morbidity and mortality.

THE RISKS ASSOCIATED WITH OBESITY

While the literature on relative risks associated with obesity is complicated, and well beyond the scope of this paper, Garner and Wooley (1991) have suggested consideration of a number of points often absent from reviews on the risks of obesity:

1) Improvements in cardiovascular risk factors (e.g. cholesterol, free fatty acid, triglycerides, blood pressure, plasma glucose) are used to justify weight loss; however, it needs to be acknowledged that these rebound to initial and sometimes even higher levels with weight regain.

2) There are studies suggesting that the health risk factors do not appear to translate into higher all-cause death rates in mild to moderate obesity.

3) There are few studies indicating that mortality risk is actually reduced by weight loss, and some suggesting that weight loss increases the risk of death.

4) Many studies indicate that the group most at risk for premature death is the underweight rather than average weight or moderately obese groups, although there has never been a national health campaign to stimulate weight gain among adults below "desirable weights."

5) Some studies indicate that a high stable weight or even gradual gaining over the years may be much healthier than maintaining or losing weight (cf. Reubin, Muller, & Sorkin, in press).

6) Morbidity and mortality risks commonly attributed to obesity have never been adequately separated from those associated with a common practice among the obese, namely dieting.

7) Even if it were proven that the health risks associated with obesity were significant, it is not at all clear how this justifies offering a solution that is ineffective for most obese people, namely dietary and behavioral interventions.

It is important to separate the arguments for dieting to reverse the obese state from those advocating modifying the quality of food intake or losing small amounts of weight aimed specifically at reversing health risks (cf. Garner & Wooley, 1991). It is possible to remaining heavy, yet to change the quality of dietary intake by reducing fat and sodium, without reducing overall caloric intake. Although data are lacking, it is reasonable to assume that the prospects of maintaining small amounts of weight loss or making qualitative dietary changes are better than reaching the traditional goal of "ideal body weight".

WHY DIETS DO NOT "WORK": RECOGNITION OF THE IMPLICATIONS OF BIOLOGICAL FACTORS ACCOUNTING FOR TREATMENT FAILURES

It is no longer a mystery why diets have such a poor long-term record of success. Indeed the failure of traditional treatments seems to be rooted in the biology of weight regulation which appears to militate against most obese people becoming or remaining thin by "normalizing" their food intake. Studies of the genetics of obesity (cf. Meyer & Stunkard, 1993), dietary obesity (cf. Sclafani, 1993), the biology of weight regulation (cf. Keesey, 1993), and the physiology of energy metabolism (Ravussin & Swinburn, 1993) lend varying degrees of support for the following points. 1) Displacement of body weight usually results in metabolic adaptations designed to "defend" the body weight normally maintained. 2) Body weight "defense" occurs in obese as well as nonobese animals. 3) Genetic factors play a major role in who will become obese when exposed to a palatable diet. Although environmental factors such as diet palatability, exercise, smoking, climate and certain drugs appear to influence the absolute levels at which body weight is regulated, these have not translated into major breakthroughs in the area of obesity treatment (Stunkard, 1993). Earlier theories attributing obesity to overconsumption have yielded to explanations favoring decreased energy expenditure in the obese (Kessey, 1993). Improved technology has led to the observation that some obese under-report food intake and over-report physical activity (Lichtman et al., 1992). However, even in this recent study, the 6 women labeled as "diet resistant" were not really "overconsuming" since their average total caloric intake was only 2386 kcal per day. This is somewhat less than the average daily caloric intake of non-obese women described as "large eaters" (George, Tremblay, Depres, Landry, Allard, LeBlanc, & Bouchard, 1991). Thus, it must be emphasized that successful weight loss and maintenance for most obese people appears not to be accomplished by "normalizing eating patterns" but rather by chronic caloric restriction.

ALTERNATIVES TO TRADITIONAL WEIGHT-LOSS PROGRAMS?

It is very difficult for a person who spent years fighting his or her weight to suddenly accept the notion that significant weight loss is unrealistic. Recommending abandoning the traditional weight loss goal has been criticized as a pessimistic, nihilistic and even irresponsible view. A common objection to raising doubts about the universal mandate for weight reduction is that this may unleash an epidemic of obesity. It could be argued that promoting "self-acceptance" among the obese might lead them to relax their dietary vigilance and gain weight. However, there is little evidence for these contentions. It is hard to imagine that the level of diet-preoccupation could be further raised among women living in this country over the past two decades, precisely the same time-frame associated with an increase in the body weights for young women (Garner et al., 1980). The literatures on the biology of weight regulation and the genetic basis for obesity suggest that the vast majority of individuals need not worry about becoming obese. Moreover, contrary to the relentless declarations by the weight loss industry, for those who are heavier than average, improvements in health and self-image do not have to wait for a thinner physique. Even modest exercise has a profound effect on health and longevity appears to have a profound effect on longevity (Blair et al., 1989). Fitness plans that are geared for diminutive body sizes may be inappropriate for those who are obese and there are now exercise programs designed specifically for large women (Lyons & Bugard, 1990). Changes in eating patterns aimed at reducing the consumption of dietary fat, sodium and alcohol may have a positive effect on health without requiring weight-loss (cf. Garner & Wooley, 1991). There also may be circumstances in which small amounts of weight-loss may be lead to enduring health benefits and this should be an area of vigorous research.

IMPLICATIONS IN DEFINING SOCIALLY AND PSYCHOLOGICALLY ACCEPTABLE BODY WEIGHTS

The arguments raised thus far have implications for the definition of socially and psychologically "desirable" or "acceptable" weights. In lieu of effective solutions to obesity, the rational and humane definition of "socially and psychologically acceptable weights" should include all weights along the weight spectrum. Psychological health and social desirability are not inherent to weight but are a reflection of the cultural climate in which the individual lives. The psychological and social consequences of weight can be changed, either by modifying weight, or by modifying the social stigma and the exceptional discrimination to which the obese are exposed. To the degree that obesity is not readily reversible, this trait should be considered like traits denoting membership in other minority groups that may have social as well as medical disadvantages. Rather than continuing to offer the obese ineffective treatments, there should be greater emphasis on exploring treatments designed to improve the self-esteem, self-acceptance, quality of life and health obese individuals without requiring prolonged or severe caloric restriction. There should be greater efforts to deal with discrimination and low self-esteem in affected persons in a manner consistent with that applied to other minority groups. This involves moving toward a definition of "acceptable" weights that respects diversity, and that does not exclude most obese individuals. Fat discrimination, affecting opportunities in housing, college admission, employment, job advancement, marriage and medical assistance, may be one of the most often overlooked civil rights issues in America today because it is mistakenly believed that obesity is simply a voluntary condition brought on by poor self-control.

In sum, traditionally, the only type of treatment offered to obese people has focused on reversing the obese state. It is either stated or implied that maintenance of significant weight loss is a realistic goal and that failure to maintain weight-loss does no harm. Both of these assumptions are inconsistent with much of what we know. There is evidence that binge-eating, wide fluctuations in body weight, negative mood changes and certain health problems may be a consequence of self-initiated and professionally led diet programs. Many obese people feel that they cannot exercise, feel good about themselves or be healthy unless they attain an "ideal body weight". This is a particularly destructive trap since treatment is not effective in the long-term. It is being increasingly recognized that health, fitness and well being can be achieved by those who are obese without significant weight loss. This has clear implications for policy regarding "acceptable" body weights. It calls for greater respect for body-weight diversity and for protection against discrimination rather than the demand that the obese simply "try harder" to achieve what has proven to be an unreasonable goal.

REFERENCES

Andersen, T., Stokholm, K., Backer, O., & Quaade, F. (1988). Long-term (5-year) results after either horizontal gastroplasty or very-low-calorie diet for morbid obesity. International Journal of Obesity, 12, 277-284.

Bennett, W. I. (1987). Dietary treatments of obesity. In R. J. Wurtman, & J. J. Wurtman (Ed.), Human obesity (pp. 250-263). New York: The New York Academy of Sciences.

Binnie, G.A.C. (1977). Ten-year follow-up of obesity. Journal of the Royal College of General Practitioners, 27, 492-495.

Bjorvell, H., & Rossner, S. (1985). Long term treatment of severe obesity: Four year follow up of results of combined behavioral modification programme. British Medical Journal, 291, 379-382.

Blair, S.N., Kohl, H.W., III, Paffenbarger, R.S., Clark, D.G., Cooper, K.H., & Gibbons, L.W. (1989). Physical fitness and all-cause mortality. A prospective study of healthy men and women. JAMA, 262, 2395-2401.

Brownell, K.D. (1982). Obesity: Understanding and treating a serious, prevalent, and refractory disorder. Journal of Consulting and Clinical Psychology, 50, 820-840.

Brownell, K. D. & Wadden, T.A. (1992). Etiology and treatment of obesity: understanding a serious, prevalent, and refractory disorder. Journal of Consulting and Clinical Psychology, 60, 505-517.

CFR (Code of Federal Regulations, Title 21, revised, 1993), 201.100 (d)(1). Office of the Federal Register, Washington, DC.

Foreyt, J.P. & Goodrick, G.K. (1992). Living without dieting. Houston TX: Harrison Publishing.

Garner, D.M. (1993). Eating disorders and what to do about obesity (editorial). International Review of Psychiatry, 5, 9-12.

Garner, D.M., Garfinkel, P.E., Schwartz, D.M., & Thompson, M.M. (1980). Cultural expectations of thinness in women. Psychological Reports, 47, 483-491.

Garner, D.M., Rockert, W., Olmsted, M.P., Johnson, C.L., & Coscina, D.V. (1985). Psychoeducational principles in the treatment of bulimia and anorexia nervosa. In D.M. Garner & P.E. Garfinkel (Eds.), Handbook of psychotherapy for anorexia nervosa and bulimia (pp. 513-572). New York: Guilford Press.

Garner, D.M. & Wooley, S.C. (1991). Confronting the failure of behavioral and dietary treatments of obesity. Clinical Psychology Review, 11, 729-780.

George, V., Tremblay, A., Depres, J.P., Landry, M., Allard, L., LeBlanc, C. & Bouchard, C. (1991). Further evidence for the presence of "small eaters" and "large eaters" among women. American Journal of Clinical Nutrition, 53, 425-429.

Graham, L.E., II, Taylor, C.B., Hovell, M.F., & Siegel, W. (1983). Five-year follow-up to a behavioral weight-loss program. Journal of Consulting and Clinical Psychology, 51, 322-323.

Hall, A. & Stewart, R. (1989). Obesity: time for sanity and humanity. The New Zealand Medical Journal, 102, 134-136.

Hovell, M.F., Koch, A., Hofstetter, C.R., Sipan, C., Faucher, P., Dellinger, A., Borok, G., Forsythe, A., & Felitti, V.J. (1988). Long-term weight loss maintenance: Assessment of a behavioral and supplemented fasting regimen. American Journal of Public Health, 78, 663-666.

Jordan, H.A., Canavan, A.J., & Steer, R.A. (1985). Patterns of weight change: The interval 6 to 10 years after initial weight loss in a cognitive-behavioral treatment program. Psychological Reports, 57, 195-203.

Keesey, R.E. (1993). Physiological regulation of body energy: implications for obesity. In: A. J. Stunkard & T. A. Wadden (Eds.) Obesity Theory and Therapy 2nd Edition, (pp. 77-96). New York: Raven Press.

Keys, A., Brozek, J., Henschel, A., Mickelson, O., & Taylor, H.L. (1950). The biology of human starvation. Minneapolis: University of Minneapolis.

Lyons, P. & Burgard, D. (1990). Great Shape. The first fitness guide for large women. Palo Alto CA: Bull Publishing Co.

Kramer, F.M., Jeffery, R.W., Forster, J.L., & Snell, M.K. (1989). Long-term follow-up of behavioral treatment for obesity: Patterns of weight regain among men and women. International Journal of Obesity, 13, 123-136.

Kuczmarski, R.J. (1992). Prevalence of overweight and weight gain in the United States. Journal of the American Dietetic Association, 89, 1259-1264.

Lichtman, S.W., Pisarska, K., Berman, E.R. et al., (1992). Discrepancy between self-reported and actual caloric intake and exercise in obese subjects. New England Journal of Medicine, 327, 1893-1998.

Marcus, M.D., & Wing, R.R. (1987). Binge eating among the obese. Annals of Behavioral Medicine, 9, 23-27..

Marketdata Enterprises. The U.S. weight loss and diet control market, Lynbrook, NY: Marketdata Enterprises, March, 1989.

Meyer, J.M. & Stunkard, A. J. (1993). Genetics and human obesity. In: A. J. Stunkard & T. A. Wadden (Eds.) Obesity Theory and Therapy 2nd Edition, (pp. 137-149). New York: Raven Press.

Murphy, J.K., Bruce, B.K., & Williamson, D.A. (1985). A comparison of measured and self-reported weights in a 4-year follow-up of spouse involvement in obesity treatment. Behavior Therapy, 16, 524-530.

Perri, M.G. & Nezu, A.M. (1993). Preventing relapse following treatment for obesity. In: A. J. Stunkard & T. A. Wadden (Eds.) Obesity Theory and Therapy 2nd Edition. (pp. 287-299). New York: Raven Press.

Perri, M.G., McAllister, D.A., Gange, J.J., Jordan, R.C., McAdoo, W.G., & Nezu, A.M. (1988). Effects of four maintenance programs on the long-term management of obesity. Journal of Consulting and Clinical Psychology, 56, 529-534.

Perri, M.G., Nezu, A.M., Patti, E.T., & McCann, K.L. (1989). Effect of length of treatment on weight loss. Journal of Consulting and Clinical Psychology, 57, 450-452.

Pirke K.M., & Ploog, D. (1987). Biology of human starvation. In P.J.V. Beumont, G.D. Burrows, & R.C. Casper (Eds.), Handbook of Eating Disorders Part 1: Anorexia and Bulimia Nervosa (pp. 79-102). New York: Elsevier.

Ravussin, E. & Swinburn, B.A. (1993). Energy metabolism. In: A. J. Stunkard & T. A. Wadden (Eds.) Obesity Theory and Therapy 2nd Edition, (pp. 97-123). New York: Raven Press.

Reubin, A., Muller, D.C. & Sorkin, J.D. (in press). Long-term effects on change in body weight on all-cause mortality. Annuals or Internal Medicine.

Rothblum, E.D. (1990). Women and weight: fad and fiction. Journal of Psychology, 124, 5-24.

Sclafani, A. (1993). Dietary obesity. In: A. J. Stunkard & T. A. Wadden (Eds.) Obesity Theory and Therapy 2nd Edition, (pp. 125-136). New York: Raven Press.

Stalonas, P.M., Perri, M.G., & Kerzner, A.B. (1984). Do behavioral treatments of obesity last? A five-year follow-up investigation. Addictive Behaviors, 9, 175-183.

Stunkard, A.T. (1993). Introduction and overview. In: A. J. Stunkard & T. A. Wadden (Eds.) Obesity Theory and Therapy 2nd Edition, (pp. 1-10). New York: Raven Press.

Stunkard, A.J. & Penick, S.B. (1979). Behavior modification in the treatment of obesity: The problem of maintaining weight loss. Archives of General Psychiatry, 36, 801-806.

Wadden, A.T. (1993). The treatment of obesity: an overview. In: A. J. Stunkard & T. A. Wadden (Eds.) Obesity Theory and Therapy 2nd Edition, (pp. 197-217). New York: Raven Press.

Wadden, A.T. & Stunkard, A.J. (1993). Psychosocial consequences of obesity and dieting: research and clinical findings. In: A. J. Stunkard & T. A. Wadden (Eds.) Obesity Theory and Therapy 2nd Edition, (pp. 163-177). New York: Raven Press.

Wadden, T.A., Stunkard, A.J., & Liebschutz, J. (1988). Three-year follow-up of the treatment of obesity by very low calorie diet, behavior therapy, and their combination. Journal of Consulting and Clinical Psychology, 56, 925-928.

Wadden, T., Stunkard, A.J., & Smoller, J. (1986). Dieting and depression: A methodological study. Journal of Consulting and Clinical Psychology, 6, 869-871.

Wooley, S.C. and Garner, D.M. (1991). Obesity treatment: The high cost of false hope. Journal of the American Dietetic Association, 91, 1248-1251.

REASONABLE WEIGHTS: DETERMINANTS, DEFINITIONS AND DIRECTIONS

Gary D. Foster

University of Pennsylvania
School of Medicine
Pittsburgh, PA 19104

INTRODUCTION

Traditionally, the goal of any weight loss effort has been simple and straight-forward: reduce to ideal weight. Establishing goals based on reasonable rather than ideal weights (Brownell & Wadden, 1991; 1992) is a dramatic paradigm shift with implications for how treatment is selected, delivered, and evaluated. Such a fundamental shift requires theoretical specificity and empirical strength. The purpose of this chapter is to review the concept of a reasonable weight from several perspectives. First, the emergence of a reasonable weight from within the historical context of obesity treatment will be described. Second, the rationale for abandoning the use of ideal weights will be presented. Third, the various factors that influence the determination of a reasonable weight will be reviewed. Finally, suggestions for further research will be presented.

HISTORICAL PERSPECTIVE

Modest Beginnings

Since the idea of a reasonable weight is a relatively recent one, it is useful to place it within the history of obesity treatment over the last 35 years. Stunkard and McLaren-Hume's (1959) seminal and bleak review provided an ominous beginning for obesity treatment. In short, they concluded that among the few patients who completed treatment, few lost weight and even fewer maintained it. It was no wonder that Stuart's (1967) paper describing an effective behavioral treatment for obesity was met with such enthusiasm. It prompted a flurry of treatment outcome studies in the 1970's that demonstrated behavioral treatments produced weight losses of approximately 4 kg in 10 weeks, and most of that weight loss was maintained at a one-year follow-up (Wadden, 1993). Although this was a significant improvement since 1959, a 4 kg weight loss, no matter how well maintained, was thought to be of limited value for patients weighing over 100 kg.

Obesity Treatment, Edited by D.B. Allison
and F.X. Pi-Sunyer, Plenum Press, New York, 1995

Aggressive Approaches

The 1980's were characterized by calls for treatments that would increase the magnitude of weight losses (Brownell, 1982; Brownell & Wadden, 1986; Foreyt, 1981). More aggressive approaches (e.g., very low calorie diets and pharmacotherapy) were combined with behavior therapy to achieve larger weight losses that could be well maintained. This approach was fueled, in part, by the assumption that medical benefits and patient satisfaction would increase with larger weight losses. Although these aggressive approaches doubled the weight losses of more conservative treatments, long-term results were not clinically different from more traditional behavioral approaches (Brownell & Stunkard, 1981; Wadden et al., 1989). By the end of the 1980's, suggestions to "push the limits of treatment" included the recognition of physiological limits in some patients (Brownell & Jeffery, 1987).

Moderation

The aggressive zeitgeist of the 1980s has been firmly supplanted by a theme of moderation in the 1990s (Brownell & Wadden, 1991; 1992; Foreyt & Goodrick, 1992; Foster & Kendall, submitted; Wilson, 1994). This dramatic change in philosophy was prompted by a confluence of scientific and cultural developments. Scientifically, the medical benefits of modest weight loss and the physiological determinants of body weight (described below) suggested more moderate goals. Culturally, the high visibility of celebrities' large weight losses and regain increased popular pessimism about the permanence of significant weight loss. Preliminary data about the potential hazards of yo-yo dieting (Lissner et al., 1991) prompted professionals (Garner & Wooley, 1991), lay advocacy groups (e.g., National Association to Aid Fat Acceptance), and the popular press (Kolata, 1992; O'Neil, 1992) to suggest that dieting may do more harm than good. This climate of popular and professional revolt lead to the increased scrutiny of commercial weight loss programs by city (New York City Department of Consumer Affairs, 1991), state (Michigan Department of Public Health, 1990), and federal (NIH Technology Assessment Conference Panel, 1992; U.S. House of Representatives, 1990) agencies. It was within this scientific and sociocultural context that the concept of a reasonable weight was proposed (Brownell & Wadden, 1991; 1992).

RATIONALE

The shift from ideal to reasonable weights requires a rationale that is clinically based and empirically derived. Several factors support such a shift.

Physiological Limits

The first is a body of research over the last decade suggesting the importance of various physiological factors (e.g., genetics, resting metabolic rate, adipose tissue development) in the regulation of body weight and weight change (Meyer & Stunkard, 1993; Ravussin & Swinburn, 1992; Sjostrom, 1993). These data dispel popular beliefs that weight is under total environmental control and suggest that the effect of the typical exhortation to "eat less and exercise more" will be greatly constrained by biological factors (Wilson, 1994). It is likely that physiological factors provide upper and lower limits within which environmental factors exert influence. Assuming that all patients should seek an ideal weight ignores the existence of these physiological boundaries and may lead to unrealistic expectations.

Cultural Pressures

The significant increase in knowledge about the biological determinants of weight has not tempered the intense cultural pressure to be thin, especially for women (Brownell, 1991). Within this sociocultural context, treatment programs should attempt to attenuate rather than exacerbate the pain of obesity. Establishing ideal weights as attainable, reinforces, at least implicitly, that "thinner is better" and that excess weight can be "corrected" solely by patients' behaviors. Setting more moderate weight loss goals and acknowledging the arbitrary nature of cultural ideals are consistent with efforts to enhance body image, improve self-esteem, and decrease weight preoccupation (Cash, 1991; Foreyt & Goodrick, 1992). Abandoning the quixotic quest for the "ideal" weight underscores that weight should not be a barometer of self-esteem, discipline, willpower or any other moral or personality variable.

Inappropriate Standards

A third reason for considering goals other than ideal weight is the inappropriateness of height-weight tables. The most frequently used are the Metropolitan Life Insurance Tables (1984) which define ideal weights, adjusted for height, as those associated with the lowest mortality based on life insurance actuarial data. Harrison (1985) has described the methodological and conceptual shortcomings of these and other height-weight databases that limit their validity and generalizability. It is unclear, for example, how the experiences of an insured population are representative of obese persons who are often denied life insurance. Even ignoring these limitations, the definition of an ideal weight does not mean that everyone is capable of attaining it. This distinction between ideal and reasonable is common in treating other medical conditions. It would be unusual, for example, to suggest that all diabetics attain a serum glucose of 80-120 mg/dl or that all hypertensives attain a blood pressure of 110/70. Rather, goals are based on individual patient factors (e.g., baseline values, comorbidity) and a consideration of empirical findings (e.g., degree of risk reduction, benefits and risks of treatment).

Medical Consequences

Perhaps the most compelling rationale for reexamining goal weights is that many obesity-related conditions, such as diabetes, hypertension, hyperlipidemia, and sleep apnea, can be significantly improved with even modest (5-10%) weight loss (Goldstein, 1992; Heymsfield, in press; Kanders & Blackburn, 1992; Pi Sunyer, 1993). These clinically significant changes occur when many patients are still considerably overweight. Goldstein (1992) argued that modest weight loss also confers a decrease in mortality risk (e.g., a 5% reduction in weight confers a 12% reduction in mortality risk for a male with a BMI of 40). Further, research in the last decade (Sjostrom, 1993) has demonstrated that the location of excess body fat, rather than the actual amount, is a more important mediator of medical risk. Thus, reductions of fat in specific areas (e.g., intra-abdominally) may be more important than overall changes.

Behavioral demands. A common sense rationale for adopting more reasonable goals is that modest changes in behavior and weight will be easier to maintain than dramatic ones (Brownell & Wadden, 1992; Goldstein, 1992). There are no data to directly assess this question, but the notion is generally supported by Kayman, Bruvold & Stern's (1990) finding that successful maintainers did not completely eliminate favorite foods, while those who relapsed attempted to follow very restrictive diets. Further indirect support is provided by Wadden, Foster & Letizia (1994) who found that a structured weight maintenance program was more effective following a 12 kg weight loss than a 22 kg weight loss, although factors other than the amount of weight loss may have accounted for the differences. Even without convincing data, there is no doubt that the behavioral demands of weight maintenance (intake and activity) will increase as weight decreases. Since reductions in energy expenditure are roughly proportional to decreases in body weight (Ravussin & Swinburn, 1993), the more weight patients lose, the lower their maintenance requirements will be.

Faulty Assumptions

The continued use of ideal weights is based on two faulty assumptions. One is that weight is the sole indicator of treatment efficacy. Our ability to easily measure weight has resulted in an overemphasis on weight, itself, rather than on the deleterious consequences associated with it. A second faulty assumption is the belief that all overweight people, at least of the same height, are the same. This assumption is reinforced by programs that employ a single approach across a wide variety of patients, expecting that all persons of the same height can attain the same weight. This inattention to heterogeneity is a principal reason that Brownell & Wadden (1991) have suggested setting more reasonable goals.

DETERMINANTS OF A REASONABLE WEIGHT

Establishing the inappropriateness of ideal weights is considerably easier than suggesting specific alternatives. We are faced with difficult decisions about what standards to use. Should goals be determined idiographically or nomothetically? Do practitioners or patients decide what is reasonable? This section will review determinants of a reasonable weight from the perspectives of professionals and patients.

Professional Perspective

Medical risk. From a professional standpoint, attempts to define reasonable outcomes should be based on a philosophy of treatment and a review of empirical findings. Although a detailed philosophy of treatment is beyond the scope of this chapter, the serious medical consequences associated with obesity constitute the driving force to treat it. Empirically, it is clear that there is significant heterogeneity in the biology and behavior of obese persons. Thus, a reasonable weight should be anchored to changes in medical risk but moderated by biological and behavioral differences. Using medical outcomes as the primary reference for reasonable weights is difficult because the measurement of medical risk is more complex than standing on a scale. A medical emphasis also raises unanswered questions about the treatment of obese individuals who present without clinically manifest illness. VanItallie & Lew (1992) have suggested clinically useful guidelines for assessing pre-treatment risk in obese patients, and Atkinson (1993) has suggested using changes in glucose intolerance, blood pressure, hyperlipidemia, and sleep apnea as indicators of medical improvement.

Behavioral demands. Behavioral requirements are the most limiting factor in attaining or maintaining any weight. Independent of how medically beneficial a particular weight may be, it must be evaluated with the context of the patient's behavioral repertoire and biological predisposition. Weight loss requires a significant allocation of time, energy, and money as patients attempt to change long-standing eating and exercise habits. As with any aspect of human performance, it may be impossible to maintain extreme changes for prolonged periods of time. The same behavioral tasks (e.g., attending sessions, increasing physical activity, decreasing fat intake) may become increasingly difficult as treatment progresses and/or weight decreases. Without minimizing the demands of weight loss, the maintenance of weight loss is even more difficult (Wadden, in press).

Patients may need to experiment in order to find a "comfort zone" in which they can maintain weight with consistent but not extraordinary effort. Rather than deciding upon a final goal before treatment, it may be more prudent to set smaller proximal goals which signal the need to examine the behavioral costs and benefits of further weight loss. Such an approach enables patients to take "breaks" and practice weight maintenance skills rather than blindly pursuing some predetermined goal. Emphasis should be on the management of a healthy weight rather than the attainment of an ideal one. This emphasis on management, rather than cure, is consistent with the treatment of other chronic conditions.

Psychosocial consequences. There is a disturbing lack of data on the psychosocial effects (positive or negative) of weight loss (Foster & Wadden, in press a). It is likely that a reasonable weight will be one associated with positive psychosocial consequences, but it is equally important to consider any adverse changes that are observed in a minority of cases (Foster & Wadden, in press b; O'Neill & Jarrell, 1992). Clinically, it may be useful to inquire about the psychosocial effects of previous weight loss efforts, with particular attention to any untoward reactions.

Patient's Perspective

The factors reviewed above are based on a treatment model in which a professional unilaterally determines treatment goals. While this approach may be appropriate for treatments that are provided by professionals (e.g., radiation, angioplasty), obesity treatment is provided by patients. They change eating and exercise habits. Thus, their views of what is reasonable will greatly affect their motivation and evaluations about treatment.

Sociocultural factors. Broad factors such as cultural ideals of beauty (Rodin, 1993), socioeconomic status (Sobal & Stunkard, 1989), and ethnicity (Kumanyika, 1993) will moderate determinations of what is reasonable. More specific contextual factors include the weights of family and friends, the amount of support required from others, the effect of weight change on social relationships, and feedback from others.

Perceptions. Many of the factors considered under the professional determinants must also be assessed from the patient's perspective. It is possible, for example, that patients and practitioners have very different notions about the various benefits and costs of treatment. For example, a 10% reduction in body weight may be a favorable outcome for practitioners, but it is likely to be unacceptable to 150 kg patient who expected to lose 75 kg. Patients' perceptions of the behavioral demands, health benefits, and psychosocial changes will greatly affect their motivation to continue treatment. Unfortunately, there has been little or no attention given to these important perceptions.

Expectations. Patients will have a variety of expectations regarding short- and long-term weight control (Wadden & Foster, 1992). These expectations and the degree to which they are met will likely affect self-efficacy and relapse (Brownell, et al., 1986). Expectations may be linked to the reason for seeking treatment, previous dieting history, or individual cognitive styles. The specific nature of patients' expectations and the likelihood of their occurrence should be evaluated carefully before treatment (Wadden & Foster, 1992).

Goal setting. Virtually all patients entering a weight control program have decided upon some goal weight. Despite its obvious importance to patients, we know little about how an actual number is selected. One study suggests that most patients begin treatment seeking an ideal weight (Miller & Eggert, 1992) while anecdotal reports suggest that patients select weights based on professional advice, ideal weight charts, weight lost during last diet, a weight at a particular landmark (e.g., wedding, pre-pregnancy), physical comfort, clothing size, or a particular number (e.g., below 200). Understanding the process of how patients select particular goals may provide insights for methods to help patients accept more modest goals.

The patient factors described above are not meant to be exhaustive, but they point to the necessity of considering patients' views in the determination of a reasonable weight. Continuing to ignore the patients' perspective will diminish the clinical utility of professionally based guidelines.

DEFINITIONS

The number and variety of factors that affect practitioners' and patients' determinations of a reasonable weight precludes a specific definition at this time. Given the lack of definitive data, what should clinicians suggest as alternatives to ideal weights?

Clinical Formula

Wadden (Sandoz Nutrition, 1988) suggested a formula based on weight history and age. The starting point for the formula is an adult weight that has been maintained for at least one year. This base weight is then increased by .5 kg for each year the patient is above 21 years of age. This formula was developed for clinical use and has not been evaluated empirically. Cormillot and Fuchs (1991) retrospectively described a "possible" weight in a clinical sample of 176 women who had maintained weight losses for at least 6 months and were weight stable. Regression analyses revealed that a "possible weight" was defined by adjusting ideal weight upward as follows: 1 kg for each 10 kg current weight is above ideal; 1 kg for each decade of obesity, and 1 kg for each decade over 20 years of age. Many patients' "possible" weights stabilized only after some weight regain, and were, on average, 9 kg greater than ideal weights. This study is not without methodological limitations, but they are the only data, to my knowledge, that empirically defined an other than ideal weight.   It can be argued that substituting any formula for ideal weight still ignores individual differences. As the authors of these formulas suggest, no one formula will be appropriate for all patients and each formula may be subject to error in some individuals. Their value lies in increasing patient acceptance for non-ideal weights and giving clinicians a springboard to discuss more reasonable goals. Moreover, they provide researchers and clinicians a definitive formula for empirical evaluation.

General Guidelines

Several less specific guidelines have suggested as alternatives to an ideal weight. Atkinson (1993) has suggested that among many variables reviewed, actual change (kg) in body weight should not be used as a criteria for success in the treatment of obesity. He suggested three broad categories of "minimum", "intermediate" and "full" success that are anchored to body size, body fat, weight maintenance, medical complications, and psychosocial problems. This approach is not without methodological difficulties, but it does appropriately shift our focus to a more broad based assessment. Foster & Kendall (under review) suggested that a 10% reduction in initial weight is an appropriate goal for all patients, principally because of its medical benefits. Independent of treatment method, most patients are able to reduce body weight by 10%. They suggest, at each successive 5% interval, that practitioners and patients jointly assess the benefits and risks of further weight loss. Brownell and Wadden (1992) suggested that a reasonable weight be no lower than an adult weight (above age 21) that has been maintained for at least one year. Higher weights may be more appropriate after considering family weight history, behavioral demands, and appearance concerns.

FUTURE DIRECTIONS

Many of the presumed benefits of a reasonable weight (less behavioral demand, increased self-efficacy, improved maintenance) have not been directly tested. Some studies, for example, suggested that extending treatment to achieve personally meaningful goal weights improved weight maintenance (Wolfe, 1992), while others found that longer treatment had no significant effect on weight loss or weight maintenance (Perri et al., 1989; Wadden, Foster & Letizia, 1994). None of these studies, however, was designed to assess the effects of different goal weights.

Methodological Difficulties

There are two primary challenges to conducting research on the determination or benefits of a reasonable weight. The first is that many of the proposed determinants of a reasonable weight are not amenable to straightforward measurement. Assessing the behavioral demands of long-term weight control, for example, requires operationalized criteria as well as reliable and valid measures. Patients' perceptions are similarly difficult to assess. Assessment of physiological measures is limited by high expense and low accessibility to most clinicians. Research is also hampered by the large number of factors and their significant variability and interaction. This heterogeneity within and between patients may obscure expected differences based solely on goal weight. These problems do not preclude meaningful research, but they underscore the need for multidimensional assessments in large samples.

Proposed Studies

Descriptive studies. Given our limited fund of knowledge about the factors that determine a reasonable weight, descriptive studies can provide specific areas for more controlled investigations. One approach is to examine the correlates of weight stability. These stabilizations may represent weight plateaus during weight loss or a weight that has been maintained for at least one year after weight loss. The biobehavioral context in which these weights occur may increase our understanding about the combination of factors that affect both weight loss and weight maintenance. It is possible, for example, that weight loss may slow due to behavioral fatigue, while weight maintenance is more affected by physiological parameters. Another approach is to study the various characteristics of persons who are successfully maintaining significant weight losses (Colvin & Ohlson, 1983). How do maintained weights differ from ideal weights? What are the physiological characteristics of those who successfully maintain weight loss and how do they perceive the behavioral demands of long-term weight control? Such studies can avoid the problems of selective sampling by studying persons who have not maintained weight loss to determine which factors distinguish the two groups.

Controlled studies. The primary focus of controlled investigations should focus on whether adopting more reasonable goal weights has any effect on long-term weight maintenance. In such trials, patients would be randomly assigned to various goal weights based on findings from descriptive studies. If physiological factors are important, for example, one group may be assigned to a weight based on initial resting metabolic rate. If a patient's individual experience is important, a goal weight may be based on a previous weight that was maintained. Without such data, goals based on ideal weight, clinical formula, or a 10% reduction in body weight seem appropriate for evaluation. Investigators will need to assess the variety of other factors (described above) that may mediate or moderate the effects of a different goal weight.

Process of patient acceptance. Within both descriptive and controlled trial, special attention should be paid to the factors that govern patients' views about reasonable weights. Patient acceptance of these goals is critical given that patients provide and evaluate treatment. It may be that certain factors govern initial goal setting (e.g., current health status, body dissatisfaction, appearance, physical symptoms, special event) while other factors (experience of behavioral demands, cognitive styles, life stressors, unmet expectations) modify these goals.

SUMMARY

Although the concept of a reasonable weight is "both sensible and humane" (Wilson, 1994), there is little research to support its presumed non-medical benefits. Recent research suggests that a shift from ideal to reasonable weights is supported by the significant heterogeneity in behavioral and biological determinants of weight. Specific definitions of a reasonable weight are hampered by its multiple determinants which are not easily assessed. Descriptive and controlled studies which include assessments of patients' perceptions may hasten the transition from principle to practice. Specifically, research is needed to determine whether reasonable weights are truly beneficial for long-term weight control and what techniques may be most effective for helping patients accept more modest outcomes.

REFERENCES

Atkinson, R.L. (1993). Proposed standards for judging the success of the treatment of obesity. Annals of Internal Medicine, 119, 677-680.

Brownell, K.D. (1991). Dieting and the search for the perfect body: where physiology and culture collide. Behavior Therapy, 22, 1-12.

Brownell, K.D. (1982). Obesity: Understanding a treating a serious, prevalent and refractory disorder. Journal of Consulting and Clinical Psychology, 50, 820-840.

Brownell, K.D., & Jeffery, R.W. (1987). Improving long-term weight loss: Pushing the limits of treatment. Behavior Therapy, 18, 353-374.

Brownell, K.D., Marlatt, G.A., Lichtenstein, E., & Wilson, G.T. (1986). Understanding and preventing relapse. American Psychologist, 41, 765-782.

Brownell, K.D., Stunkard, A.J. (1981) Couples training, pharmacotherapy, and behavior therapy in the treatment of obesity. Archives of General Psychiatry, 38, 1233-1239.

Brownell, K.D., & Wadden, T.A. (1986). Behavior therapy for obesity: Modern approaches and better results. In K. D. Brownell & J. P. Foreyt (Eds)., Handbook of eating disorders: Physiology, psychology and treatment of obesity, anorexia, and bulimia (pp. 180-197). New York: Basic Books.

Brownell, K.D., & Wadden, T.A. (1991). The heterogeneity of obesity: Fitting treatments to individuals. Behavior Therapy, 22, 153-177.

Brownell, K.D., & Wadden, T.A. (1992). Etiology and treatment of obesity: Understanding a serious, prevalent and refractory disorder. Journal of Consulting and Clinical Psychology, 60, 505-517.

Cash, T.F. (1991) Body image therapy: A program for self-directed change. New York: Guilford Press.

Colvin, R.H. & Olson, S.B. (1983) A descriptive analysis of men and women who have lost significant weight and are highly successful at maintaining weight loss. Addictive Behaviors, 8, 287-295.

Cormillot, A. & Fuchs, A. (1991) Possible weight. In Y. Oomura, S. Tarui, S. Inoue, & T. Shimazu (eds) Progress in obesity research 1990. (pp. 663-664) London: John Libbey.

Foreyt, J.P., Goodrick, G.K., Gotto, A.M. (1981). Limitations of the behavioral treatment of obesity. Journal of Behavioral Medicine, 4, 159-174.

Foreyt, J.P. & Goodrick, G.K. (1992) Living without dieting. Houston, TX: Harrison Publishing.

Foster, G.D. & Kendall, P.C. (under review). The realistic treatment of obesity: Changing the scales of success.

Foster, G.D. & Wadden, T.A. (in press, a). Social and psychological effects of weight loss. In K.D. Brownell & C.G. Fairburn (Eds.) Comprehensive handbook of eating disorders and obesity. New York: Guilford Press

Foster, G.D. & Wadden, T.A (in press, b) The psychology of obesity, weight loss and weight regain. In G.L. Blackburn & B. Kanders (Eds) Obesity: Pathophysiology, psychology and treatment. NY: Chapman and Hall.

Garner, D.M. & Wooley, S.C. (1991). Confronting the failure of behavioral and dietary treatments for obesity. Clinical Psychology Review, 11, 729-780.

Goldstein, D.J. (1992) Beneficial effects of modest weight loss. International Journal of Obesity, 16, 397-416.

Harrison, G.G. (1985). Height-weight tables. Annals of Internal Medicine, 103, 989-993.

Heymsfield, S.B. (in press). Defining the weight necessary to achieve substantial health gains. In F.X. Pi Sunyer & D.B. Allison (Eds). Obesity treatment: Establishing goals, improving outcomes, and establishing the research agenda. NY: Plenum Press.

Kanders, B.S. & Blackburn, G.L. (1992). Reducing primary risk factors by therapeutic weight loss. In T.A. Wadden, T.B. Van Itallie (Eds.), Treatment of the seriously obese patient (pp. 213-230). NY: Guilford.

Kayman, S. Bruvold, W., & Stern, J.S. (1990). Maintenance and relapse after weight loss in women: Behavioral aspects. American Journal of Clinical Nutrition, 52, 800-807.

Kolata, G.L. (1992) Do diets work? New York Times, November 22, p. 1.

Kumanyika, S.R. (1993). Special issues regarding obesity in minority populations. Annals of Internal Medicine. 119, 650-654.

Lissner, L., Odell, P.M., D'Agostino, R.B., Stokes, J., Kreger, B.E., Belanger, A.J., & Brownell, K.D. (1991). Variability of body weight and health outcomes in the Framingham population. New England Journal of Medicine, 324, 1839-1844.

Metropolitan Life Insurance Company (1984). 1983 Metropolitan height and weight tables. Statistical Bulletin of New York Metropolitan Life Insurance Company, 64, 2-9.

Meyer, J.M. & Stunkard, A.J. (1993). Genetics and human obesity. In: A.J. Stunkard & T.A. Wadden (Eds) Obesity: Theory and therapy. (pp. 137-150) New York: Raven Press.

Miller, W.C. & Eggert, K.E. (1992). Weight loss perceptions, characteristics, and expectations of an overweight male and female population. Medicine, Exercise, Nutrition and Health, 1, 42-47.

Michigan Department of Public Health (1991) Toward safe weight loss. Lansing, MI: Author.

NIH Technology Assessment Conference Panel (1993). Methods for voluntary weight loss and control. Annals of Internal Medicine. 119, 764-770.

New York City Department of Consumer Affairs (1991). A weighty issue: Dangers and deceptions of the weight loss industry. NY: Author.

O'Neill, M. (1992) A growing movement fights diets instead of fat. New York Times, April 12, p. 1.

O'Neil P.M., Jarrell M.P. (1992) Psychological aspects of obesity and dieting. In T.A. Wadden, T.B. Van Itallie (eds) The treatment of the seriously obese patient, (pp. 252-272). New York: Guilford Press.

Perri, M.G., Nezu, A.M., Patti, E.T., McCann, K.L. (1989). Effect of length of treatment on weight loss. Journal of Consulting and Clinical Psychology, 57, 450-452.

Pi-Sunyer, F.X. (1993). Short-term medical benefits and adverse effects of weight loss. Annals of Internal Medicine, 119, 722-726.

Ravussin, E. & Swinburn, B.A. (1993) Energy metabolism. In A.J. Stunkard & T.A. Wadden (Eds) Obesity: Theory and therapy. (pp.97-123) New York: Raven Press.

Rodin, J. (1993). Cultural and psychosocial determinants of weight concerns. Annals of Internal Medicine, 119, 643-645.

Sandoz Nutrition (1988). Weight and lifestyle inventory. Minneapolis, MN: Author.

Sobal, J. & Stunkard, A.J. (1989). Socioeconomic status and obesity: A review of the literature. Psychological Bulletin, 105, 260-275.

Sjostrom, L. (1993). Impacts of body weight, body composition, and adipose tissue distribution on morbidity and mortality. In: A.J. Stunkard & TA Wadden (eds) Obesity: Theory and Therapy (pp. 13-41). New York: Raven Press.

Stuart, R.B. (1967). Behavioral control of overeating. Behavior Research and Therapy, 5, 357-365.

Stunkard, A.J., & McLaren-Hume, N. (1959). The results of treatment for obesity. Archives of Internal Medicine, 103, 79-85.

U.S. House of Representatives, Committee on Small Business, Subcommittee on Regulation, Business Opportunities, and Energy. (1990). Deception and fraud in the diet industry: Part I. (pp.101-150). Washington, D.C.: U.S. Government Printing Office.

Van Itallie, T.B. & Lew, E.A. (1992) Assessment of morbidity and mortality risk in the overweight patient. In T.A. Wadden, T.B. Van Itallie (eds) The treatment of the seriously obese patient (pp. 3-32) New York: Guilford.

Wadden, T.A. (in press). Characteristics of successful weight loss maintainers. In F.X. Pi Sunyer & D.B. Allison (Eds). Obesity treatment: Establishing goals, improving outcomes, and establishing the research agenda. NY: Plenum Press.

Wadden, T.A. (1993). The treatment of obesity: An overview. In: A.J. Stunkard & TA Wadden (eds) <u>Obesity: Theory and Therapy</u> (pp. 197-217). New York: Raven Press.

Wadden, T.A., & Foster, G.D. (1992). Behavioral assessment and treatment of markedly obese patients. In T.A. Wadden, T.B. Van Itallie (Eds.), <u>Treatment of the seriously obese patient</u> (pp. 290-330). NY: Guilford.

Wadden, T.A., Foster, G.D., & Letizia, K.A. (1994). One year behavioral treatment of obesity: Comparison of moderate and severe caloric restriction and the effects of weight maintenance therapy. <u>Journal of Consulting and Clinical Psychology, 62</u>, 165-171.

Wadden, T.A., Sternberg, J.A., Letizia, K.A., Stunkard, A.J., & Foster, G.D. (1989). Treatment of obesity by very low calorie diet, behavior therapy and their combination: A five-year perspective. <u>International Journal of Obesity, 13</u>, 39-46.

Wilson, G.T. (1994). Behavioral treatment of obesity: Thirty years and counting. <u>Advances in Behavior Research and Therapy, 16</u>, 31-75.

Wolfe, B.L. (9992). Long-term maintenance of weight loss following attainment of goal weight: A preliminary investigation. <u>Addictive Behaviors, 17</u>, 469-477.

IS WEIGHT STABILITY ITSELF A REASONABLE GOAL?

Andrew M. Prentice

Dunn Clinical Nutrition Centre
Hills Road
Cambridge, United Kingdom CB2 2DH

INTRODUCTION

The answer to whether weight stability is a reasonable goal depends first and foremost on the degree and type of a patient's obesity. "Yes - if you're slim!" would be a simple facetious response, and one which is not entirely irrelevant to a conference on obesity treatment since many slightly overweight people seek treatment for a perceived, but in fact non-existent, problem. Weight stability is almost certainly the optimal goal for such people since unnecessary attempts at weight loss may trigger abnormal attitudes to food which could precipitate much greater problems than those associated with mild overweight. Also inherent within this first answer is the reminder that prevention is better than cure. This message is becoming ever more important in the light of emerging evidence, summarised below, that weight loss may be undesirable, even in the obese.

The answer also depends on to whom you put the question. Life insurance companies will focus on mortality as their criterion of 'reasonableness', government departments on reducing the cost burden on their health budget, employers on reduced absenteeism and improved productivity, surgeons on reduced risk of post-operative complications, and general physicians on factors such as reduced blood pressure or improved glucose tolerance. But perhaps most importantly the patient will probably have a completely different agenda including improved looks, self-image and hence mental well-being, and will continue to seek treatment even if it carries an increased risk of premature mortality since the risk is often considered remote. To most *patients* weight stability is certainly *not* a reasonable goal.

In addressing this question it is useful to make a number of initial assumptions: a) that it is accepted that obesity does represent a significant independent risk factor for a number of serious diseases and for early death especially at a body mass index (BMI) >30 kg/m^2. (The question of whether there is any 'safe' obesity, for instance with low waist/hip ratio, is considered elsewhere in this conference.); b) that it is accepted that weight gain in definitely undesirable in someone who is average to overweight (see for example Mason *et al.* 1990); and c) that for cosmetic and other minor reasons true weight loss is always judged to be successful and desirable at least by the patient. This paper will therefore address only the potential benefits of weight loss and of weight cycling, and will concentrate on major endpoints, especially mortality.

WEIGHT LOSS, RISK FACTORS AND MORBIDITY

There is an abundant literature demonstrating that moderate weight loss can have significant palliative effects on a wide range of obesity-induced metabolic and physical dysfunctions. The evidence has recently been extensively reviewed by Kanders & Blackburn (1992) who recommend that '..... 10-20% weight loss can ameliorate most obesity-related diseases.' Few people would dispute that in terms, for instance, of glucose tolerance or osteoarthritis weight loss is preferable to weight stability even if some of the weight lost is subsequently regained. Perhaps the only disease in which there has been a perception that weight loss might actually be detrimental in the short term is gall stone formation. However, Kanders & Blackburn (1992) conclude that '.... with careful monitoring and appropriate treatment, weight loss can reduce the risk of gallstone formation.'

WEIGHT LOSS AND MORTALITY

Compared to the large amount of evidence linking obesity to increased mortality there is a surprisingly small amount of prospective or retrospective data on the question of whether weight loss has a beneficial impact on survival. Much of the data that does exist is confounded by at least one of the following factors: a) the possibility that weight loss is due to pre-existing disease at the time of enrollment into the study;   b) inadequate control for smoking;   c) the fact that actuarial data on patients offered reduced premiums after weight loss may be biased by the fact that they have to pass a new medical examination (thus being selected for good health) whereas the control group do not;   and d) that voluntary versus involuntary weight loss is not

Table 1. Summary of studies reporting beneficial effect of weight loss on longevity.

Citation	Sample size		Deaths	Effect on mortality
Dublin (1953)	M	600	33	16 - 37% reduction
	F	1700	165	20 - 39% "
Society Actuaries (1960) reduction	M	?	450	15 - 36%
Society Actuaries (1980)	M	1900	35	'quite favourable'
Hammond & Garfinkel (1969)	M	359k	12965	CHD: 11% reduction
				Stroke: 6% "
	F	446k	5963	CHD: 1% "
				Stroke: 6-25% "
Wannamathee & Shaper (1990)	M	7272	357	10% reduction
Lean et al. (1992)	M		146	3-4 mo survival/kg lost
	F		117	

Adapted from Williamson & Pamuk (1993)

distinguished. Factors (a) and (b) would tend to underestimate benefit, factor (c) tends to overestimate. The effect of (d), which is of particular interest in the present context, is unknown but it is usually assumed to underestimate benefit.

Williamson & Pamuk (1993) have reviewed the results of a search which yielded only 6 relevant data sets. Their summary of the pertinent results is shown in Table 1. Note that the first three (insurance company) studies may be biased towards a favourable response by the effect of the additional medical. The Cancer Prevention Study I reported by Hammond & Garfinkel (1969) represents by far the biggest study. Stroke and CHD mortality were analysed by age, gender, initial body weight (<90, 90-109, 110-119, >120% mean weight) and 5-year weight loss (<10, 10-19, 20+ lbs). In only six cells were the CHD or stroke mortality significantly reduced and in four of these the effect was rather trivial. Weight loss was never effective in groups <110% of mean weight for the population, or in groups losing more than 20 lbs. The anticipated benefits of weight loss were therefore not clearly apparent. Likewise the benefits seen in the last two studies in Table 1 were not substantial and are open to some methodological queries. Williamson & Pamuk (1993) conclude that: ' Taken as a whole, the evidence from these 6 studies that weight loss in obese persons increases longevity is equivocal.' Two further important studies have been published since the above review was prepared.

Pamuk *et al.* (1992) reported on the relationship between weight loss and survival in 4690 men and women in the NHANES I Epidemiologic Follow-up Study, 1971-1987. Effects of pre-existing disease were minimised by restricting the follow-up to those who survived a minimum of 5 years after the initial survey. All cause, CVD and non-CVD mortality was

Table 2. Summary of results from the NHANES I Epidemiologic Follow-up Study relative risk of death over 10 y follow-up.

	Weight loss (%)	≤ 26	Maximum BMI 26 to <29	>29
Men				
All causes	<5	1.0	0.9	1.5
	5 to <15	1.1	1.3	1.2
	>15	1.8	2.1	2.0
C V D	<5	1.0	1.0	1.9
	5 to <15	1.0	1.7	1.4
	>15	1.3	1.9	2.5
Non C V D	<5	1.0	0.9	1.0
	5 to <15	1.2	1.0	1.0
	>15	2.1	2.4	1.6
Women				
All causes	<5	1.0	0.8	1.5
	5 to <15	1.5	1.4	1.8
	>15	2.7	1.9	2.8
C V D	<5	1.0	0.7	1.8
	5 to <15	1.8	1.9	2.4
	>15	2.9	2.7	3.3
Non C V D	<5	1.0	0.9	1.3
	5 to <15	1.4	1.0	1.3
	>15	2.2	1.1	2.3

From Pamuk *et al.* (1992).

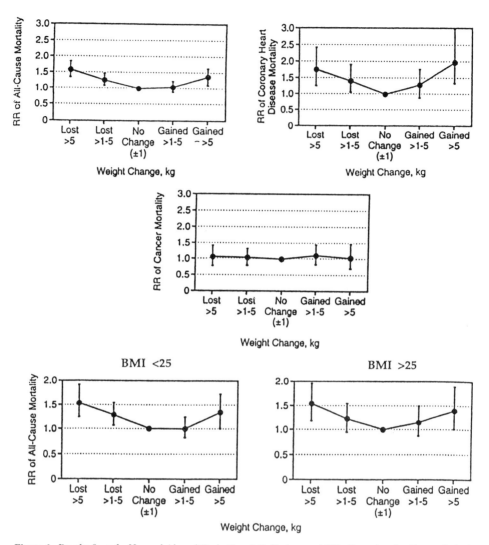

Figure 1. Results from the Harvard Alumni Study (Lee & Paffenbarger. 1992. Reproduced with permission)

analysed according to weight loss (<5, 5 to <15, >15%) and maximum BMI (<26, 26 to <29, >29 kg/m²) in men and women separately (Table 2). The relative risk of death over a 10 year follow-up increased significantly with BMI but also *increased* with weight loss in almost all BMI and gender groups. The increase for CVD tended to be greater than for non-CVD disease thus further minimising the likelihood that the effects were caused by extant cancers.

Lee & Paffenbarger (1992) reported on all cause, CVD and cancer mortality in 11,703 male Harvard alumni according to categories of weight change (lost >5, lost 1-5, no change, gained 1-5, gained >5 kg). Once again early mortality was excluded. All cause and CVD mortality was lowest in the weight stable group and increased progressively with increasing weight gain and weight loss (Figure 1). Cancer mortality was not related to change.

In summary, the evidence for a protective effect of weight loss against premature death is not convincing, and there is persuasive new evidence that weight loss might actually be detrimental by a mechanism as yet unexplained. By these criteria weight stability might well be a reasonable or even preferable goal in favour of elusive and potentially harmful weight loss.

WEIGHT CYCLING, RISK FACTORS AND MORBIDITY

There are rather few data concerning the possible impact of weight cycling on risk factor profile and on morbidity. Rodin *et al.* (1990) reported a slight association between weight cycling and increased waist/hip ratio, but the direction of the association is not clear. Jeffrey *et al.* (1992) found that weight cycling was not associated with an elevation of any of a number of standard CHD risk factors which they studied. However, Phinney (1992) claims that Jeffrey may have missed the real culprit and reports evidence that weight loss and weight cycling might cause a critical imbalance in unsaturated fatty acid ratios which could increase risk of CHD.

WEIGHT CYCLING AND MORTALITY

In the past few years there has been considerable interest in a number of reports that weight cycling might be associated with increased mortality. These have recently been reviewed by Lissner & Brownell (1992). Table 3 shows that three out of seven studies find a significant positive association between weight cycling and all cause mortality, and four out of seven for CVD mortality. The studies with positive findings tend to be the more statistically robust and it is difficult to dismiss the results on methodological grounds.

Table 3. Summary of epidemiological associations between weight cycling and mortality.

Study	Group	Trend	Significance
All-Cause Mortality - Positive Associations			
Gothenburg	- men	Positive	p = .003
	- women	Positive	p = .03
Framingham	- men	Positive	p = .0001
	- women	Positive	p = .0001
MRFIT	- SI smokers	Positive	p = .01
All-Cause Mortality - No Associations			
Western Electric		Positive	NS
Baltimore		Positive	NS
Charleston		Positive	NS
MRFIT	- UC smokers	Positive	NS
	- nonsmokers	Negative	NS
Cardiovascular Disease - Positive Associations			
Gothenburg	- men	Positive	p = .02
Framingham	- men	Positive	p = .0001
	- women	Positive	p = .05 to .005
MRFIT	- all	Positive	p = .001
	- SI smokers	Positive	p = .001
	- UC smokers	Positive	p = .02
Western Electric		Positive	p < .05
Cardiovascular Disease - No Associations			
Baltimore		Positive	NS
Zutphen		Negative	NS
MRFIT	- nonsmokers	Negative	NS

Adapted from Lissner & Brownell (1992).

The Framingham study probably represents the best example (Lissner *et al.* 1991). Weight variability in 1376 men and 1804 women measured over eight biennial study cycles together with recall of weight at 25 years was used to compute weight level, weight change (increasing or decreasing trend) and weight variability (coefficient of variation). Mortality was assessed over a 32 year follow-up period with exclusion of early deaths. In both men and women weight variability was positively associated with total and CHD mortality: in the men the associations were extremely strong. Weight change was also *negatively* associated with mortality implying that people whose weight tended to decrease had an increasing risk of death, although the original authors make little of this point.

At present there are few suggestions about possible mechanisms, but there seems to be a general acceptance that there must be some validity to the findings. However, as with the weight loss studies it has not been possible to separate out weight cycling which arises from voluntary as opposed to involuntary weight loss.

CONCLUSIONS

There is undoubtedly cause for concern about possible detrimental effects of weight loss, although as yet none of this can be definitely ascribed to intentional attempts at weight loss. This concern must be added to the risk/benefit analysis performed at the outset of any treatment programme. It strengthens the view held by many that weight stability is a reasonable goal for anyone with BMI <30 kg/m^2. For the massively obese (BMI >40 kg/m^2) the equation probably still lies heavily in favour of weight loss, but for those with BMI 30-40 kg/m^2 the decision has been complicated and cannot really be resolved without reference to the individual patient's profile of obesity-related disorders. The evidence concerning weight cycling suggests that even greater efforts should be made to avoid weight regain after successful periods of loss.

Finally, the 'Dangerous to be fat - dangerous to lose it' Catch-22 faced by the obese patient reinforces the view that programmes of prevention will ultimately be much more useful than programmes of treatment.

ACKNOWLEDGEMENTS

I am most grateful to Dr. D. H. Williamson for helpful correspondence

REFERENCES

Dublin, L.I. & Marks, H.H. (1951). Mortality among insured overweights in recent years. Transactions of the Association of Life Insurance Medical Directors of America, 35, 235-263.

Hammond, E.C. & Garfinkel, L. (1969). Coronary heart disease, stroke, and aortic aneurysm. Archives of Environmental Health, 19, 167-182.

Jeffrey, R.W., Wing, R.R., French, S.A. (1992). Weight cycling and cardiovascular risk factors in obese men and women. American Journal of Clinical Nutrition, 55, 641-644.

Kanders, B.S. & Blackburn, G.L. (1992). Reducing primary risk factors by therapeutic weight loss. In Treatment of the Seriously Obese Patient. Wadden, T.A. & van Itallie, T.B. eds. New York, The Guildford Press, pp 213-230.

Lean, M.E.J., Powrie, J.K., Anderson, A.S., Garthwaite, P.H. (1990). Obesity, weight loss and prognosis in type 2 diabetes. Diabetic Medicine, 7, 228-233.

Lee, I-M & Paffenbarger, R.S. (1992). Change in body weight and longevity. JAMA, 268, 2045-2049.

Lissner, L. & Brownell, K.D. (1992). Weight cycling, mortality, and cardiovascular disease: A review of epidemiologic findings. In Obesity, Bjorntorp, P., Brodoff, B.N. eds. Philadelphia, JB Lippincott Company, pp 653-661.

Lissner, L., Odell, P.M., D'Agostino, R.B., Stokes, J., Kreger, B.E., Belanger, A.J., Brownell, K.D. (1991). Variability of body weight and health outcomes in the Framingham population. New England Journal of Medicine, 324,1839-1844.

Manson, J.E., Colditz, G.A., Stampfer, M.J., et al. (1990) A prospective study of obesity and risk of coronary heart disease in women. New England Journal of Medicine, 322, 882-889.

Pamuk, E.R., Williamson, D.H., Madans, J., Serdula, M.K., Kleinman, J.C., Byers, T. (1992). Weight loss and mortality in a national cohort of adults, 1971-1987. American Journal of Epidemiology, 136, 686-697.

Phinney, S.D. (1992). Weightcycling and cardiovascular risk in obese men and women. American Journal of Clinical Nutrition, 56,781.

Rodin, J., Radke-Sharpe, N., Rebuffé-Scrive, M., Greenwood, M.R.C. (1990). Weight cycling and fat distribution. International Journal of Obesity, 14, 303-310.

Society of Actuaries (1959). Build and blood pressure study 1959 (Vol 1). Society of Actuaries, Chicago. March 1960: 117-120.

Society of Actuaries (1979). Build study 1979 (Vol 1). Society of Actuaries and Association of Life Insurance Medical Directors of America, Chicago. March 1980: 117.

Wanamethee, G. & Shaper.A.G. (1990). Weight change in middle-aged British men: implications for health. European Journal of Clinical Nutrition, 44,133-142.

Williamson, D.F. & Pamuk, E. (1993). A review of the evidence that weight loss is associated with increased longevity. Annals of Internal Medicine, in press.

REGRESSION CHANGE MODELS WITH INCOMPLETE REPEATED MEASURES DATA IN OBESITY RESEARCH

J. J. McArdle [1] and D. B. Allison [2]

[1]Department of Psychology
University of Virginia
Charlottesville, Virginia 22963

[2]Obesity Research Center
St. Luke's/Roosevelt Hospital Center
Columbia University College of Physicians & Surgeons
New York, New York 10025

INTRODUCTION

Human beings are dynamic organisms. We exist in time and space and change in many ways in space-time. Questions about these changes represent some of the most important questions in obesity research. We ask questions about what changes occur, such as, "How variable are people's weights over time?" We ask questions about the causes of changes, such as, "What factors cause people's weights to vary over time?" We ask questions about the effects of these changes, such as, "How do changes in weight affect longevity?"

All too often, we reconstruct our time varying data into data appropriate for traditional statistical procedures developed for other reasons. Worse yet, we also force our questions about change into the procrustean beds of these traditional statistical procedures and lose sight of the dynamic answers we seek. Fortunately, more flexible statistical methods and procedures have been and are being developed (for overviews, see Nesselroade & Baltes, 1979; Collins & Horn, 1991). These procedures allow us to model change in highly flexible manners and on an individual level; to ask what factors determine (or at least predict) the parameters of these models; and finally, to take advantage of what is frequently seen as a shortcoming of this type of data, namely, data points collected at different time points for different subjects.

In this paper, we provide a brief introduction to these methods including an example of their use with a sample data set. We analyze data from the Obesity Research Center (NY) treatment program on Body Mass Index and Electro-Cardiogram QT interval for a sample of 68 persons studied over approximately six months on up to five occasions of measurement. In these analyses we calculate individual regression models, examine dynamic characteristics of these models, and examine additional predictors of changes in these variables. We wish to

Obesity Treatment, Edited by D.B. Allison
and F.X. Pi-Sunyer, Plenum Press, New York, 1995

stress that the data here are presented only for illustrative purposes. In actual practice, more sophisticated and alternative models would certainly be considered.

The simple regression techniques presented here provide a basic overview of dynamic models for incomplete repeated measures data. More complex modeling techniques, such as pedigree analysis, multilevel models, or random coefficient models are not presented. Readers interested in more details on these complex models should see the papers by David Rindskopf and Robert Elashoff in this volume, or other sources listed in the references here (Bock, 1989; Collins & Horn, 1991; McArdle & Hamagami, 1991; Bryk & Raudenbush, 1992).

METHODS

Subjects

All data used here were obtained from the Obesity Research Center at St. Luke's/Roosevelt Hospital. In a treatment study 68 obese individuals participated in a partial liquid diet treatment program to lose weight. These individuals were 62% female and 28% male, and were between 23 and 64 years of age (mean=44, sd=12) at the initial time of measurement.

Measures

A wide variety of measurements were made on each individual, including: (1) Body Mass Index (BMI) = kg/meters^2. The BMI is used here as a proxy measure of fatness; (2) Adjusted QT Interval (AQT) = the QT segment of the EKG, corrected for the RR interval using the Framingham equation (i.e., AQT = QT + .154 [1-RR]) averaged over three occasions within each measurement. The AQT is associated with an increased risk for malignant ventricular arrhythmias and sudden cardiac death. (3) Other measures, such as Waist-to-Hip ratios and

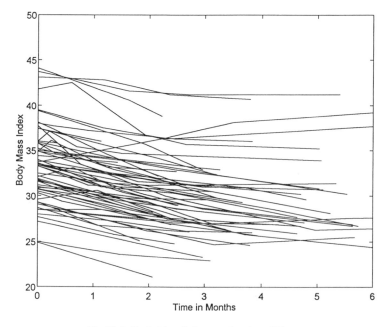

Fig. [1a]: Body Mass Index as a function of Time

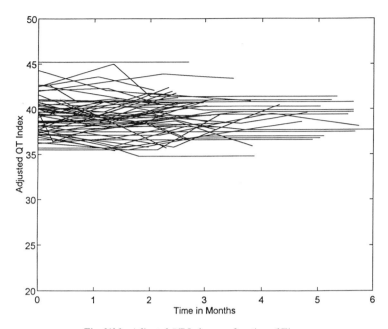

Fig. [1b]: Adjusted QT Index as a function of Time.

Blood Serum Electrolytes were also measured but are not used here.

Longitudinal measurements on each person took place over a six month interval. The number of occasions of measurement (NumRep) varied for each person (N): (1) M=1 on N=4, (2) M=2 on N=10, (3) M=3 on N=24, (4) M=4 on N=24, (5) M=5 on N=1 persons. The interval of time (T) between measurements also varied but it was measured. Figures [1a] and [1b] are plots of the individual scores (BMI and AQT) as a function of the time of measurement. Each single line plotted over time represents a set of scores for each of the 68 persons in the study. Figure [1a] shows the overall pattern of BMI scores going down over time, and Figure [1b] shows the overall pattern of AQT scores staying mostly constant over time.

Planned Analyses

The analyses of these data will be based on simple regression techniques for time dependent data. A three part series of models are described in Table [1]. In the first set of models [1a] we fit a linear regression model for the prediction of the outcome scores (either BMI or AQT) as a function of the time (T) since initial treatment. This time-based model is fitted separately to the scores for each individual (n), and two regression coefficients are saved: i.e., (1) the $LEVEL_n$ score and (2) the $SLOPE_n$ score. In all cases, the $ERROR_n$ some can be calculated and, in some cases, more complex regression models (e.g., polynomial, exponential, etc.) might be needed.

In a second set of analyses, we try to predict individual differences in the $SLOPE_n$ scores as a function of the previous $LEVEL_n$ scores and other measured scores. The basic difference equation formulation is presented in Table [1b] and in the path diagrams of Figure [2]. Figure [2a] shows the individual SLOPE-AQT score as a function of the individual LEVEL-AQT score and a constant (drawn here as a triangle), including the usual regression error term (e). Figure [2b] adds another variable to this equation. In the first relationship we include the prediction of individual SLOPE-AQT from individual LEVEL-BMI scores. We also include a second

Table 1. Simple Dynamic Regression Models for Incomplete Repeated Measures Data

---

[1a]: **Fitting Individual Regression Models**
For n = 1 to N, and t = 0 to T(n),
SCORE(t,n) = LEVEL(n) + SLOPE(n) TIME(n) + ERROR(t,n) where,
T(n) = the total number of repeated observations for person n,
SCORE(t,n) is the individual score at time t,
TIME(n) is the time delay of trial t since the initial treatment,
LEVEL(n) is the intercept term for each person,
SLOPE(n) is the slope term for each person, and
ERROR(t,n) is the random error term.

[1b]: **Fitting Difference Models to Individual Model Coefficients**
SLOPE(n) = A(0) + A(1) LEVEL(n) + A(2) EXOGENOUS(n) + ERROR(n) where, for n = 1 to N,
A(0) = the intercept term,
A(1) = the regression coefficient for SLOPE on LEVEL variables,
A(2) = the regression coefficient for SLOPE on EXOGENOUS variables, and
ERROR(n) = the individual SLOPE random residual term.

[1c]: **The Dynamic Interpretation of Regression Coefficients (see Coleman, 1968)**
SLOPE(n) = D(1) [EQUILIBRIUM(n) - LEVEL(n)] + ERROR(n)
  = D(1) EQUILIBRIUM(n) - D(1) LEVEL(n) + ERROR(n)
    = D(1) [A(0) + A(2) EXOGENOUS(n)] - D(1) LEVEL(n) + ERROR(n)
    = [D(1) A(0)] + [D(1) A(2)] EXOGENOUS(n) - D(1) LEVEL(n) + ERROR(n)
    = D(0) + D(2) EXOGENOUS(n) - D(1) LEVEL(n) + ERROR(n)
where, for n = 1 to N,
D(1) = -A(1) or exp[A(1)t] = the dynamic aspect of the process, the lack of dependence of the SCORE on past history, the resistance of the system against change, or the speed of adjustment to an equilibrium determined by the EXOGENOUS variables;
D(2) = A(2)/|A(1)| = the coefficient for the equilibrium value of the SCORE as a function of the EXOGENOUS variables.
D(0) = 0 or A(0)/|A(1)| = the average first difference of all SLOPEs.

---

regression model for the prediction of the other difference variable, SLOPE-BMI, from both the LEVEL-BMI and the LEVEL-AQT. The error terms in these equations, e_1 and e_2, are allowed both variance and covariance. The final diagram [2c] adds several other demographic variables to these difference equations, including SEX and AGE at the initial testing time.

In a final set of analyses the resulting coefficients from these regression models will be reinterpreted in terms of "system dynamics." This will include a direct expression of the model in the re-expression of terms first defined by Coleman (1968) and others (e.g., Rosenfeld, 1980; Nielsen & Rosenfeld, 1981; Tuma & Hannan, 1984; Arminger, 1987). These interpretations include terms such as "the rate towards equilibrium" and the "equilibrium point." Details of these re-expressions are presented in Table [1c]. We will also plot the trajectories implied by these coefficients using the now common "solution-space" and "phase-space" plots of the model parameter predictions over time (as in McArdle, Boker & Hamagami, 1993).

Standard linear regression procedures will be used here in all calculations, although we do recognize there are some advantages to a full structural model equation analyses (see Arminger, 1987; McArdle, Boker & Hamagami, 1993). Logit transformations of the BMI and AQT variables were calculated to rule out artifacts of percentage scores. However, all such transformations produced virtually identical results for all models presented here (R=.99). (Table 1, Figure 2)

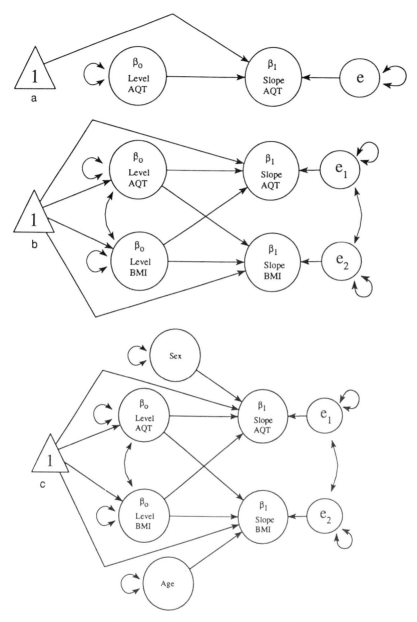

Figure 2a]: Path diagram of Levels and Slopes
2b]: Adding a Second Predictor
2c]: Adding Exogenous Predictors

RESULTS

Descriptive Statistics

In the first level of analysis all individual LEVEL and SLOPE regressions were calculated for each of the N=68 subjects. Of course, a SLOPE score could not be calculated for the four persons who only had one data point. To present a simple description of these data, Figure [3] is a display of the individual LEVEL and SLOPE scores for both BMI and AQT variables plotted against the individual Age at initial testing. The variables are fairly evenly

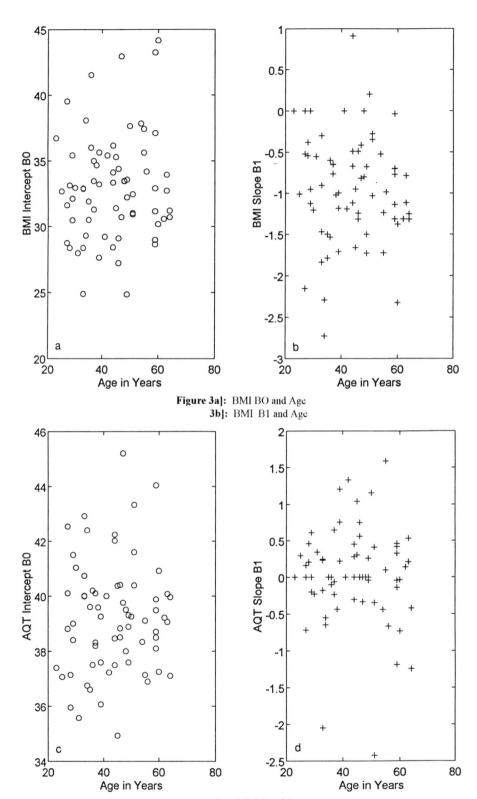

Figure 3a]: BMI BO and Age
3b]: BMI B1 and Age

Figure 3c]: AQT BO and Age
3d]: AQT B1 and Age

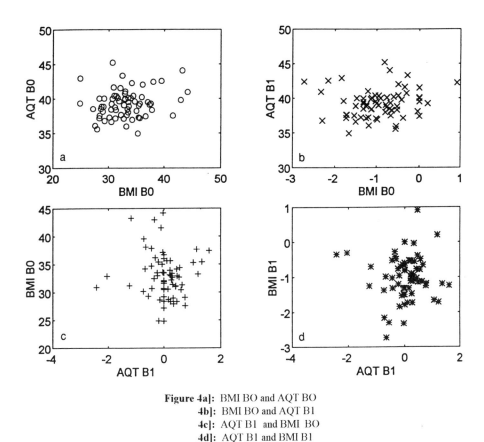

Figure 4a]: BMI BO and AQT BO
4b]: BMI BO and AQT B1
4c]: AQT B1 and BMI BO
4d]: AQT B1 and BMI B1

Table 2. Descriptive Statistics from St. Luke's Treatment Study (Notes N=68; Asterisk indicates parameter is significantly different than zero at the p< .05 level).

[2a]: Means and Standard Deviations

	L-BMI	S-BMI	L-AQT	S-AQT	Sex	Age	NumRep
Means	33.0*	-1.02*	39.2*	0.03	.279	43.7	3.23
(SDs)	(4.0)	(.62)	(2.0)	(.68)	(.452)	(11.6)	(1.04)

[2b]: Product-Moment Correlations

	L-BMI	S-BMI	L-AQT	S-AQT	Sex	Age	NumRep
LEVEL-BMI	1.00						
SLOPE-BMI	-.11	1.00					
LEVEL-AQT	.20	.10	1.00				
SLOPE-AQT	-.08	.01	-.34*	1.00			
Sex	-.02	-.03	-.34*	-.24	1.00		
Age	.11	.06	.07	-.06	.19	1.00	
NumRep	.16	.27	-.06	-.10	.11	.19	1.00

distributed across this range and no systematic relationships are seen with Age. Figure [4] gives four bivariate plots of the LEVEL (or B_0) and SLOPE (or B_1) variables among themselves. Once again, no strong relationships or extreme outliers are seen in these plots.

The first set of results are summarized in Table [2]. In Table [2a] we list the means and

59

standard deviations for the individual regression parameters, and in Table [2b] we list the correlation coefficients among these parameters. Of some importance here are the means for the SLOPE scores. The BMI scores have a significant downward trend (mean = -1.02) for the group over time, but there is substantial individual variation (sd=.62) in this trend. In contrast, the AQT scores exhibit no trend (mean = 0.03 ns) for the group over time, but there is also substantial individual variation (sd=.68) around this average. Only two correlations are significant: The SLOPE and LEVEL of the AQT scores (r=-.34) and the SLOPE-AQT and Sex variables (r=-.34). These correlations will be examined further using regression models below.

Dynamic Regression Analyses

The two most important dependent variables in these analyses are SLOPE-AQT and SLOPE-BMI. The results of three different regression models fitted to each of these variables is presented in Tables [3].

The first model of Table [3a] shows a significant negative relationship (-.11) between the SLOPE and LEVEL of AQT, and the overall equation is significant as well (R^2=.11). The second equation adds the LEVEL-BMI to this prediction, but neither the coefficient nor change of explained variance is significant. The third equation adds the exogenous variables Sex and Age to the equation, and the coefficient for Sex is significant (-.61) as is the change in the explained variance (up to R^2=.26).

A dynamic interpretation of this AQT equation is now possible. The overall mean changes indicate that the group AQT does not change over this time. However, the D(1)=.11 indicates a statistical significance of past history on AQT changes, but the small size of the effect indicates that the system is relatively open to change. The progress towards an equilibrium point is admittedly slow but significant. The lack of any effect from the BMI means that BMI is not a component of this AQT dynamic system. In contrast, the significant negative effect of Sex means the Females (Sex=0) have generally higher SLOPE-AQT that the Males (Sex=1). One possible interpretation of this is that the equilibrium point of AQT is reached faster in Females than in Males.

Table 3. Regression Results from St. Luke's Treatment Study (Notes: N=68; Asterisk indicates parameter is significantly different than zero at the p< .05 level).

[3a]: SLOPE-AQT Regression Model Results

| | Raw Linear Regression Coefficients | | | | | Explained |
	Constant	L-AQT	L-BMI	Sex	Age	Variance
Model 1	4.4*	-.11*	----	----	----	11% *
Model 2	4.4*	-.11*	-.00	----	----	12% *
Model 3	6.4*	-.16*	.00	-.61*	-.00	26% *

[3b]: SLOPE-BMI Regression Model Results

| | Raw Linear Regression Coefficients | | | | | Explained |
	Constant	L-BMI	L-AQT	Sex	Age	Variance
Model 1	-.46	-.02	----	----	----	1%
Model 2	-1.8	-.02	-.04	----	----	3%
Model 3	-2.0	-.02	.04	-.02	-.00	3%

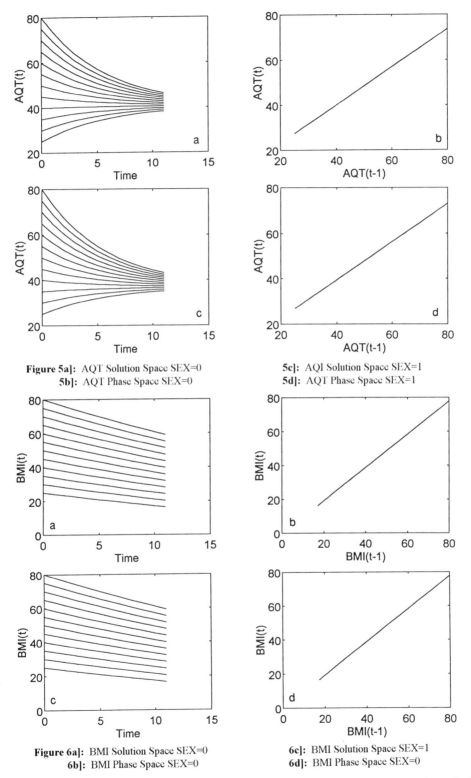

Figure 5a]: AQT Solution Space SEX=0
5b]: AQT Phase Space SEX=0

5c]: AQI Solution Space SEX=1
5d]: AQT Phase Space SEX=1

Figure 6a]: BMI Solution Space SEX=0
6b]: BMI Phase Space SEX=0

6c]: BMI Solution Space SEX=1
6d]: BMI Phase Space SEX=0

Figure [5] gives two dynamic portraits of the parameters of the model 3 equation. Figure [5a] is labelled the "Solution Space" because here we plot the expected trajectory over time for

Females with different starting values of AQT (at t=0). For Females we see the extremes values converging back towards the equilibrium point near the middle. Figure [5b] is labelled the "Phase Space" of the parameters, and here we plot the relations between consecutive points AQT(t) and AQT(t-1) for individuals starting at different initial levels. This is a straight line indicating no unusual dynamic features at all. Figure [5c] and [5d] give the same plots of the Male equations, and the overall trajectories are virtually identical to the Females.

The equations of Table [3b] tell a different story for the SLOPE-BMI variable. Basically, no coefficient is significant here in any of the three models. The BMI is essentially a variable with no dynamic characteristics at all. Figure [6] shows the expression of these parameters in terms of both solution and phase spaces. The clear result for BMI is that it is going down over time, but neither the previous BMI, AQT, Sex or Age, have anything to do with this process, and this process is not moving towards any stable equilibrium point.

DISCUSSION

These data analyses were presented for illustrative purpose, but they do highlight some interested issues. For example, these dynamic results have demonstrated that there is no dynamic relationship between the BMI and AQT, either for LEVEL or SLOPE variables. If replicated, this result would challenge the need for weight loss to control EKG problems. Furthermore, the Electro-Cardiogram AQT variable appears to have some individual dynamics but AQT is not changing on the average. Somewhat paradoxically, the Body Mass Index is going down on the average, but BMI does not appear to be reaching toward any consistent point of stability or equilibrium. Without this kind of stable dynamic, it is hard to see how the BMI weight loss can be retained for any clear period of time. However, we must emphasize again that these results are based on a small limited data set which limited the complexity of models we with which we could experiment.

These kinds of interpretations need to be examined with more subjects, more occasions of measurements, and using more variables. Perhaps it is also obvious that we can deal with incomplete or sparse data sets by modeling "change as an individual characteristic." In this and other future experiments we need to consider other threats to the validity of these interpretations, including non-random selection effects and obtrusiveness of measurement. From this perspective we can also create more optimal experiments, including the possibility of using varying or random time-lags (see McArdle, Boker & Hamagami, 1993). Nevertheless, it is clear that mean changes over time are not the only important feature of the group and individual dynamic processes. For these reasons, a clear dynamic model must be defined as part of the experimental design.

Questions about change are ubiquitous in obesity research. In etiological studies we may ask how some genetic, physiological, psychological, or social factor leads to continued growth of adipose stores until obesity is reached. In treatment research, we ask how much do people lose, who loses, and how are these losses related to changes in psychological, physical, and social functioning. In epidemiological research we ask how people's weights change with age and how these changes affect morbidity and mortality.

Somewhere around 100 years ago without knowing about DNA, Mendel was out planting pea plants and, without having oral glucose tolerance Tests available Minkowski was (so the story goes) tasting dog urine to find out about diabetes. And roughly around that same time Sir Ronald Fisher in Rothamstad was inventing the analysis of variance because he didn't have a computer and it was a bit cumbersome to do many t-tests. One hundred years later, we are pleased to see that Rudy Liebel is not planting peas and Xavier Pi-Sunyer is not tasting dog urine. Unfortunately, many of us are still stuck in not knowing what to do beyond the analysis of variance. Thus, it is nice to see that in the 1990's, some more advanced statistical methods available to us. It is hoped that methods described herein increase the researchers armamentarium for successfully tackling such weighty issues as raised above.

ACKNOWLEDGEMENTS

We thank Steven M. Boker and Michael C. Neale for their thoughtful comments on earlier drafts of this manuscript.

REFERENCES

Arminger, G. (1987). Linear stochastic differential equation models for panel data with unobserved variables. In N.B. Tuma (Ed.), Sociological Methodology, 1987. San Francisco: Jossey-Bass, pp. 187-212.

Bryk, A.S., & Raudenbush, S.W. (1993). Hierarchical Linear Models: Applications and Data Analysis Methods. Newbury Park: SAGE Press.

Coleman, J. S. (1968). The mathematical study of change. In H.M. Blalock, Jr., and A. Blalock (Eds.), Methodology in social research. pp. 428-478. New York: McGraw-Hill.

Collins, L. M., & Horn, J. L. (Eds.) Best Methods for the Analysis of Change. Washington DC: APA Press

Nesselroade, J. R., & Baltes, P. B. (1979). Longitudinal research in the study of behavior and development. New York: Academic Press.

Tuma, N. B., & Hannan, M. T. (1984). Social dynamics: Models and Methods. New York: Academic Press.

Bock, R. D. (Ed.) (1984). Multilevel analysis of educational data. New York: Academic Press.

McArdle, J.J., Boker, S.M., & Hamagami, F. (1993). A Dynamic--Structural Analysis of the Theory of Fluid and Crystallized Intelligence from Incomplete Life--Span and Time--Lag Data. The Psychometric Society Annual Meetings, June 18, 1993.

McArdle, J.J., & Hamagami, F. (1992). Modeling incomplete longitudinal and cross-sectional data using latent growth structural models. Experimental Aging Research, 18 (3). 145-167.

Neilsen, F., & Rosenfeld, R.A. (1981). Substantive interpretations of differential equation models. American Sociological Review, 46, 159-174.

Rosenfeld, R. A. (1980). Race and sex differences in career dynamics. American Sociological Review, 45, 583-609.

ARE THERE PEOPLE WHO DO NOT NEED TO LOSE WEIGHT: THE ROLE OF BODY FAT DISTRIBUTION AND IMPLICATIONS FROM DIABETES RESEARCH

Steven M. Haffner

University of Texas Health Science Center at San Antonio
Division of Clinical Epidemiology
Department of Medicine
7703 Floyd Curl Drive
San Antonio, TX 78284-7873

INTRODUCTION

A number of studies indicate that both overall adiposity and upper body adiposity predict the incidence of non-insulin dependent diabetes mellitus (Ohlson, Larrson, Svardsudd, Welin, Ericksson, Wihelmson, Bjorntorp, & Tibblin, 1985; Haffner, Stern, Mitchell, Hazuda, & Patterson, 1990; Bergstorm, Newell-Morris, Leonetti, Shuman, Wahl, & Fujimoto, 1990; Lundgran, Bengtsson, Blohme, Lapidus, & Sjostrom, 1989). The mechanism of the increased risk of overall adiposity and an adverse body fat distribution is increased insulin resistance and the resultant hyperinsulinemia (Kissebah, Vydelingum, Murray, Evans, Jartz, Kalkhoff, & Adams, 1982; Krotkiewski, Bjorntorp, Sjostrom, & Smith, 1983). Relatively few studies have been large enough to examine whether the effect of obesity and body fat distribution are additive in their effect on diabetes. Since the effect of an adverse body fat distribution may be greater than the effect of overall adiposity on insulin resistance (Ibid.), we postulated that obese individuals with a favorable body fat distribution might be relatively spared from the risk of diabetes in the 8-year follow-up of the San Antonio Heart Study.

METHODS

The San Antonio Heart Study is a population-based study of diabetes and cardiovascular disease in Mexican Americans and non-Hispanic whites. From 1979 to 1982 we randomly sampled households from several San Antonio census tracts: two low-income (barrio) census tracts, two-middle income (transitional) census tracts (approximately half Mexican American and half non-Hispanic whites) and a cluster of suburban census tracts (10% Mexican American and non-Hispanic whites) (Stern, Rosenthal, Haffner, Hazuda, & Franco, 1984). All men and non-pregnant women 25-64 years of age residing in the randomly selected households were eligible for the study. One thousand two-hundred eighty-eight Mexican Americans and 929 non-Hispanic whites attended on-clinic examination. The overall response rate was 63.9%. Mexican Americans were defined as individuals whose ancestry and cultural traditions derived from a Mexican national origin (Hazuda, Comeaux, Stern, Haffner, Eifler, & Rosenthal, 1986). A detailed description of the 1979-1982 survey was published previously (Stern, Rosenthal, Haffner, Hazuda, & Franco, 1984).

At the baseline examination, blood specimens were obtained after a 12-14 hour fast and two hours after administration of a 75-g glucose equivalent load (Glucola, Ames, Elkhart, IN). Plasma glucose concentrations were measured with an Abbott bichromatic analyzer (South Pasadena, CA). Anthropometric measurements (height, weight, and subscapular and triceps skinfold thickness) were made after each participant had removed his or her shoes and upper garments and donned an examination gown. The triceps skinfold thickness was measured posteriorly over the right triceps muscle midway between the aromial and olecranon processes with the subjects arm hanging relaxed at the side. The subscapular skinfold thickness was also measured on the right side just below the inferior angle following the natural contour of the skin. Body mass index (BMI) was calculated as weight (kg) divided by height squared (m2). The ratio of subscapular-to-triceps skinfold thickness (STR) was chosen as a measure of central adiposity.

In October 1987, an 8-year follow-up study was begun to determine the incidence of NIDDM and cardiovascular disease. The overall response rate was 81%. This report is restricted to the 1,477 subjects who were free of diabetes at the baseline examination in 1979-1982 and who attended the medical examination 8 years later. At the follow-up examination (Haffner, Mitchell, Hazuda, & Stern, 1991), plasma glucose was measured in the fasting and 2 hours after the administration of 75 gm glucose equivalent load (Koladex or Orangedex, Custom Laboratories, Baltimore). The methods used for glucose and anthropometric measurements were identical to those used in the baseline examination. Diabetes mellitus was diagnosed according to the World Health Organization Criteria (fasting plasma glucose criteria >7.8 mmol/l and/or 2-hr plasma glucose >11.1 mmol/l) (World Health Organization, 1985).

The effect of obesity and body fat distribution was evaluated by a test for trend (SAS Institute Inc, 1988). Multiple logistic regression analysis (Dallal, 1988) was used to estimate the odds ratio (OR) associated with each risk factor adjusted for all other risk factors. The ranking of subscapular-to-triceps ratio was done separately in each sex.

RESULTS

The 8-year incidence of non-insulin dependent diabetes mellitus was 5.3% (80/1477). The incidence of NIDDM increased both with an adverse body fat distribution and with greater overall adiposity (Table 1). These effects were statistically independent. The effect of obesity was similar in subjects with both a favorable and unfavorable body fat distribution.

We next fit multiple logistic regression models for the incidence of NIDDM with age, gender, BMI, STR, and ethnicity as independent main effect. First order interaction terms of BMI x STR, BMI x Gender, STR x Gender and STR x Ethnicity were also modelled. Except for the interaction of STR x Gender (p=.041), the other interaction terms were not statistically significant (p>0.100). Thus this confirms earlier work from our group (Haffner, Mitchell, Hazuda, & Stern, 1991) of greater effect on body fat distribution on the incidence of NIDDM in women than in men.

We next fit separate logistic regression models in subjects with high and low STR separately (Table 2). In both groups a five unit change in BMI significantly predicted the

Table 1. Incidence of Diabetes by Body Fat Distribution and Obesity

| | Body fat distribution[*] | | |
	low	high	RR
Body Mass Index (kg/m2)			
low (<25)	5/315 (1.6%)	5/178 (2.8%)	1.77
medium (25-30)	6/248 (2.4%)	11/246 (4.5%)	1.85
high (>30)	15/177 (8.5%)	38/315 (12.1%)	1.42
Overall	26/738 (3.4%)	54/739 (7.3%)	2.07
RR (high/low)	5.34	4.29	

*high and low subscapular-to-triceps skinfold ratios were determined by the median split for men and women separately.

Abbreviations: RR = relative risk

Table 2. Multiple Logistic Regression for the Incidence of NIDDM

Independent Variable	OR	95% CI	p-value
Low STR subjects			
Age (change 10 years)	1.85	(1.21,2.82)	.004
BMI (change 5 units kg/m2)	1.69	(1.21,2.35)	.004
STR (change 0.23 units)	3.17	(1.52,6.64)	.002
Gender (women/men)	1.23	(0.73,1.80)	.114
Ethnic (MA/NHW)	1.83	(0.76,4.33)	.184
High STR subjects			
Age (change 10 years)	1.31	(0.99,1.74)	.058
BMI (change 5 units kg/m2)	2.16	(1.70,2.74)	<.001
STR (change 0.23 units)	1.08	(0.92,1.26)	.346
Gender (women/men)	2.10	(0.96,4.61)	.066
Ethnic (MA/NHW)	1.34	(0.68,2.67)	.407

Abbreviations: NIDDM = non-insulin dependent diabetes mellitus; OR = odds ratio; CI = confidence interval; BMI = body mass index; STR = ratio of subscapular-to-triceps skinfolds; MA = Mexican American; NHW = non-Hispanic white

incidence of NIDDM (low STR: OR=1.69, 95% CI=1.21; and high STR: OR=2.16, 95% CI=1.70, 2.74).

DISCUSSION

We have shown in this report that both overall adiposity as measured by body mass index and an unfavorable body fat distribution as measured by the ratio of subscapular of triceps skinfold, are independent predictors of the incidence of NIDDM. Our results thereby confirm earlier Swedish studies in men (Ohlson et al., 1985) and women (Haffner et al., 1990) and

Japanese American men (Bergstorm et al, 1990). In stratified analysis, Ohlson et al. (1985) found an increase of diabetes with higher BMI in the highest two tertiles of WHR but not in the lowest tertile of WHR. Lundgren et al. (1989) found an effect of BMI in the highest two quintiles of WHR but not in the lower quintiles of WHR. We have also shown that the effect of unfavorable body fat distribution is at least as great in lean subjects as in obese subjects. Thus data is consistent with cross-sectional results showing a strong effect of BMI on the prevalence of NIDDM in subjects with low as well as high waist-to-hip ratio in Mexican Americans in San Antonio (Haffner, Mitchell, Stern, Hazuda, & Patterson, 1992).

Landin et al. did not find an effect of WHR on insulin concentrations and insulin resistance in lean premenopausal women (Landin, Krotkiewski, & Smith 1989; Landin, Lonnroth, Krotkiewski, Holm, & Smith, 1990). However, they did find an effect of WHR in obese premenopausal women in metabolic ward studies. Our data in the current report as well as in an earlier cross-sectional study (Haffner, Mitchell, Stern, Hazuda, & Patterson, 1992) found a strong effect of WHR on risk of NIDDM in both lean and obese men and women. Bonora et al. (1992) has shown the effects of total body fat content and fat topography are different in lean and obese premenopausal women. In lean women (n=18), total body fat content was related inversely to both total and non-oxidative glucose disposal during the insulin clamp, whereas no relationship was found between glucose disposal (overall, oxidative and non-oxidative) and WHR, STR or visceral fat. In contrast, in obese women (n=18), no relationship was observed between total body content and any measure of insulin-mediated glucose disposal. However, both WHR and visceral fat were inversely related with overall, oxidative and non-oxidative glucose disposal rates during the insulin clamp. In contrast in 87 Finnish men, a similar effect of WHR on glucose disposal was observed in both lean and obese men (Haffner, Karphapaa, Mykkanen, & Laakso, submitted for publication). Body mass index was significantly associated with overall whole-body glucose disposal (r=-.30), oxidative (r=-.21) and also with non-oxidative glucose disposal (r=-.25). Waist-to-hip ratio was also significantly associated with overall (r=-.54), oxidative (r=-.23) and non-oxidative (r=-.50) glucose disposal. After adjustment for BMI, WHR continued to be significantly related to overall (r=-.42) and non-oxidative (r=-.20) glucose disposal but not with glucose oxidation. The latter pattern is important since although defects in both glucose oxidation and non-oxidative glucose disposal exist in subjects with established NIDDM (DeFronzo, 1988), non-diabetic relatives of subjects with non-insulin dependent diabetes have decreased non-oxidative glucose disposal but normal glucose oxidation (Eriksson, Fransilla-Kallunki, Ekstrand, Saloronta, Widen, Scholin, & Groop, 1987; Gulli, Ferrannini, Stern, Haffner, & DeFronzo, 1992). This study suggests that perhaps upper body adiposity might comprise an early lesion associated with non-oxidative glucose disposal in the prediabetic state.

Our study suggests an independent effect of both overall adiposity and an unfavorable body fat distribution in the etiology of non-insulin dependent diabetes mellitus. Although upper body adiposity is strongly associated with the incidence of NIDDM, even obese subjects with an increased upper body adiposity are at risk compared to lean subjects with similar body fat distribution.

REFERENCES

Bergstorm, R.W., Newell-Morris, L.L., Leonetti, D., Shuman, W.P., Wahl, P.W., Fujimoto, W.Y. (1990). Association of elevated fasting C-peptide levels and increased intra-abdominal fat distribution with development of NIDDM in Japanese American men. Diabetes,39, 104-111.

Bonora, E., Del Prato, S., Bonadonna, R., et al. (1992). Total body fat distribution and fat topography are associated differently with in vivo glucose metabolism in non-obese and obese non-diabetic women. Diabetes, 41, 1151-1159.

Dallal, G. (1988). Logistic: A logistic regression package for the IBM PC. Statistician, 42,272, abstract.

DeFronzo, R.A. (1988). Lilly Lecture 1987. The triumvirate: Beta cell, muscle, liver: A collusion responsible for NIDDM. Diabetes,37, 667-687.

Eriksson, J., Fransilla-Kallunki, A., Ekstrand, A., Saloronta, C., Widen, E., Scholin, C., Groop, L. (1987). Early metabolic defects in persons at increased risk for non-insulin dependent diabetes mellitus. New England Journal of Medicine, 321, 337-343.

Gulli, G., Ferrannini, E., Stern, M., Haffner, S.M., DeFronzo, R.A. (1992). The metabolic profile of NIDDM is fully established in glucose intolerant offspring of two Mexican American parents. Diabetes, 41, 1575-1586.

Haffner, S.M., Karphappaa, P., Mukkaneen, L., Laakso, M. (Submitted for publication). Insulin resistance, body fat distribution and sex hormones in men.

Haffner, S.M., Mitchell, B.D., Hazuda, H. P., Stern, M.P. (1991). Greater influence of central adipose tissue on incidence of non-insulin dependent diabetes in women than men. American Journal of Clinical Nutrition,53, 1312-1317

Haffner, S.M., Mitchell, B.D., Stern, M.P., Hazuda, H.P., Patterson, J.K. (1992). Public health significance of upper body adiposity for non-insulin dependent diabetes mellitus in Mexican Americans.16, 177-184.

Haffner, S.M., Stern, M.P., Mitchell, B.D., Hazuda, H.P., Patterson, J.K. (1990). Incidence of type II (non-insulin dependent diabetes) mellitus in Mexican American predicted by fasting insulin and glucose levels, obesity and body fat distribution. Diabetes,39, 283-288.

Hazuda, H.P., Comeaux, P.J., Stern, M.P., Haffner, S.M., Eilfer, C.W., Rosenthal, M. (1986). A comparison of three indicators for identifying Mexican Americans in epidemiologic research: Methodological findings from the San Antonio Heart Study. American Journal of Epidemiology, 127, 96-112.

Kissebah, A.H., Vydelingum, N., Murray, R., Evans, D.J., Kalkhoff, R.K., Adams, P.W. (1982). Relationship of body fat distribution to metabolic complications of obesity. Journal of Clinical Endocrinology and Metabolism,54,254-260.

Krotkiewski, M., Bjorntorp, P., Sjostrom, L., Smith, U. (1983). Impact of obesity on metabolism in men and women: Importance of regional adipose distribution. Journal of Clinical Investigation, 72,1150-1162, 1983.

Landin, K., Krotkiewski, M., Smith, U. (1989). Importance of obesity for the metabolic abnormalities associated with an abdominal fat distribution. Metabolism,38, 572-576.

Landin, K., Lonnroth, P., Krotkiewski, M., Holm, G., Smith, U. Increased insulin resistance and fat cell lipolysis in obese but not lean women with high waist/hip ratio. European Journal of Clinical Investigation, 20: 530-535.

Lundgren, H., Bengtsson, C., Blophme, G., Lapidus, L. Sjostrom, L. (1989). Adiposity and adipose tissue distribution in relation to the incidence of diabetes in women: Results from a prospective population study in Gothenburg, Sweden. International Journal of Obesity, 13: 413-423.

Ohlson, L.O., Larrson, B., Svardsudd, K., Welin, L., Ericksson, H., Wihelmson, L., Bjorntorp, P., Tibblin, G. (1985). The influence of body fat distribution on the incidence of diabetes mellitus. 13.5 years of follow-up of the participants in the study of men born in 1913. Diabetes, 34, 1055-1058.

SAS Institute Inc. (1988). SAS/STAT user's guide. Release 6.03. Cary, NC. SAS Institute Inc.

Stern, M.P., Rosenthal, M., Haffner, S.M., Hazuda, H.P., Franco, L.J. (1984). Sex difference in the effects of sociocultural status on diabetes and cardiovascular risk factors in Mexican Americans: The San Antonio Heart Study. American Journal of Epidemiology, 120, 834-851.

World Health Organization. (1985). Diabetes mellitus. (WHO technical report series 727). Geneva: World Health Organization.

THE EFFECT OF CENTRAL FAT DISTRIBUTION ON CARDIOVASCULAR DISEASE

F. Xavier Pi-Sunyer

Obesity Research Center
St. Luke's/Roosevelt Hospital
Columbia University
New York, NY 10025

The effect of fat distribution on cardiovascular disease has become a question of great interest in the last decade. As long ago as 1956, Vague , in writing about masculine (central) and feminine (peripheral) fat distribution, suggested that atherosclerotic risk was higher in those with a central fat distribution (Vague, 1956). He was a clinical endocrinologist, rather than an epidemiologist, and his observation received little initial attention. However, the effect of fat distribution on cardiovascular disease has become a question of great interest in the last decade. This is because evidence has accumulated that where the fat is located is important with regard to its health effects. Much of this impact is independent of the amount of the fat itself. The evidence which attributes health risk for cardiovascular disease to central fat distribution will be reviewed in this article.

Epidemiologists generally study morbidity, mortality, or both. In their studies, the definition of cardiovascular disease has generally included myocardial infarction, angina pectoris, and stroke. In epidemiologic studies, fat distribution has been generally defined by anthropometric measurements. These have generally been the waist/hip ratio or else skinfold thicknesses. Either single markers of central fat, such as the subscapular skinfold, have been used or, more commonly, ratios of central to peripheral skinfolds. Of these, the most commonly used have been the subscapular to triceps, or a sum of central to peripheral skinfolds. More recently, simply waist circumference has been used in some studies. More sophisticated measures of central fat, such as computed tomography (CT) scans or magnetic resonance imaging (MRI) have been utilized by some investigators. The advantage of these imaging techniques is that they can determine the amount of visceral fat and compare that to subcutaneous fat at the same "cut" or level of a CT or MRI scan. Because of their expense, however, they have been rarely used.

A number of cross-sectional studies have associated central fat distribution with risk factors for cardiovascular disease. For example, Krotkiewsky et al (1983) reported that hypertension, hyperinsulinemia, glucose intolerance, and hypertriglyceridemia were found more readily in men and women with a more central (or masculine) fat distribution, as measured by the W/H ratio. Kissebah et al (1982), Hartz et al (1984), and Szathmary and Holt (1983) have shown similar results with different groups also studied cross-sectionally.

As a result of such cross-sectional prevalence studies, it became important to do longitudinal incidence studies of the effect of central fat distribution on cardiovascular disease. Larsson et al (1984) reported on the influence of body fat distribution on the risk of cardiovascular disease (ischemic heart disease and stroke) and death from all causes. They reported the effect of obesity and, independently, of central or abdominal fat distribution as measured by the waist to hip ratio (W/H). Even though the associations with the W/H ratio were not significant in multivariate analysis when blood pressure and serum cholesterol concentration were taken into account, W/H was more closely related to risk than was weight. Surprisingly, the highest risk for CHD occurred in those men in the highest tertile for W/H but the lowest tertile for BMI.

In the Framingham study, at the 22 yr point, truncal obesity, as expressed by subscapular skinfold thickness, was found to be a better predictor of coronary heart disease than was obesity per se as measured by either BMI or waist circumference (Higgins et al, 1983; Stokes et al, 1985). In the Honolulu Heart Program, a 12 year follow-up of 7692 men showed that subscapular skinfold thickness has a greater impact on coronary heart disease (CHD) than did BMI (Donahue et al, 1987). While there was an independent effect of subscapular skinfold thickness on CHD risk after adjustment for BMI and other CHD risk factors, this was not true of BMI after similar corrections. In the Paris Prospective Study (Ducimitiere et al, 1985), 7746 men were followed from 5 to 9 years for angina pectoris, myocardial infarction, and sudden death. Subscapular, axillary, and subumbilical skinfold thickness was used as a measure of central fat and the sum of 4 skinfolds in the thigh were used as a measure of peripheral fat distribution. The ratio of the first sum to the second sum showed a greater risk than any individual skinfold. This risk was still significant when usual CVD risk factors were factored out. In such an analysis, BMI was not a risk factor. However, it must be pointed out that a large study which followed over 6000 men and women showed no effect between W/H ratio and incidence of cardiovascular disease (Gillum, 1987).

Lapidus et al (1984) in a study of 1462 women aged 38-60 years who were followed for 12 years in Sweden, found that W/H ratio was a predictor for myocardial infarction, angina, stroke, and death. BMI only predicted myocardial infarction. Hartz et al (1990) found a relationship between W/H ratio and angiographically determined cardiovascular disease. A more recent study by Thompson et al (14) using skinfolds for a measure of central fat, also found a relationship between central fat distribution and cardiovascular disease.

Further studies have been done cross-sectionally on specific risk factors for cardiovascular disease. Despres et al (1988) studied central obesity in relation to prevalence of dyslipidemia. The relative distribution of subcutaneous fat, as reflected by the trunk to extremity skinfolds (T/E) ratio, and the absolute amount of subcutaneous abdominal fat, obtained by the measurement of abdominal skinfold thickness, were significantly correlated with serum triglycerides, HDL-cholesterol, and the HDL-cholesterol /total cholesterol ratio. Analysis of variance on the T/E ratio and on BMI showed significant and independent effect of the two on the lipid measurements. Ostlund et al (1990) used the W/H ratio to show an inverse correlation between that measurement of central fat and HDL_2 levels, while they could find no such relationship with BMI.

Anderson et al (1988) showed a correlation between increasing W/H ratio and total cholesterol, HDL-cholesterol, triglycerides, and apoprotein B. Similar findings were found by Seidell et al (1989) in a group of women. Freedman et al (1990) also reported such results.

Studies have been done using skinfold ratios as a measure of central to peripheral fat distribution. Bonithon-Kopp et al (1991) used such a ratio and found a relationship to apoprotein A and Haffner et al (1987) found increased triglycerides.

There are a number of studies that have related central fat distribution to high blood pressure. Most have used the W/H ratio as a measure of central fat. Among these are Hartz et al (1984), Kalkhoff et al (1983), Weinsier et al (1985), White et al (1986), Gillum et al (1987), Williams et al (1987), Tonkelaar et al (1989), Landin et al (1989), Cassano et al (1990), Bonithon-Kopp et al (1990). In addition, others have used skinfolds as a measure of central fat and again have related it to high blood pressure. These include studies by Blair et al (1984) and Pouliot et al (1990).

More recently, an effort has been made to differentiate between the effect of subcutaneous central fat accumulation and visceral (or intra-abdominal) fat accumulation. The clarification of this phenomenon has been complicated by the fact that it is very difficult to measure visceral fat: it has required computerized tomography (CT scan) or magnetic resonance imaging (MRI). Both of these techniques are expensive, but adequate surrogate markers have not been developed to date. As a result, the studies that have been done have been small and cross-sectional in nature.

Both Peiris et al (1989) and Fujioka (1987) have described increased health risk for diabetes and cardiovascular disease from visceral rather than sub-cutaneous central fat accumulation. Also, Kanai et al (1990) showed a positive effect of increasing blood pressure with increased visceral obesity in women, using CT scans to measure central visceral fat.

In summary, body fat distribution has been found to be related to cardiovascular health risk. This effect is independent of BMI and, in some studies, has been found to be a stronger predictor of disease (Pi-Sunyer, 1983). Although the effect has not been found in all studies where it has been looked for, the preponderance of data support a strong association. It is likely that with a better diagnostic differentiation of abdominal fat into visceral vs. subcutaneous fat, more clear information will accrue on the impact of each of these deposits on cardiovascular disease.

REFERENCES

Anderson, A., Sobocinski, K., Freedman, D., Barboriak, J., Rimm, A., & Gruchow, H. (1988). Body fat distribution, plasma lipids, and lipoproteins. Arteriosclerosis, 8, 88-94.

Blair, D., Habicht, J., Sims, F., Sylvester, D., & Abraham, S. (1984). Evidence for an increased risk for hypertension with centrally located body fat and the effect of race and sex on this risk. American Journal of Epidemiology, 119, 526-40.

Bonithon-Kopp, C., Raison, J., Egloff, M., Guy-Grand, B., & Ducimetiere, P. (1991). Skinfold and body circumferences as measures of body fat patterning in a French female active population: relationships with the metabolic risk profile. Journal of Clinical Epidemiology, 44, 475-82.

Brenner, B.M., Garcia, D.L., & Anderson, S. (1988). Glomeruli and blood pressure. Less of one, more of the other? American Journal of Hypertension., 1, 335-47.

Cassano, P., Segal, M., Vokonas, P., & Weiss, S. (1990). Body fat distribution, blood pressure, and hypertension. A prospective cohort study of men in the Normative Aging Study. Annals of Epidemiology, 1, 33-48.

Despres, J.P., Tremblay, A., Perusse, L., Leblanc, C., & Bouchard, C. (1988). Abdominal adipose tissue and serum HDL-cholesterol association independent from obesity and serum triglyceride concentration. International Journal of Obesity, 12, 1-13.

Donahue, R.P., Abbot, R.D., Bloom, E., Reed, D.M., & Yano, K. (1987). Central obesity and coronary heart disease in men. Lancet, 1, 821-4.

Ducimetiere, P., Richard, J. Cambien, F., Avous, P., & Jacqueson, A. Relationship between adiposity measurements and the incidence of coronary heart disease in a middle-aged male population - the Paris Prospective Study I. American Journal of Clinical Nutrition, 4, 31-8.

Freedman, D., Jacobsen, S., Barboriak, J., Sobocinski, K., Anderson, A., Kisseba,h A., Sasse, E, & Gruchow, H. (1990). Body fat distribution and male female differences in lipids and lipoproteins. Circulation, 8, 1498-1506.

Fujioka, A., Matsuzawa, Y., Tokunaga, K., & Tarui, S. (1987). Contribution of intra-abdominal fat accumulation to the impairment of glucose and lipid metabolism in human obesity. Metabolism, 26, 54-9.

Gillum, R. (1987). The association of body fat distribution with hypertension, hypertensive heart disease, coronary heart disease, diabetes and cardiovascular risk factors in men and women aged 18-79 years. Journal of Chronic Diseases, 40, 421-8.

Haffner, S., Stern, M., Hazuda, H., Pugh, J., & Patterson, J. (1987). Do upper-body and centralized adiposity measure different aspects of regional body fat distribution? Diabetes, 36, 43-51.

Hartz, A., Rupley, D., & Rimm, A. (1984). The association of girth measurements with disease in 32,856 women. American Journal of Epidemiology, 119, 71-80.

Hartz, A., Grubb, B., Wild, R., Van Nort, J., Kuhn, E., Freedman, D., & Rimm, A. (1990). The association of waist-hip ratio and angiographically determined coronary artery disease. International Journal of Obesity, 14, 657-65.

Hubert, H.B., Feinleib, M., McNamara, P.H., & Castelli, W.P. (1983). Obesity as an independent risk factor for cardiovascular disease: a 26-year followup of participants in the Framingham Heart Study. Circulation, 67, 968-977.

Kalkhoff, R., Hartz, A., Rupley,.D., Kissebah, A., & Kelber, S. (1983). Relationship of body fat distribution to blood pressure, carbohydrate tolerance, and plasma lipids in healthy obese women. Journal of Laboratory and Clinical Medicine, 102, 621-7.

Kanai, H., Matsuzawa, Y., Kotani, K., Keno, Y., Kobatake, T., Nagai, Y., Fujioka, S., Tokunaga, K., & Tarui, S. (1990). Close correlation of intra-abdominal fat accumulation to hypertension in obese women. Hypertension, 16, 484-90.

Kissebah, A.H., Vydelingum, N., Murray, R., Evans, D.J., Hartz, A.H., Kalkhoff, R.K., & Adam,s P.W. (1982). Relation of body fat distribution to metabolic complications of obesity. Journal of Clinical Endocrinology and Metabolism, 54, 254-60.

Krotkiewski, M., Bjorntorp, P., Sjostrom, L., & Smith, U. (1983). Impact of obesity on metabolism in men and women. Journal of Clinical Investigations, 72, 1150-62.

Landin, K., Krotkiewski, M., & Smith, U. (1989). Importance of obesity for the metabolic abnormalities associated with an abdominal fat distribution pattern. Metabolism, 33, 68-75.

Lapidu,s L., Bengtsson, C., Larsson, B., Pennert, K., Rybo, E., & Sjostrom, L. (1984). Distribution of adipose tissue and risk of cardiovascular disease and death: a 12 year folllow up of participants in the population study of women in Gothenburg, Sweden. British Medical Journal, 289, 1257-61.

Larsson, B., Svardsudd, K., Welin, L., Wilhemsen, L., Bjorntorp, P., & Tibblin, G. (1984). Abdominal adipose tissue distribution, obesity, and risk of cardiovascular disease and death: 13 year follow-up of participants in the study of men born in 1913. British Medical Journal, 288, 1401-4.

Ostlund, R.E. Jr., Staten, M., Kohrt, W.M., Schultz, J., & Malley, M. (1990). The ratio of waist-to-hip circumference, plasma insulin level, and glucose intolerance as independent predictors of the HDL2 cholesterol level in older adults. New England Journal of Medicine, 322, 229-34.

Peiris, A., Sothmann, M., Hoffman, R., Hennes, M., Wilson, C., Gustafson, A., & Kissebah, A. (1989). Adiposity, fat distribution, and cardiovascular risk. Annals of Internal Medicine, 110, 8-?

Pi-Sunyer, F.X. (1993). Medical hazards of obesity. Annals of Internal Medicine, 119, 655-60

Pouliot, M., Despres, J., Moorjani, S., Lupien, P., Tremblay, A., & Bouchard, C. (1990). Apolipoprotein E polymorphism alters the association between body fatness and plasma lipoproteins in women. Journal of Lipid Research, 31, 1023-9.

Seidell, J., Cigolini, M., Duerenberg, P., Oosterlee, A., & Doorbos, G. (1989). Fat distribution, androgens, and metabolism in nonobese women. American Journal of Clinical Nutrition, 50, 269-73.

Stokes, J., Garrison, R., & Kannel, W.B. (1985). The independent contribution of various indices of obesity to the 22-year incidence of coronary heart disease: the Framingham Heart Study. In Vague,J. ed. Metabolic Complications of Human Obesity. Amsterdam: Elsevier , 49-57.

Szathmary, E.J.E., & Holt, N. (1983). Hyperglycemia in Dogrib Indians of the Northwest Territories, Canada: Association with age and a centripetal distribution of body fat. Human Biology, 55, 493-515.

Thompson,C.,Ryu ,J, Craven,T., Kahl, F, & Crouse J. (1991). Central adipose distribution is related to coronary atherosclerosis. Arteriosclerosis and Thrombosis, 11, 327-33.

Tonkelaar, I., Seidell ,J., Van Noord, P., Baanders-vanHalewijn, E., Jacobus, J., & Bruning, P. (1989). Factors influencing waist/hip ratio in randomly selected pre- and post-menopausal women in the DOM-project (preliminary results). International Journal of Obesity, 13, 817-24.

Vague, J. (1956). The degree of masculine differentiation of obesities: a factor determining predisposition to diabetes, atherosclerosis, gout, and uric calculus disease. American Journal of Clinical Nutrition, 4, 20-34.

Weinsier, R., Norris, D., Birch, R., Bernstein, R., Wang, J., Yang, M., Pierson, R., & VanItallie, T. (1985). The relative contribution of body fat and fat pattern to blood pressure level. Hypertension, 7, 578-85.

White, M., Pereira, L., & Garner, J. (1986). Association of body mass index and waist0hip ratio with hypertension. Canadian Medical Association Journal, 135, 313-20.

Williams, P., Fortmann ,S., Terry, R., Garay, S., Vranizan, K., Ellsworth, N., & Wood, P. (1987). Association of dietary fat, regional adiposity, and blood pressure in men. JAMA, 257, 3251-6.

IS SELF-ACCEPTANCE A REASONABLE GOAL?

Susan C. Wooley

University of Cincinnati
College of Medicine
Cincinnati, OH 45267-0559

For several decades evidence has accumulated on the genetic and constitutional determinants of obesity and the inefficacy of diets in producing lasting weight loss (for review see Stunkard & Penick, 1979; Wooley, Wooley & Dyrenforth, 1979; Foreyt, Goodrich & Gotto, 1981; Bennett, 1984, 1987; Garner & Wooley, 1991; Brownell, 1991; Wilson, in press). In recent years, these findings have been joined by data suggesting that weight loss and the virtually inevitable weight regain which follows not only fails to lastingly improve health but may instead risk physical and mental health (for review see Andrews, 1980; Keys, 1980; Ernsberger & Haskew, 1987; Garner & Wooley, 1991; Wooley & Garner, 1991; Prentice, this volume). Such findings, while far from conclusive, make the already perplexing question of whether to abandon dietary treatments of obesity more pressing still.

Data supporting the above assertions have been extensively reviewed elsewhere and will not be reiterated. It is the premise of this argument that the question before us is not one which will be decided by further research unless and until a fundamental discovery allows us to address for the first time the underlying biological causes of obesity. While a strong argument exists for expanding basic research on obesity, applied research has reached a point of diminishing returns. Further data is unlikely to materially alter our dilemma: how to balance the possible benefits of successful weight loss by the few against the costs of failed treatment to the many and how to think about a problem steeped in social and political as well as medical significance.

Even to approach these questions requires a degree of detachment and a shift in perspective. One may wonder whether a field has the ability to evaluate itself, especially when a paradigm shift would essentially dissolve it. Many of the field's renowned researchers have invested a lifetime in developing and testing treatments for obesity. A moratorium on dieting would change not only their future but their past, imparting a new and profoundly discouraging meaning to the cumulative body of work which is our field. Although as scientists we strive for objectivity and detachment, we are human; capable of imbuing events with meaning, we must struggle with the meanings that change would entail.

History has shown that the scientific method is no guarantee against catastrophic errors in perspective. In <u>The Mismeasure of Man</u>, cultural anthropologist Steven Jay Gould (1981) reminds us of many such errors, including T. X. Huxley's "scientific" argument for the intellectual inferiority of blacks. Such error is not, of course, random as Barbara Ehrenreich and Deirdre English (1978) make clear in a history of medical advice to women that locates the offered "remedies" in a sociocultural context in which female inferiority was jealously, if often unwittingly, guarded. We must now ask whether our own views are shaped by equally invisible and powerful social forces.

Reluctance to abandon futile treatments of obesity has been linked by many thoughtful observers to cultural change, particularly the historic shift in female roles in this century. (e.g., Orbach, 1978; Wooley & Wooley, 1979; Dyrenforth, Wooley & Wooley, 1980; Chernin, 1986; Steiner-Adair, 1986; Wolf, 1990; Silverstein, in press.) Since the distribution of body fat is the most readily visible marker of gender, it is perhaps not surprising that it should carry a great psychic charge at such a time of change. The rearrangement of gender relations has already influenced psychiatry, its long-standing theories dissolving as increasing numbers of symptoms have been found to be direct sequelae of such covert phenomena as physical and sexual abuse. Many female maladies are now understood in ways that were impossible even 20 years ago, without benefit of the discoveries and reconceptualizations brought about by feminism.

The stigmatization of obesity damages women, for whom eating disorders have replaced hysteria as the disease most symptomatic of their prejudicial treatment. As the drive for thinness continues to escalate in the culture, and in individuals influenced by it, body disparagement has become a problem so widespread among women that it is addressed in virtually all contemporary analyses of female psychology. And yet, as a field, we have absented ourselves from this dialogue, as though we alone were exempt from the great cultural influences of our day.

We have done a poor job of encouraging dissent within the field with the result that much of the debate has taken place in the mass media. Sometimes critics of obesity treatment have been charged with irresponsibly endangering the health of the individuals they dissuade from dieting. The sheer number of proponents for obesity treatment tends to silence the few critics, as do recurrent calls for "consensus." In his acceptance speech for the Leo G. Reeder award in medical sociology, Marshall Becker (1993) warned of the dangers of consensus, citing the efforts of Richard Carleton, Chairman of the National Cholesterol Education Program, to silence critics. "Let's not confuse. Let's coalesce. Let's speak with the same voice," urged Carleton. As a New York Times editorial (1990) retorted, "[That's] not how science works. Eminent authorities can err en masse, especially when they coalesce and suppress confusion..."

We must recognize that the "problem" of "fatness" looks very different from different vantage points. To researchers and practitioners concerned primarily with obesity, the significance of body fat is its association with certain health risks and with negative social consequences believed to be immutable. Yet even the modest shift in perspective to that of a researcher or practitioner in eating disorders casts the matter in a radically different light since the "treatment" of one "disease" constitutes the major risk factor for the other. These differences in perspective occur among groups sharing a common education and practicing in the same disciplines, often on the same corridors of the same buildings. Obviously, the differences become greater as one considers the perspectives of academic feminists, political activists and the grass roots self-help and size-acceptance movements.

Meaningful dissent is hindered by the absence of a common language among these differing groups. Objections to obesity treatment often fail less because they challenge prevailing views than because they violate the format of discourse. Only data-based presentations on the failure of dieting are given a place in the field's dialogue, but they are unlikely to produce change because they remain within the paradigm, inviting questions about particulars and calls for additional clarifying research, a process that keeps the field alive and well. Meanwhile, criticism from other perspectives glances off the field, failing to engage its members because it is not "of them."

As argued by Thomas Kuhn, in his well-known analysis of paradigm shifts, change rarely occurs through the conversion of influential persons holding a dominant view, but through their attrition and replacement by younger persons attracted to a different model. By this view, the war on obesity might be lost, not in combat, but by its failure to recruit new warriors -- an outcome that is unlikely given the current economic incentives for maintaining the status quo but highly probable should government regulation limit the profits from obesity treatment. It is doubtful that many would be drawn to a helping role which helps so few and is therefore inherently unrewarding.

We will probably continue, for a while at least, to believe that it is possible to prevent obesity without encouraging weight preoccupation. But it is the same set of attitudes and behaviors which we hope simultaneously to encourage and discourage and, increasingly, the same population groups targeted for these contradictory messages: the young, especially young females. One might easily find prevention programs for obesity and for eating disorders delivering diametrically opposed advice, one urging children to attend more carefully to diet and exercise and the other urging decreased concern. Increasingly, we will be forced to confront these contradictions as the emphasis in both fields shifts to prevention and early intervention.

What, it might be asked, <u>would</u> we do if we stopped treating obesity? We would have a conversion problem for one of the country's major industries. There are many appropriate alternatives: 1) Increase funding for basic research on the pathogenesis of obesity. 2) Assist obese people in achieving goals which might be attainable: alterations of diet and exercise patterns known to improve health; enhancement of body image and self-esteem; diagnosis and treatment of eating disorders where these exist; diagnosis and treatment of psychological disorders where these exist; and the establishment of stable eating patterns disrupted by chronic dieting. Several recent programs have found beneficial effects of such alternative treatment methods (e.g., Ciliska, 1990; Polivy & Herman, 1992). 3) Adapt the sophisticated behavioral technologies developed to treat obesity to the modification of such health-endangering habits as smoking. 4) Redirect resources which have long gone into the weight loss industry to remediable social conditions known to influence disease. As Levin (cited in Becker, 1993) has noted, even a small increase in education or economic level for an individual or population has a much greater impact on health than all our health resources combined. Used for early childhood education, for example, the money spent on diet products and services would go a long way toward relieving the human suffering caused by poverty. At a time when our nation is struggling to meet the most basic health needs of its population, it is a tragic waste to pour precious resources into a futile undertaking.

REFERENCES

Andres, R. (1980). Effect of obesity on total mortality. International Journal of Obesity, 12, 277-284.

Becker, M. (1993). A medical sociologist looks at health promotion. Journal of Health & Social Behavior, 34 (March), 1-6.

Bennett, W.I. (1984). Dieting. Ideology versus physiology. Psychiatric Clinics of North America, 7, 321-334.

Bennett, W.I. (1987). Dietary treatments of obesity. In R. J. Wurtman & J.J. Wurtman (Eds.), Human obesity (pp. 250-263). New York: The New York Academy of Sciences.

Brownell, K.D. (1991). Dieting and the search for the perfect body: Where physiology and culture collide. Behavior Therapy, 22, 1-12.

Chernin, K. (1986). The hungry self: Women, eating and identity. London: Virago Press.

Ciliska, D. (1990). Beyond dieting. New York: Branner/Mazel.

Dyrenforth, S.R., Wooley, O.W., Wooley, S.C. (1980). A woman's body in a man's world: A review of findings on body image and weight control. In J. R. Kaplan (Ed.) A woman's conflict: The special relationship between women and food (pp. 30-57). New Jersey: Prentice-Hall, Inc.

Editorial. (1990, March 3). Fats, fads, fasts, fallacies. New York Times.,p. 14.

Ehrenreich, B. & English, D. (1978). For her own good: 150 years of the experts' advice to women. New York: Anchor Press/Doubleday.

Ernesberger, P. & Haskew, P. (1987). Health implications of obesity: An alternative view. Journal of Obesity and Weight Regulation, 6, 58-137.

Foreyt, J.P., Goodrick, G.K. & Gotto, A.M. (1981). Limitations of behavioral treatment of obesity: Review and analysis. Journal of Behavioral Medicine, 4, 159-174.

Garner, D.M., Wooley, S.C. (1991). Obesity treatment: The high cost of false hope. <u>Journal of the American Dietetic Association, 91</u>, 1238-1251.

Gould, S.J. (1981). <u>The mismeasure of man</u>. New York: W. W. Norton.

Keys, A. (1980). Overweight, obesity, coronary heart disease and mortality. <u>Nutrition Reviews, 38</u>, 297-307.

Orbach, S. (1978). <u>Fat is a feminist issue: The anti-diet guide to permanent weight loss</u>. New York and London: Paddington Press.

Perlick, D., Silverstein, B. (in press). The faces of female discontent. In P. Fallon, M. Katzman, S. Wooley, Eds. <u>Feminist perspectives on eating disorders</u>. New York: Guilford Press.

Polivy, P. & Herman, C.P. (1990). Undieting: A program to help people stop dieting. <u>International Journal of Eating Disorders, 11</u>, 3, 261-268.

Prentice, A.M. (in press). Is weight stability itself a reasonable goal? In <u>Proceedings of Obesity Treatment: Establishing Goals, Improving Outcomes and Reviewing the Research Agenda</u>. New York: Plenum Press.

Steiner-Adair, C. (1986). The body politic: Normal female adolescent development and development of eating disorders. <u>Journal of the American Academy of Psychoanalysis, 14</u>, 95-114.

Stunkard, A.J., Penick, S.B. (1979). Behavior modification in the treatment of obesity: The problem of maintaining weight loss. <u>Archives of General Psychiatry, 36</u>, 801-806.

Wilson, G.T. (in press). Behavioral treatment of obesity: Thirty years and counting. <u>Advances in Behavior Research & Therapy</u>.

Wolf, N. (1990). <u>The Beauty Myth</u>. London: Chatto & Windus Ltd.

Wooley, O.W., Wooley, S.C., Dyrenforth, S.R. (1979). Obesity and women II: A neglected feminist topic. <u>Women's Studies International Quarterly, 2</u>, 81-92.

CULTURAL FACTORS IN DESIRABLE BODY SHAPES AND THEIR IMPACT ON WEIGHT LOSS AND MAINTENANCE

Shiriki Kumanyika

Center for Biostatistics and Epidemiology
Pennsylvania State University
Hershey PA, 17033

"Cultural factors" refers to societal attitudes, beliefs, norms or values common to a particular demographic group or population or to the determinants of these beliefs. In the U.S. literature on obesity and weight control the cultural reference point is typically the mainstream culture, for example, as expressed in the mass media, in fashion magazines, or in the physical attributes of female beauty queens (Wiseman, Gray, Mosimann, & Ahrens, 1992; Rodin, 1991; Bowen, Tomoyasu, & Cauce, 1991). The predominant view is that obesity or large body size is undesirable and negatively stigmatized. The ideal tends to be thin rather than simply non-obese.

While the existence of these cultural attitudes in American society is generally accepted, the degree to which they are applied to or embraced by various demographic or racial/ethnic groups is variable (Sobal, & Stunkard, 1989; Kumanyika, 1993; Rand, & Kuldau, 1990). The slender ideal is more likely to be applied to women as a criterion of physical attractiveness and appears to be more central to the self-concept of women than men. Among women, the slender ideal appears to be most important for women of higher socioeconomic status and to Caucasian women. The association of these cultural attitudes with weight loss and maintenance for a given individual are difficult to pinpoint, however, since a preoccupation with being thin is not necessarily associated with success at weight control.

When sought in samples of individuals not confined to those presenting for obesity treatment, evidence that demographic groups in American society differ, on the degree of fidelity to the slender body ideal can be elicited, so long as the interview approach is sufficiently unbiased to permit this evidence to emerge. Findings suggestive of a lesser impact of the prevailing negative cultural attitudes towards obesity in African American communities comes from studies of children, adolescents, young- and older adults (Allan, Mayo, & Michel, 1993; Desmond, Price, Hallinan, & Smith, 1989; Grita, & Crane, 1991; Emmons, 1992; Kaplan, & Wadden, 1986; Klem, Klesges, Bene, & Mellon, 1990; Rucher, & Cash, 1992; Stevens, Kumanyika, Keil, & Becker, in press; Wing, Adams-Campbell, Marcus, & Janney, 1993; Thomas, & James, 1988)). These findings include a lesser preoccupation with dieting, less dietary restraint, a lesser tendency to define being overweight as problematic, negative attitudes about being too thin, some ability to disassociate from the media image of a slender ideal body size, a lack of association of obesity with poor health, less centrality of body image in one's overall self concept, and a multi-dimensional perspective on body size in which the definition of normal may be quite broad and in which body proportions, strength, health status, and the ability to command respect modify evaluation of overall size per se.

However, as a cautionary note, the more mixed picture of obesity-related attitudes in African American communities is just that--a mixed picture. It cannot be interpreted simplistically as a uniformly positive view of obesity or as evidence of a lack of motivation to lose weight. The latter impression is clearly contradicted by the high prevalence of dieting reported by African American women in national surveys (Piani, & Schoenborn, 1993; Williamson, Serdula, Anda, Levy, & Byers, 1992). The blending of cultural views in American society may lead to the concurrent influence of several, not necessarily consistent attitudinal perspectives.

Although there is continued allegiance to paradigms that assume relatively uniform susceptibility to the prevailing view that obesity is bad and thinness is good, receptivity to a more diverse view is increasing. This may be due, in part, to the increased interest solving the puzzle of obesity in high risk minority groups such as African American women (Bowen, Tomoyasu, & Cauce, 1991; Allan, Mayo, & Michel, 1993; Kumanyika, Wilson, & Guilford-Davenport, 1992; Kumanyika, 1986). The prevalence of obesity in African American women aged 45 to 74 years is approximately 60 percent and is associated with a high burden of obesity-related morbidity (e.g., hypertension, diabetes, heart disease) (Kumanyika, 1986). This creates a strong mandate to identify effective obesity treatment approaches for African American women and lends importance to findings which may provide clues as to how to do this. Results of clinical trials suggest indirectly that cultural factors (e.g., tolerance for overweight) may negatively impact upon the weight control efforts of black women. Intensive weight reduction programs provided for the purpose of hypertension prevention or treatment indicate less weight loss in African American women than white women (Kumanyika, Obarzanek, Stevens, Hebert, & Whelton, 1991; Wylie-Rosett, Wasertheil-Smoller, Blaufox, et al. 1993).

Attempts to explain obesity-tolerant attitudes draw upon anthropological or sociological reports describing scenarios wherein having excess fat symbolizes a physiological and economic advantage (Brown, & Konner, 1987). Such scenarios apply, for example, in cases of inadequate or inconsistent food availability and high rates of infectious diseases, cases where thinness, rather than obesity, would be indicative of poor health. The high prevalence of obesity in most U.S. minority populations can be discussed in this context. Patterns of obesity in association with socioeconomic status in developing countries tend to be opposite to those in industrialized countries in that the poor are thin and the affluent are fat (Sobal, & Stunkard, 1989).

Historical examples of the idealization of plumper physiques are cited to establish that the current positive view of thinness has not always been in force in the reference cultures of white Americans (Weigley, 1984). Relatively tolerant attitudes towards obesity have been reported in older Americans (Harris, & Furakawa, 1986). Recognition that views of obesity in a minority group such as African American women may differ from those in the mainstream may actually enhance recognition that the views within the mainstream are more diverse than those expressed by or attributed to people in treatment programs. This diversity of motivation may help to explain some of the current enigmas about the lack of long term efficacy of programs which may assume a more uniform motivation.

Several research directions related to cultural influences on obesity treatment can be suggested. One is to develop a more systematic conceptual framework for assessing and characterizing desirable body size or body shape. Several terms and variables are currently used: 1) desired or ideal weight; 2) self-perception as overweight; 3) the degree of dissatisfaction with body weight; 4) perceived attractiveness; 5) perceived health status in relation to weight; and 6) self-concept in relation to weight. The redundancy or lack of it among these variables needs clarification. Concepts of acceptable body size, functional aspects of being overweight, and positive associations of overweight and health should be expanded to better characterize some of the less well-recognized attitudes that have emerged in qualitative research.

The mechanisms whereby cultural attitudes influence weight control outcomes are another important area for elucidation in future research. Cultural meanings and values about body size operate in concert with cultural attitudes about eating and activity. Motivations for weight control influence the ultimate outcomes through pathways involving the knowledge, skills, and resources needed to actually achieve goals for which one is motivated.

Directions for research related to prevention and treatment models should include attempts to explicitly incorporate cultural attitudes and the determinants of these attitudes into the theoretical framework rather than relying only on models of individual or family behavior. Identifying implicit cultural assumptions in current treatment models will be an important first step along these lines (Kumanyika, Morssink, & Agurs, 1992).

REFERENCES

Allan, J. D., Mayo, K., & Michel, M. (1993). Body size values of white and black women. Research in Nursing and Health, 16, 323-333.

Bowen, D. J., Tomoyasu, N., & Cauce, A.M. (1993). The triple threat: A discussion of gender, class, and race differences in weight. Women and Health, 17, 123-143.

Brown, P.J., & Konner, M. (1987). An anthropological perspective on obesity. Annals of the New York Academy of Sciences, 499, 29-46.

Desmond, S.M., Price, J.H., Hallinan, C., & Smith, D. (1989). Black and white adolescents' perceptions of their weight. Journal of School Health, 59, 353-358.

Emmons, L. (1992). Dieting and purging behavior in black and white high school students. Journal of the American Dietetic Association, 93, 306-312.

Gritz, E.R., & Crane, L.A. (1991). Use of diet pills and amphetamines to lose weight among smoking and non-smoking high school seniors. Health Psychology, 10, 330-335.

Harris, M.B., & Furakawa, C. (1986). Attitudes toward obesity in an elderly sample. Journal of Obesity and Weight Regulation, 5, 5-16.

Kaplan, K.M., & Wadden, T.A. (1986). Childhood obesity and self-esteem. Journal of Pediatrics, 109, 367-370.

Klem, M.L., Klesges, R.C., Bene, C.R., & Mellon, M.W. (1990). A psychometric study of restraint: The impact of race, gender, weight, and marital status. Addictive Behaviors, 15, 147-152.

Kumanyika, S. (1986). Obesity in black women. Epidemiologic Reviews, 9, 31-50.

Kumanyika, S. (1993). Special issues regarding obesity in minority populations. Annals of Internal Medicine, 119, 650-654.

Kumanyika, S., Morssink, C., Agurs, T. (1992). Models for dietary and weight change in African American women: Identifying cultural components. Ethnicity and Disease, 2, 166-175.

Kumanyika, S., Obarzanek, E. Stevens, V.J., Hebert, P.R., & Whelton, P.K. (1991). Weight-loss experience of black and white participants in NHLBI-sponsored clinical trials. American Journal of Clinical Nutrition, 53, 1631S-1638S.

Kumanyika, S., Wilson, J., & Guilford-Davenport, M. (1992). Weight-related attitudes and behaviors of black women. Journal of the American Dietetic Association, 93, 416-442.

Piani, A.L., Schoenborn, C.A. (1993). Health Promotion and Disease Prevention, United States, 1990: Vital and Health Statistics 10 (185). DHHS Publication No. (PHS) 93-1513.

Rand, C.S.W., & Kuldau, J.M. (1990). The epidemiology of obesity and self-defined weight problem in the general population: Gender, race, age, and social class. International Journal of Eating Disorders, 9, 329-343.

Rodin, J. (1993). Cultural and psychosocial determinants of weight concerns. Annals of Internal Medicine, 119, 635-643.

Rucker, C.E., & Cash, T.F. (1992). Body images, body-size perceptions, and eating behaviors among African American and white college women. International Journal of Eating Disorders, 12, 291-299.

Sobal, J., & Stunkard, A.J. (1989). Socioeconomic status and obesity: A review of the literature. Psychological Bulletin, 105, 260-275.

Stevens, J., Kumanyika, S., Keil, J.E., & Becker, L.H. (in press). Body image and eating restraint in elderly men. Obesity Research.

Thomas, V.F., & James, M.D. (1988). Body image, dieting tendencies, and sex role traits in urban black women. Sex Roles, 18, 523-529.

Weigley, E.S. (1993). Average? Ideal? Desirable? A grief overview of height-weight tables in the United States. Journal of the American Dietetic Association, 84, 417-423.

Williamson, D.F., Serdula, M.K., Anda, R.F., Levy, A., & Byers, T. (1992). Weight loss attempts in adults: Goals, duration, and rate of weight loss. American Journal of Public Health, 82, 1251-1257.

Wing, R.R., Adams-Campbell, L.L., Marcus, M.D., & Janney, C.A. (1993). Effect of ethnicity and geographical location on body weight, dietary restraint, and abnormal eating attitudes. Obesity Research., 1, 193-198.

Wiseman, C.V., Gray, J.J., Mosimann, J.E., & Ahrens, A.H. (1992). Cultural expectations of thinness in women: An update. International Journal of Eating Disorders, 11, 85-89.

Wylie-Rosett, J., Wassertheil-Smoller, Blaufox, D. et al. (1993). Trial of Antihypertensive Intervention and Management: Greater efficacy with weight reduction than with a sodium-potassium intervention. Journal of the American Dietetic Association, 93, 408-415.

WHY SHOULD PATIENTS BE MATCHED TO TREATMENTS, HOW MAY IT OCCUR, AND HOW CAN IT BE STUDIED?

John Garrow

Department of Human Nutrition
Charterhouse Square
London, United Kingdom EC1M 6BQ

WHAT WE KNOW ABOUT OBESITY

A main objective of this workshop is to answer the question: "What else do we need to know?" However it is convenient to state here some propositions the truth of which I believe has been established. The evidence for this view is set out elsewhere (Garrow 1988).

1. Health risks associated with obesity start to be evident somewhere in the range of Quetelet's Index (or Body Mass Index) 25 to 30 kg/m^2. Above 30 kg/m^2 the threat to longevity and health rises quite steeply.
2. The association of obesity with risk of heart disease (which is the main cause of the excess mortality among obese people) is stronger among young adults than among men aged 50 years or more.
3. For a given amount of total body fat intra-abdominal fat carries a greater risk than subcutaneous fat, probably because free fatty-acids released from intra-abdominal adipocytes cause greater insulin insensitivity than similar lipolysis in subcutaneous sites. However we have no means by which we can significantly alter the rate at which fat is lost from different sites in the same person.
4. The prevalence of obesity (defined as > 30 kg/m^2) is increasing among both men and women in all age groups in the UK, and probably in other developed and developing countries also. If the present trend continues obesity may overtake cigarette smoking as an important cause of avoidable ill-health.
5. The excess weight in obese people comprises about 75% of fat and 25% of fat-free tissue. This mixture has an energy value of 7000 kcal/kg.
6. Change in energy stores can be accurately predicted by the difference between energy input and output. A rate of loss of 1 kg/week of adipose tissue (as defined in 5. above) therefore requires an average daily energy deficit of 1000 kcal/day, and *pro rata*.

If the above statements are accepted it appears that the effective treatment of obesity

Obesity Treatment, Edited by D.B. Allison
and F.X. Pi-Sunyer, Plenum Press, New York, 1995

should be very simple, by reducing the energy intake (ie. dieting). This is not the case because the people who seek medical help for obesity have selected themselves by their inability to diet effectively. I believe that, among omnivorous mammals, obesity is the natural consequence of longevity and affluence. Observation of domestic pets will show that if they are given access ad libitum to palatable food, and protected from their natural predators, they will usually become obese. This is true even of the rat fed on laboratory chow: it has an increased life expectancy if its food intake is restricted. It is not surprising that man in affluent countries tends to become obese unless food intake is voluntarily restricted. I contend, therefore, that middle-aged normal-weight people are testimony to the fact that dieting controls obesity. Among obese people this has not worked: to find the reason for this failure and to help to correct it is one of the three main tasks for anyone treating obesity. The other two are to help the obese person to maintain weight at a desired level, and (where necessary) to restore the self-esteem of the formerly obese person. In what follows a plan is suggested by which these aims may be achieved, but the strategy is not the same for every obese patient, which is why treatments should be matched to patients.

SUCCESS REQUIRES MOTIVATION AND TECHNIQUE

We may fail to acquire a skill - to play a musical instrument, to learn a foreign language, to lose weight, or maintain weight loss - for reasons which fall into two categories which for brevity I shall call "motivation" and "technique". These are separate categories, but they interact. If a person does not much want to acquire a skill, then the most expert coaching will not achieve much progress, while a person who desperately wants to succeed may fail to do so as a result of bad advice. However the enthusiasm of the coach will not long survive indifference from the person being coached, and motivation to succeed will be eroded by continual failure.

The obvious reason why obese patients should be matched to treatments is that some are chiefly lacking in motivation, some chiefly lack technique, and some lack both. Successful treatment must address the area where the deficiency lies.

Jeremiads about the ineffectiveness of obesity treatment (e.g., Garner & Wooley 1991) draw attention to the high failure rate when a given treatment protocol is applied to a group of "obese patients". This is not surprising if the group is a heterogeneous one, with different needs, some of which are not addressed by the treatment under review. Obese patients can be arbitrarily but conveniently categorized according to the severity of their obesity by bands of "desirable" weight from 20-25 kg/m^2, and Grade I, II and III obesity which are separated by boundaries at 30 kg/m^2 and 40 kg/m^2 respectively (Garrow 1988). They can also be categorized, independently and less objectively, according to their desire to lose weight. Figure 1 shows a simplified scheme in which Grade II and III obese are lumped together as "obese", and motivation is reduced to a two-point scale in which the individual does, or does not, wish to lose weight. This is an absurd oversimplification, but it will serve to illustrate the confusion which arises when these distinctions are totally ignored.

The background state in Fig 1 is "normal weight and happy with it", and I will assume that this is the preferred state for virtually everyone if that is possible. Arrow (a) indicates people passing from "obese and wanting to lose weight" to the preferred state. Arrow (b) indicates people who are not obese (they may be in the desirable range, or Grade I), but who want to lose weight, passing to the preferred state. This may be achieved by reassurance, with or without modest weight loss. Arrow (c) indicates the special case of patients with anorexia nervosa, who are probably <20 kg/m^2, with whom this Workshop is not directly concerned. Since arrows (a), (b) and (c) all result in people achieving the preferred state I assume that there will be general agreement that these transitions are desirable.

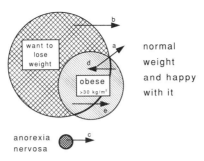

Figure 1. Venn diagram to indicate that some obese patients do, and some do not, want to lose weight. Arrows (a) (b) and (c) indicate desirable transitions to a state of being of normal weight and happy with it. Either flow (d) or (e) is preferable, depending on the belief that flow (a) is, or is not, possible.

However there is controversy concerning arrow (d) which indicates obese people who were previously not wanting to lose weight developing this desire. If you believe (as I do) that transition (a) is desirable and possible, then you will consider (d) desirable, since it is equivalent to providing obese people with motivation, without which they will not achieve the desirable transition (a). However if, like Garner and Wooley, you believe that (a) is virtually impossible then (d) would merely cause dissatisfaction, and the reverse process (e) would be beneficial, since obese people would then be more content with their lot.

IS SUSTAINED WEIGHT LOSS METABOLICALLY IMPOSSIBLE?

Garner & Wooley (1991) say (p 742) "There is consistent evidence from both human and animal studies that weight loss in the obese leads to reductions of 15-30% in energy requirements". There are 11 papers cited in support of this statement, of which 8 concern studies on human patients. Three papers report changes in metabolic rate when patients are changed from a high to a low energy diet. Bray (1969) found a 15% decrease in energy expenditure among massively obese patients when they had been changed from a diet supplying 3500 kcal/day to one supplying 450 kcal/day, at a stage when their weight had decreased by only 6.6%. Donahoe et al. (1984) found a decrease of 8.4% in metabolic rate in 10 female subjects who were on a diet supplying 800 kcal/day for 6 weeks, when their weight had decreased by only 4%. Finer et al. (1986) used a very low calorie diet (about 300 kcal/day) to achieve a 24% weight reduction among 5 female patients whose metabolic rate fell by 19.3%, and weight loss of 27.3% among 6 male patients whose metabolic rate fell by 25.3%. It is well known that when subjects are put into negative energy balance there is an immediate decrease of about 6% in resting metabolic rate, even when there has been negligible weight loss (Dauncey 1980, Garrow and Webster 1989). (There is a similar increase in resting metabolic rate with positive energy balance, even before significant weight has been gained). Added to this the thermic effect of feeding is about 10% of energy ingested, so a change from 3500 to 500 kcal would be expected to cause a decrease of about 300 kcal/day in this thermic effect. It is therefore not correct to ascribe changes in energy expenditure after large shifts in energy intake to "weight loss": the effect of weight loss is a change of about 12 - 15 kcal/day for 1 kg weight change.

Two of the papers cited by Garner and Wooley report changes in metabolic rate after weight loss when the measurements were made in energy balance both before and after weight loss. Thus Barrows et al. (1987) found a decrease of 16.5% in metabolic rate for a decrease of 20.5% in body weight, and Elliott et al. (1989) a decrease of 14.7% in metabolic rate for a decrease of 25.5% in body weight. The reference to Ravussin et al. (1982) seems to be an error, since that paper does not deal with changes in metabolic rate with weight change, but Ravussin et al. (1985) report a 'v7 decrease of 9.2% in metabolic rate for a decrease of 11.3% in body weight. The change in energy requirements in the last three papers mentioned agree with our previous calculation (Garrow and Webster 1989) that the long-term effects of weight loss is a decrease of 12-15 kcal/day per kg weight change. The actual values are 14.0, 9.2 and 13.4 kcal/kg weight change respectively.

Two of the papers cited by Garner and Wooley have not yet been discussed, since they used different methods from those mentioned above. Liebel and Hirsch (1984) made a retrospective analysis of the energy intake which was found to maintain weight within a limit of 0.5 kg over 7 days in obese patients before and after weight loss, but this does not provide a very accurate estimate of energy requirements. Geissler et al. (1987) measured the energy expenditure of post-obese subjects and weight-matched lean volunteers, who were fed the diet which they claimed was their maintenance requirement. In the event the post-obese patients had an intake of 1298 kcal and an output of 1601 kcal, so they were studied while in negative energy balance. The lean volunteers were fed 1945 kcal but expended only 1882 kcal, so they were studied under conditions of positive energy balance. In these circumstances it is not possible to ascribe the 11.4% smaller energy expenditure in the post-obese patients to a metabolic adaptation to weight loss.

Certainly substantial weight loss is associated with a decrease in energy requirements: it would be astonishing if this were not so. The crucial question is whether an obese person who reduces from, say, 100 kg to 70 kg then has a lower energy requirement for weight maintenance than a person of similar age, sex and body composition who has always been at 70 kg. The analysis of Dore et al. (1982) indicates that, provided the weight loss is not achieved by excessively severe dieting, the post-obese patient is not metabolically disadvantaged.

The most dramatic demonstration that weight loss continues indefinitely if the negative energy balance is maintained comes from the report of Bortz (1969). He had the unusual opportunity to study in a metabolic ward a massively obese man who was maintained on a diet supplying 800 kcal/day for two years, during which time his weight decreased by 500 lb (227 kg). No measurements of energy expenditure were made during this study, but from the rate of weight loss we can make a rough calculation of the energy deficit. During the first 100 days of dieting the weight loss was approximately 50 kg, and between 600 - 700 days of dieting it was approximately 20 kg. The weight loss of 190 kg between the mid-points of these periods (ie. day 50 to 650) would be expected to decrease energy expenditure by about 2300 kcal/day, which agrees well with the change needed to explain the change in the rate of weight loss which was observed. Thus the evidence does not support the popular view that "dieting makes you fat" because the metabolic rate falls so dramatically as an adaptation to dietary restriction. There are, of course, many people who, having lost a substantial amount of weight, believe that their requirements for weight maintenance were subsequently abnormally low. I have spent many years investigating patients with this complaint, and have never found the decrease was greater than that which would be expected on the basis of the principles set out above. Tremblay et al. (1991) have recently reported such a case, and shown that the reported low energy intake was not confirmed by calorimetry.

The converse problem has been investigated by Webb and Annis (1983). They studied energy balance and weight gain in two groups of subjects who were overfed by 1000 kcal/day for 30 days. One group were lean subjects (mean weight 74.2 kg) who reported that they were "hard gainers" who had little tendency to gain weight with increased energy intake. The other group were overweight (86.8 kg) who reported that they gained weight very easily with overfeeding. In the event weight gain (2.5 and 2.2 kg respectively) was similar in the two groups, as were other parameters of energy balance.

To summarize: I will now discuss the treatment of obese patients on the basis that:

a. those >30 kg/m^2 are at significant health risk, particularly if they are young.
b. diets do not work in obese people because they do not have the motivation and/or technique to diet effectively, and not because they differ metabolically from lean people.
c. an average energy deficit of 1000 kcal/day will in the long term cause a weight loss of 1 kg/week. A rate of weight loss in the range 0.5-1.0 kg is usually appropriate. Loss of 1 kg in weight will normally cause a decrease in maintenance energy requirements of 12-15 kcal/day. Obese people 'v7 initially have higher-than-normal energy requirements, and after weight loss their reduced energy requirements are not different from stable-weight controls of similar age, sex and body composition.
d. in view of b. and c. above it can be predicted that weight lost by obese patients will be regained unless something prevents this weight regain.
e. obese people tend to have a low self-esteem, which may be a result of the disabilities associated with obesity, or disappointment with repeated failures to lose weight, or unsympathetic management by health professionals.

AN ALGORITHM FOR MATCHING TREATMENT TO PATIENTS

Figure 2 describes a flow system by which patients may be matched to appropriate treatments. First it is necessary to establish if the patient is obese (>30 kg/m^2). If so, the path down the right side of the diagram applies. If they have a sound diet plan, and lose weight at an appropriate rate, it is only necessary to provide encouragement while the patient decreases to an appropriate target weight. If the patient is not obese the path on the left of the diagram applies, but young (< 35 year old) patients should be encouraged to achieve a weight of <25 kg/m^2.

The problem usually concerns the obese patient who, despite good dietary advice, does not lose weight at the appropriate rate. The possibilities are either that the patient is accurately observing the diet, or not. If the patient believes that his or her energy intake is (say) 1000 kcal/day, but no weight is lost over a period of months, this must mean that total energy output is also approximately 1000 kcal/day, which has never yet been documented for an obese adult. If the facilities for 24-hour calorimetry are available energy output can be measured, and the hypothesis that requirements are only 1000 kcal/day can be tested and (in my experience) invariably refuted. Often (but not invariably) this provides sufficient motivation for the patient

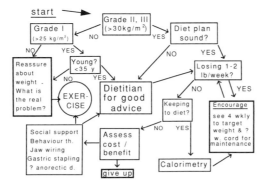

Figure 2. Flow diagram indicating pathways by which patients who want to lose weight can be allocated to appropriate treatments.

to resume more accurate compliance with the diet. Alternatively it may be agreed that the diet is not being accurately observed, for many reasons. It is the right of any patient to decide that the disadvantages of dieting outweigh the benefit which will accrue. However the skillful therapist will be able to suggest forms of social support, or behavioural procedures, or (less subtly) jaw wiring, gastric stapling or anorectic drugs, which may tip the balance and make dieting the more acceptable option.

In Figure 2 exercise is shown as an option both for obese and non-obese people. This is because the benefits of exercise apply to both groups, and I do not regard physical exercise as a practical therapy for obesity, since the exercise tolerance of obese people is so low. However I believe it has an important role in prevention of obesity, and also in maintenance of weight loss in post-obese people.

MAINTENANCE OF WEIGHT LOSS

Maintenance of reduced weight in obese patients is very important, but difficult to achieve. It has already been noted that obese patients are a self-selected group of people who, for various reasons, are unable to diet effectively to maintain their weight in a desirable range. After weight loss their energy requirements are reduced from the former obese state, so it is obvious that if they return to "normal" eating (ie. the intake which supported the initial obese body weight) they will in time return to that weight. This is not to say that to prevent weight regain the patient must remain on a reducing diet for ever. Suppose a person taking 1200 kcal/day is losing about 800 g/week, and attains target weight. The fact that they were losing 800 g/week implies that 1200 kcal/day is 800 kcal/day less than expenditure, so in theory they should now maintain weight on an intake of 2000 kcal/day. In practice this calculation has to be slightly modified, since the increase of 800 kcal/day in intake will be associated with about 80 kcal/day extra from thermic effect of feeding, and the change from a negative energy balance to equilibrium energy balance will also increase energy expenditure by about 6% - say another 70 kcal/day. To set against this there is the probability that, on passing from a reducing to a maintenance diet, body glycogen stores will be repleted. This will cause an initial increase in body weight, just as the depletion of these stores accounts for the initial rapid weight decrease at the start of a reducing diet.

The difficulty in maintaining reduced weight in post-obese people cannot be explained purely on the basis of thermodynamics. It is not entirely clear how people who maintain "desirable" weight throughout an adult lifetime achieve this, but I believe that the ability to detect unwanted weight gain is an important factor. From time to time I have experimentally manipulated my own body weight over a range of 10 kg or so (Garrow and Stalley 'v7 1977), and it is impossible to be "blind" to weight changes of this magnitude if you wear the same pair of trousers. At the upper end of the range they will hardly fasten at the waist, and at the lower end they will hardly stay up. However the obese person who has reduced from, say, 100 kg to 70 kg is in a different situation. If weight increases to 80 kg this is not an unknown experience: indeed it is still significantly below maximum weight, and therefore not particularly alarming. On this basis I have been supplying reduced obese patients with a waist cord which sensitively and reliably monitors unwanted weight gain (Garrow and Gardiner 1981, Garrow and Webster 1986, Garrow 1992a). The efficacy of this has not been formally tested by randomised clinical trial, but I am very impressed by the improvement in maintenance of weight loss among patients with a waist cord compared with those without one. It is obvious that people who have lost a substantial amount of weight do not want to regain it: typically they do so when life events distract their attention and they do not notice the weight regain until it has become so large that the situation is out of control and demoralising. With a waist cord this situation does not arise: the cord becomes tight so it cannot be ignored: a decision must be made either to cut the cord or to lose weight. Most patients make the latter choice.

RESTORATION OF SELF-ESTEEM

Garner and Wooley (1991) suggest restoration of self-esteem as an preferable alternative to weight loss in obese people. This seems a false antithesis. The experience of repeated failures to lose weight, and the physical and social disabilities associated with significant obesity, must contribute to the low self-esteem typically shown by obese patients. If (as I believe) it is possible for obese patients to achieve a normal weight and body composition, this will remove these disabilities, and also be an achievement of which the patient can rightly take considerable pride. Even if it is possible to restore the patients self-esteem without weight loss, the restoration of self-esteem in addition to weight loss seems an obviously preferable plan.

I entirely accept that weight loss as an alternative to restoration of self-esteem is not an acceptable policy, and it is one for which some therapists are rightly criticised. It is all too easy to fall into the "diet relationship trap" (Garrow 1992b). Initially the relationship between the obese patient and dietitian is constructive and gratifying: the diet offers the means for the patient to achieve normal weight, health and independence, so expectations are high. This happy state persists so long as weight loss continues, but sooner or later the patient comes to a follow-up appointment having failed to lose weight, or even have regained some weight. Since the patient has a rather fragile self-esteem this probably precipitates an excessively apologetic attitude of the part of the patient, who says that the time of the therapist has been wasted, it should have been spent on more important patients, and similar protestations of unworthiness. The trap is now set, and it only needs the therapist to agree that time has indeed been wasted, and that the performance of the patient is disappointing, for the trap to close. Instead of restoring the self-esteem of the patient the relationship now gives the patient further cause for further self-depreciation and despair. Anyone who has experience of prolonged support of obese patients will know how difficult it is to maintain a constructive and supportive attitude towards a diffident patient who has blown the diet. It is not helping anyone to reprimand a patient who is doing his or her best, but equally it is not helpful to be so sympathetic that the outcome is that all parties agree than dieting is impossible, and probably not helpful anyway. Steering the narrow path between this Scylla and Charybdis is a feat which few of us can consistently achieve.

CONCLUSIONS, AND ITEMS FOR THE RESEARCH AGENDA

I believe that the objectives for treatment of obese patients should be:

a. to maintain weight loss of 1-2 lb/week until 30 kg/m^2 (or 25 kg/m^2 in young people) is achieved;
b. to maintain this weight indefinitely; and
c. where necessary, to restore the self-esteem of the patient.

I have tried to indicate how these objectives may be achieved in virtually any obese patient, but since patients differ the treatment must be matched to the needs of the individual patient.

SUGGESTIONS FOR THE RESEARCH AGENDA ARE THESE:

We need to agree to what is known about the health risks of obesity (> 30 kg/m^2) and the thermodynamics of weight loss. I do not agree with Garner and Wooley (1991) that the health risks of obesity have been overstated, but I do agree that it has been wrongly implied that these risks apply to many people who are not obese (as defined above). I do not agree that "dieting makes you fat" or that there are such powerful adaptive changes in energy output that dietary treatment for obesity is doomed to failure. Promulgation of these false ideas destroys the motivation of obese people who are sensibly trying to lose weight, and therefore acts against the public interest.

I think the main weakness in present therapeutic programmes is inability to achieve maintenance of weight loss. In my own experience the waist cord is a major advance in this direction, and I would like to see this technique objectively tested by other researchers.

It would obviously be a major advance if obesity could be prevented. For reasons set out elsewhere (Garrow 1988) I believe that the best chance of achieving this is by limiting the weight gain of children who are overweight at age 5 years, so that over the next seven years the normal relationship of weight to height is achieved. This does not involve weight loss: merely a slight slowing of weight gain, which should not retard height growth. I would like to see this theory experimentally tested.

REFERENCES

Barrows, K., Snook, J.T. (1987) Effects of a high protein, very-low-calorie diet on resting metabolism, thyroid hormones, and energy expenditure of obese, middle-aged women. American Journal of Clinical Nutrition, 45, 391-398.

Bortz, W.M. (1969) A 500 pound weight loss. American Journal of Medicine, 47, 325-331.

Bray, G.A. (1969) The effect of caloric restriction on energy expenditure in obese patients. Lancet, ii:397-398.

Dauncey, M.J. (1980) Metabolic effects of altering the 24 h energy intake in man, using direct and indirect calorimetry. British Journal of Nutrition, 43, 257-269.

Donahoe, C.P., Lin, D.H., Kirschenbaum, D.S., Keesey, R.E. (1984) Metabolic consequences of dieting and exercise in the treatment of obesity. Journal of Consulting and Clinical Psychology, 52, 827-836.

Dore, C., Hesp, R., Wilkins, D., Garrow, J.S. (1982) Prediction of energy requirements of obese patients after massive weight loss. Human Nutrition: Clinical Nutrition, 36C, 41-48.

Elliot, D.L., Goldberg, L., Kuehl, K.S., Bennett, W.M. (1989) Sustained depression of the resting metabolic rate after massive weight loss. American Journal of Clinical Nutrition, 49, 93-96.

Finer, N., Swan, P.C., Mitchell, F.T. (1986) Metabolic rate after massive weight loss in human obesity. Clinical Science, 70, 395-401.

Garner, D.M., Wooley, S.C. (1991). Confronting the failure of behavioral and dietary treatments for obesity. Clinical Psychology Review, 11, 729-780.

Garrow, J.S. (1988). Obesity and related diseases, London: Churchill Livingstone, pp 329.

Garrow, J.S. (1992a). The management of obesity. Another view. International Journal of Obesity 16: suppl 2, S59-S63.

Garrow, J.S. (1992b) Treatment of obesity. Lancet, 340, 409-413.

Garrow, J.S, Gardiner, G.T. (1981) Maintenance of weight loss in obese patients after jaw wiring. British Medical Journal, 282, 858-860.

Garrow, J.S, Stalley, S.F. (1977) Cognitive thresholds and human body weight. Proceedings of the Nutrition Society, 36, 18A.

Garrow, J.S., Webster, J.D. (1986) Long-term results of treatment of severe obesity with jaw wiring and waist cord. Proceedings of the Nutrition Society, 45, 119A.

Garrow, J.S., Webster, J.D. (1989) Effects of weight and metabolic rate of obese women of a 3.4 MJ (800 kcal) diet. Lancet i, 1429-1431.

Geissler, C.A., Miler, D.S., Shah, M. (1987) The daily metabolic rate of the post- obese and the lean. American Journal of Clinical Nutrition, 45, 914- 920.

Leibel, R.L., Hirsch, J. (1984) Diminished energy requirements in reduced-obese patients. Metabolism, 33, 164-170.

Ravussin, E., Burnand, B., Schultz, Y., Jequier, E. (1982) Twenty-four hour energy expenditure and resting metabolic rate in obese, moderately obese, and control subjects. American Journal of Clinical Nutrition, 35, 566-573.

Ravussin, E., Burnand, B., Schultz, Y., Jequier, E .(1985) Energy expenditure before and after energy restriction in obese patients. American Journal of Clinical Nutrition, 41, 753-759.

Trembla,y A., Seale, J., Almeras, N., Conway, J., Moe, P. (1991) Energy requirements of post-obese man reporting a low energy intake at weight maintenance. American Journal of Clinical Nutrition, 54, 506-508.

Webb, P., Annis, J.F. (1983) Adaptation to overeating in lean and overweight women. Human Nutrition: Clinical Nutrition, 37C, 117-131.

TREATMENT OPTIONS AND THE MAINTENANCE OF WEIGHT LOSS

L. Arthur Campfield

Metabolic Diseases Research
Hoffmann - La Roche, Inc.
Nutley, NJ 07110

Obesity is a complex, prevalent and important medical problem. Multiple treatment options with documented medically significant outcomes, including safe and effective pharmacological approaches, are needed to assist patients improve compliance to voluntary life style changes that lead to success in achieving and maintaining weight reduction. These treatment options may range from short-term to long-term interventions to lifestyle changes. A interesting possibility would be interventions that lead to, or support, sustained lifestyle changes. Multiple treatment options implies matching treatments to patients. Among the possible classification categories for patients are: overweight or obese, free from associated disease or medically at risk, "successful" dieters or refractory to dietary treatment.

The problem of maintaining weight loss and the prevention of weight regain or weight maintenance is a major challenge in obesity treatment. This area will certainly receive increasing attention. However, this will require that the field agree on an operational definition of weight maintenance. The ideal of zero weight regain over any time interval of interest is not useful in practice. What is acceptable weight maintenance? Is it simply delayed weight regain or is it the maintenance of a non-zero difference between pretreatment weight and the current weight? Research on successful weight maintainers has identified some common characteristics, in particular, adherence to exercise programs. Strategies for the promotion of weight maintenance include psychosocial, exercise, diet and nutrition and behavioral modification.

Several issues related to the use of pharmacological agents in the treatment of obesity must continue to be addressed by the scientific community. First, what are the goals of treatment? The potential uses of antiobesity agents are: 1) induction of weight loss; 2) maintenance of weight loss; 3) to improve compliance to diet; 4) reduction of associated risk factors (+/- weight loss); and 5) "staged" or " downward staircase" weight loss with intermediate plateaus. A second issue is single versus multiple drug therapies and the related question of sequential or combined drug treatment. A third issue is an evaluation of the pros and cons of treatment for life. A fourth question is related to the risk/benefit analysis of obesity treatment: How little efficacy is acceptable ?

An alternative, medically oriented goal for the treatment of obesity to replace our current focus on body weight, body mass index or body fat is the concept of "metabolic fitness".

Obesity Treatment, Edited by D.B. Allison
and F.X. Pi-Sunyer, Plenum Press, New York, 1995

Metabolic fitness can be generally defined as the absence of any metabolic or biochemical risk factor for diseases associated with obesity. At least four alternative formulations of this concept can be proposed as alternative, medically oriented goals of the treatment of obesity. Ranging from the least to the most aggressive, they are: 1) medically significant reduction of risk factors; 2) restoration of abnormal risk factors to normal ranges; 3) reversal of "high normal"or "borderline" parameters; or 4) prevention of risk factors in overweight individuals. An important feature of this concept is that improvements in "metabolic fitness" may be independent of, or poorly correlated with, weight loss. This concept and its treatment goals focus on the attainment of improved health and not on some rather arbitrary body weight. Perhaps this concept may "level the playing field" for obese patients in terms of both treatment expectations and outcome assessment.

Progress toward multiple treatment options with documented outcomes will require shifts in the dominant paradigms within pharmaceutical industry, the scientific community and the regulatory agencies. We must put Occam's razor aside in favor of confronting the inherent complexity of the problem and providing a complex, effective, multifactorial treatment approach. The dominant hypotheses in drug discovery has been that a single molecule with a well defined action at the "correct" molecular or biochemical "target" should reverse most, if not all, of the pathological aspects of obesity. Over the last decade or so, a consensus appears to be growing that drugs are no longer conceived of as "magic bullets" that will induce and maintain weight loss in the absence of behavioral changes but rather as adjuncts to behavioral-based therapy.

However, significant progress toward improved treatment of obesity will require utilization of new knowledge emerging for new research to develop multiple interventions that can be sequentially or concurrently applied at multiple sites to improve the efficacy of the voluntary behavioral and life style changes made by obese patients. A scientific community focused on the etiology and consequences of obesity must also give serious attention to the goals, assessment and medical significance of therapeutic interventions in subpopulations of obese patients. More research is essential at all levels of analysis in the energy balance regulatory system. A more complete understanding of the function of critical cells, tissues, organs, organ systems and regulatory sites involved in energy balance in normal and pathological states is required. In addition, more research on interventions must be conducted and outcome assessment is essential. Obesity treatment will be improved if each basic and clinical investigator would routinely ask the following two questions when proposing and planning research: How will the results of this experiment improve the treatment of obese patients? Can I increase the impact of this experiment on obesity treatment with changes in design?

Regulatory agencies must also rely less on precedent and be open to new therapeutic approaches directed not only at inducing statistically significant weight loss but also weight maintenance, reduction of risk factors for associated conditions and the improvement of "metabolic fitness".

An additional area of research will be the optimal ways to blend behavioral and medication based approaches to obesity treatment. Among the several models are:1) separate treatments are arbitrarily combined in same patient; 2) combination tailored to patients or a "menu approach" in which one or more behavioral approaches and medication are selected; 3) an integrated, multifaceted approach in which medication supports behavioral change and helps patients to "learn to become successful" at sustaining beneficial voluntary behavioral and life style changes. An interesting possibility is that improved treatment may result if the dosing schedule for medication is not independent of the diet and exercise aspects of the treatment program. That is, it may be possible that meal contingent dosing may increase compliance to diet. It will be important to learn if rituals and routines associated with aspects of treatment can affect compliance to diet and exercise and treatment outcome.

In conclusion, additional basic and clinical research combined with these paradigm shifts and regulatory flexibility will hopefully lead to a treatment approach in which patients will "learn to become successful" at sustaining beneficial voluntary behavioral and lifestyle changes. In such an approach, pharmacological treatment would not be an end in itself but rather would be used to support, reinforce and sustain desirable behavioral changes leading to improved health.

REFERENCES

Campfield, L.A. "Simple solutions for complex problems? Occam's razor, the FDA, and the pharmacological treatment obesity" Proceedings of Seminar on Human Obesity: Current Status of Scientific and Clinical Progress, AAAS'93, Boston, MA., February 12-13, 1993.

WHY DO PEOPLE FAIL TO MAINTAIN WEIGHT LOSS?

Joseph S. Rossi

Cancer Prevention Research Center
University of Rhode Island
Providence, RI 02881-0808

For individuals faced with the task of losing weight, there are essentially two main issues: losing the weight in the first place and then maintaining the loss. In this respect, we have found that weight loss is not very different from many other problems that are refractory to change, such as smoking cessation or exercise adoption (O'Connell & Velicer, 1988; Prochaska et al., in press-b; Rossi, 1992; Rossi et al., in press-b). In confronting the problem of failure to maintain, I am struck by our readiness to place the onus of the task on the individual. Instead, I suggest that we own some of the responsibility for maintenance failure ourselves, as researchers and treatment providers. The challenge that faces us is to develop behavioral models and interventions that can encompass the wide range of attitudes, cognitions, affect, and activities that characterize individuals throughout the process of change, from initial motivation (or lack thereof), through inevitable relapse, and to eventual success.

An organizing principle that we have found especially useful, especially for the addictions but for other problem behaviors as well, is the concept of motivational readiness to change. Our studies of how people change on their own and as a result of professional intervention suggests that people move through a series of *stages of change* in their attempts to change a problem behavior (Prochaska et al., 1992a; Prochaska, 1993).

Individuals in the *precontemplation* stage of change have no intention of losing weight in the next six months. Precontemplators do not feel that their weight problem is serious enough to require behavior change, or they may deny that they have a problem. Some may be demoralized from repeated unsuccessful attempts to change. In either case, the costs of changing behavior clearly outweigh the benefits. Precontemplators often feel that they are being pressured into change by family, friends, or society in general. Coerced change is rarely successful, however, and as soon as the pressure is off, precontemplators typically revert to old behavior patterns. Defensiveness and resistance to change are the most distinctive characteristics of the precontemplation stage.

Individuals in the *contemplation* stage of change are considering change within the next six months but are not currently prepared to lose weight. Unfortunately, contemplators typically do not act on their intentions and frequently remain stuck in this stage of change for lengthy periods of time. Contemplators substitute thinking for action, constantly struggling with

Obesity Treatment, Edited by D.B. Allison
and F.X. Pi-Sunyer, Plenum Press, New York, 1995

weighing the costs and benefits of changing behavior. Indecision and lack of commitment are the most distinctive characteristics of the contemplation stage.

Individuals in the *preparation* stage of change intend to act on their weight problem in the next 30 days. Typically, they have taken some action within the past year and they have definite plans for losing weight. These are the individuals we want to recruit to our action-oriented programs and they are the most likely to benefit from such programs. Decision-making and commitment are the most distinctive characteristics of the preparation stage.

The *action* stage is the period of active engagement in changing problem behavior and is what most people, including professionals, think of as behavior change. The period of action usually lasts about six months, as this typically encompasses the period of greatest risk of relapse for many problem behaviors. A common problem for people in the action stage is that they do not give themselves enough time to deal with their problem and may give up too quickly when they do not immediately succeed. Another common problem is that many individuals do not know what constitutes a sufficient degree of behavior change. They may set goals that are impossible to reach, or they may be satisfied with changes that do not adequately reduce their risk of disease. Modification of the target behavior to an acceptable criterion and significant overt efforts to change are the most distinctive characteristics of the action stage.

After six months of continuous successful action, individuals achieve the *maintenance* stage. In this stage, people continue to work on preventing relapse and consolidate the gains made during the action stage. Situational temptations to engage in the problem behavior decline and efficacy in coping with tempting situations increases throughout this period. Maintenance is thus a continuation of the change process and not a static period. There is still a risk of relapse, and for some individuals and for some problem behaviors, maintenance may be a life long struggle. For others, the temptation to engage in the problem behavior may decline eventually to such low levels that the problem may no longer be a salient issue for them. Such individuals may be considered to have reached the *termination* stage of change. Whether a termination stage for weight control can be attained has not been established and would probably be controversial.

The stages of change have important implications for the design of intervention programs. We have found that the amount of progress people make in changing behavior is a function of their stage of change. Treatment programs that help people advance even one stage of change in a month double the chances that participants will take action in the next six months (DiClemente et al., 1991). Strategies that are effective in moving individuals from precontemplation to contemplation, or in moving contemplators to being ready for action, will not be effective in moving people to action (Prochaska et al., 1985). It is likely that the discouraging results of weight control programs are due, at least in part, to the application of action-oriented strategies to participants who are not ready for action, or to the application of interventions that move people to contemplate change but demand action-oriented outcomes as the "bottom-line" indication of success (Rossi et al., in press-c).

In our study of over 14,000 members of a Health Maintenance Organization (HMO), nearly 40% of those with a body-mass index (BMI) greater than 25 had made no attempts to lose weight in the previous 6 months. Furthermore, the majority of these individuals (51.7%) had no intention of even trying to lose weight in the next 6 months. Less than 25% of the sample was prepared to take action. Yet, most of our treatment programs are designed for people ready to take action. The majority of individuals will not succeed in such programs. In fact, they are likely not to enroll in such programs to begin with, and having enrolled, they are most likely to drop out. For example, in a series of action-oriented worksite programs conducted by some of our colleague, 80% of the participants dropped out (Prochaska et al., 1992b). This is certainly one important reason why people fail to maintain weight loss.

The problem of recruitment is a serious one. With worksite or home-based action-oriented programs, participation rates are typically 1% to 5% for smoking cessation and 3% to

10% for weight loss (Prochaska, 1993). An intensive proactive, action-oriented recruitment strategy attempted by our colleagues for smokers in a major HMO fared no better. For precontemplators, 35% signed up, but only 3% showed up, and only 2% completed the program. For smokers in contemplation and preparation, 65% signed up, 15% showed up, and 11% finished.

We have now developed a home-based expert system intervention for smoking cessation that is stage-matched. This expert system assesses an individual's stage of change and provides appropriate self-help materials designed to help the individual progress to the next stage of change (Velicer et al., 1993, in press). In a sample of 5,000 smokers recruited from an HMO and 5,000 smokers from the community recruited using random digit dialing methods, we are obtaining participation rates of approximately 75%. This has important implications for the impact of an intervention on the population. If we define program impact as effectiveness X participation, then even a strong, action-oriented program that achieves a 40% success rate but that reaches only 5% of the population will have relatively low impact (e.g., 40% X 5% = 2%). A less successful program that reaches a much greater proportion of the population can have a more substantial impact on public health (e.g., 25% X 75% = 20%).

The stages are assumed to be invariant, with individuals needing to complete the tasks and consolidate the gains of one stage before they are ready to progress to the next. For most behavior problems the majority of individuals do not progress smoothly through the stages. A cyclical pattern is most common, with individuals reaching the action or maintenance stage, then relapsing and recycling to an earlier stage of change. Relapse is an all too common phenomenon, especially among the addictions, and on any one attempt the likelihood of successful change is small. Fortunately, most relapsers do not regress all the way back to the precontemplation stage. Some of the gains made before the relapse episode are preserved, so that subsequent action attempts are more likely to be successful. For example, we have found that smokers who relapse to the contemplation stage are much better prepared to make subsequent action attempts than contemplators who have been unable to quit even for 24 hours and who are stuck in the contemplation stage (DiClemente et al., 1991). From this standpoint, we regard relapse not as a failure to maintain, but as an opportunity to learn from previous mistakes, to weed out unsuccessful change strategies and try new ones. Relapse is essential for initiating the process of recycling.

Our studies of how people change have also identified a common set of *processes of change* that mediate the transitions between the stages of change (Prochaska et al., 1992a). The processes of change are overt and covert change strategies and techniques that can be employed by professionals, such as therapists or physicians, or by people changing on their own or with the aid of self-help programs. Ten processes have been consistently replicated across a variety of problem behaviors, including consciousness raising, counterconditioning, dramatic relief, environmental reevaluation, helping relationships, reinforcement management, self liberation, self reevaluation, social liberation, and stimulus control (Prochaska & DiClemente, 1985; Rossi, 1992). The processes are hierarchically organized into two general categories: the experiential processes incorporate the cognitive, evaluative, and affective aspects of change whereas the behavioral processes include more specific, observable change strategies.

Specific transitions between stages are mediated by distinct subsets of the processes of change (Prochaska et al., 1991; Rossi et al., in press-c). In general, however, individuals in the early stages of change should emphasize the use of the experiential processes of change, whereas individuals in the later stages should emphasize the use of the behavioral processes. Our studies and those of others have shown that when individuals or treatment programs mismatch processes to stages, action attempts are likely to fail (Fitzgerald & Prochaska, 1990; Gritz et al., 1992; Ockene et al., 1992; Prochaska et al., 1985). For example, in one study of weight loss we conducted with 700 smokers, weight relapsers inappropriately continued to rely on the experiential processes of change (Rossi et al., 1991). In addition, relapsers did not use the behavioral process of counterconditioning as frequently as did successful weight loss maintainers.

The relationship between the stages and processes of change provides guidance for the development of successful intervention programs applicable not only for individuals who are ready to change a problem behavior but for the vast majority of people who are neither prepared nor motivated to change. There is an emerging consensus that matching interventions to stages of change can enhance the efficacy and generalizability of treatment programs (Baranowski, 1990; Brownell et al., 1986). We have developed interventions tailored to participant's stage of change for smoking cessation (Prochaska et al., in press-a), exercise adoption (Marcus, Banspach et al., 1992), and sun exposure (Rossi et al., in press-a) that have proved successful. We need to develop such programs for weight control.

Although the validity of the stages and processes of change model for weight control has generally been established, much more needs to be accomplished. Measurement of the stages of change for weight control is problematic in several areas, but especially in defining what constitutes an appropriate criterion for successful action. A good criterion should represent the established consensus of experts in the field. For example, the American College of Sports Medicine (1990) has recommended that healthy adults exercise at least three times a week for at least 20 minutes each time. Therefore, this criterion has been adopted as defining action for exercise (Marcus, Rossi et al., 1992). In smoking cessation it is not sufficient to reduce smoking by 50% or to switch to low tar and nicotine brands. Although such changes in smoking probably reduce some risks, health professionals have agreed that complete abstinence is necessary for sustained health benefits, and therefore, action is defined as abstinence from smoking (Velicer et al., 1992).

Unfortunately, no consensus has yet developed for what constitutes an ideal, a healthy, or even a reasonable standard for weight. The difficulty is understandable, as an acceptable criterion must take height, age, sex, and perhaps even changing cultural norms into account. The problem is further complicated in that weight control is not a specific behavior, like smoking a cigarette, but rather a goal to be reached. In addition, not all strategies employed to control weight are healthy or low risk behaviors (e.g., smoking cigarettes, purging). Successful, healthy, low-risk weight control is likely to be dependent on multiple behavior changes, including maintenance of a low fat diet and regular exercise. Whether such whole scale lifestyle change is likely to be acceptable to individuals or even effective as a means of weight control, and how to design and implement health promotion programs to change multiple behaviors are important challenges for researchers. It won't be easy. In our sample of 17,000 HMO subscribers, individuals with higher BMI scores were more likely to be in the action or maintenance stage of change for losing weight ($r = .40$). But BMI scores were essentially unrelated to stage of change for reducing dietary fat ($r = -.02$) and were negatively related to stage of change for exercise adoption ($r = -.12$). Nearly 60% of those with BMI scores less than 25 exercised regularly, but less than 40% of those with BMI scores greater than 30 did so. Less than 25% of those with BMI scores greater than 30 were taking action on both their dietary fat and exercise habits.

Interventions designed to help people lose weight have typically met with limited success and have suffered high rates of relapse and attrition (Brownell & Wadden, 1992). We need to move away from action-oriented programs that are relevant to only a small percentage of individuals and to develop stage-specific interventions that are applicable to individuals in every stage of change. Assessment of stage of change at in-take or enrollment would permit assignment to program modules that engage those processes of change effective in moving individuals to the next stage of change. The goal of such programs would be to accelerate movement through the stages of change towards eventual maintenance of a problem-free lifestyle.

REFERENCES

American College of Sports Medicine (1990). Position statement on the recommended quantity and quality of exercise for developing and maintaining cardiorespiratory and muscular fitness in healthy adults. Medicine and Science in Sports and Exercise, 22, 265-274.

Baranowski, T. (1990). Reciprocal determinism at the stages of behavior change: An integration of community, personal and behavioral perspectives. International Quarterly of Community Health Education, 10, 297-327.

Brownell, K.D., Marlatt, G.A., Lichtenstein, E., & Wilson, G.T. (1986). Understanding and preventing relapse. American Psychologist, 41, 765-782.

Brownell, K.D., & Wadden, T.A. (1992). Etiology and treatment of obesity: Understanding a serious, prevalent, and refractory disorder. Journal of Consulting and Clinical Psychology, 60, 505-517.

DiClemente, C. C., Prochaska, J. O., Fairhurst, S. K., Velicer, W. F., Velasquez, M. M., & Rossi, J. S. (1991). The process of smoking cessation: An analysis of precontemplation, contemplation and preparation stages of change. Journal of Consulting and Clinical Psychology, 59, 295-304.

Fitzgerald, T. E., & Prochaska, J. O. (1990). Nonprogressing profiles in smoking cessation: What keeps people refractory to self-change? Journal of Substance Abuse, 2, 87-105.

Gritz, E.R., Berman, B.A., Bastani, R., & Wu, M. (1992). A randomized trial of a self-help smoking cessation intervention in a nonvolunteer female population: Testing the limits of the public health model. Health Psychology, 11, 280-289.

Marcus, B. H., Banspach, S. W., Lefebvre, R. C., Rossi, J. S., & Carleton, R.A. (1992). Using the stages of change model to increase the adoption of physical activity among community participants. American Journal of Health Promotion, 6, 424-429.

Marcus, B.H., Rossi, J.S., Selby, V.C., Niaura, R.S., & Abrams, D.B. (1992). The stages and processes of exercise adoption and maintenance in a worksite sample. Health Psychology, 11, 386-395.

Ockene, J., Kristeller, J.L., Goldberg, R., Ockene, I., Merriam, P., Barrett, S., Pekow, P., Hosmer, D., Gianelly, R. (1992). Smoking cessation and severity of disease: The Coronary Artery Smoking Intervention Study. Health Psychology, 11, 119-126.

O'Connell, D., & Velicer, W. F. (1988). A decisional balance measure and the stages of change model for weight loss. International Journal of the Addictions, 23, 729-750.

Prochaska, J.O. (1993). Working in harmony with how people change naturally. Weight Control Digest, 3, 249, 252-255.

Prochaska, J.O., & DiClemente, C.C. (1985). Common processes of self-change in smoking, weight control, and psychological distress. In S. Shiffman & T. A. Wills (Eds.), Coping and substance use (pp. 345-363). New York: Academic Press.

Prochaska, J.O., DiClemente, C.C., & Norcross, J.C. (1992a). In search of how people change: Applications to addictive behaviors. American Psychologist, 47, 1102-1114.

Prochaska, J.O., DiClemente, C.C., Velicer, W.F., Ginpil, S., & Norcross, J.C. (1985). Predicting change in smoking status for self-changers. Addictive Behaviors, 10, 395-406.

Prochaska, J.O., DiClemente, C.C., Velicer, W.F., & Rossi, J.S. (in press-a). Standardized, individualized, interactive and personalized self-help programs for smoking cessation. Health Psychology.

Prochaska, J. O., Norcross, J. C., Fowler, J. L., Follick, M. J., & Abrams, D.B. (1992b). Attendance and outcome in a work site weight control program: Processes and stages of change as process and predictor variables. Addictive Behaviors, 17, 35-45.

Prochaska, J.O., Velicer, W.F., Guadagnoli, E., Rossi, J.S., & DiClemente, C.C. (1991). Patterns of change: Dynamic typology applied to smoking cessation. Multivariate Behavioral Research, 26, 83-107.

Prochaska, J.O., Velicer, W.F., Rossi, J.S., Goldstein, M.G., Marcus, B.H., Rakowski, W., Fiore, C., Harlow, L., Redding, C.A., Rosenbloom, D., Rossi, S.R. (in press-b). Stages of change and decisional balance for twelve problem behaviors. Health Psychology.

Rossi, J.S. (1992, August). Common processes of change across nine problem behaviors. Paper presented at the 100th annual convention of the American Psychological Association, Washington, DC.

Rossi, J.S., Blais, L.M., & Weinstock, M.A. (in press-a). The Rhode Island Sun Smart Project: Skin cancer prevention reaches the beaches. American Journal of Public Health.

Rossi, S.R., Rossi, J.S., Rossi-DelPrete, L.M., Prochaska, J.O., Banspach, S.W., & Carleton, R.A. (in press). A processes of change model for weight control for participants in a community-based weight loss program. International Journal of the Addictions.

Rossi, J.S., Rossi, S.R., Velicer, W.F., & Prochaska, J.O. (in press-c). Motivational readiness to control weight: The transtheoretical model of behavior change. In D.B. Allison (Ed.), Methods for the assessment of eating behaviors and weight related problems. Newbury Park, CA: Sage.

Rossi, S.R., Rossi, J.S., & Prochaska, J.O. (1991, August). Processes of change for weight control: A follow-up study. Paper presented at the 99th annual meeting of the American Psychological Association, San Francisco, CA.

Velicer, W.F., Prochaska, J.O., Bellis, J.M., DiClemente, C.C., Rossi, J.S., Fava, J.L., & Steiger, J.H. (1993). An expert system intervention for smoking cessation. <u>Addictive Behaviors, 18</u>, 269-290.

Velicer, W. F., Prochaska, J. O., Rossi, J. S., & Snow, M. G. (1992). Assessing outcome in smoking cessation studies. <u>Psychological Bulletin, 111</u>, 23-41.

Velicer, W.F., Rossi, J.S., Ruggiero, L., & Prochaska, J.O. (in press). Minimal interventions appropriate for an entire population of smokers. In R. Richmond (Ed.), <u>Interventions for smokers: An international perspective</u>. New York, NY: Williams and Wilkins.

WHAT CHARACTERIZES SUCCESSFUL WEIGHT MAINTAINERS?

Thomas A. Wadden

University of Pennsylvania School of Medicine
Department of Psychiatry
3600 Market Street-Suite 738
Philadelphia, PA 19104

INTRODUCTION

Long-term maintenance of weight loss is certainly not common but it does occur. In any study of 100 patients, a handful maintain their full weight loss 3 to 5 years later, and a significant minority maintain losses of 5 kg or more (Kramer, Jeffery, Forster, & Snell, 1989; Wadden, Sternberg, Letizia, Stunkard, & Foster, 1989). These individuals are usually overlooked, however, in the justifiably gloomy reports of the failures of dieting, and they are hard to characterize because of their few numbers.

This brief review summarizes what we know about the behavioral characteristics of weight maintainers, as determined in prospective clinical trials, as well as uncontrolled case studies. Data from clinical trials are the more reliable and are derived from measuring patient characteristics before or during treatment and then determining their association with long-term weight change (Jeffery et al., 1984).

Retrospective case studies employ a different method in which investigators identify, usually by chart review or newspaper advertisement, a sample of individuals who report that they have maintained a weight loss (Colvin & Olson, 1983). Such studies have the advantage of obtaining a large number of successful candidates but suffer shortcomings that include the unknown reliability of patients' reports of their weight and behavior, as well as the uncertain generalizability of the findings. Such investigations do provide important hypotheses to test in controlled trials.

This review begins with an examination of two treatment factors, continued care and exercise, that have been consistently shown to facilitate weight maintenance. These data are the strongest that we have because they demonstrate a clear causal relationship between a behavioral intervention and long-term weight control. This review does not discuss predictors of attrition or short-term weight loss, topics that have been covered elsewhere (Wadden & Letizia, 1992; Wilson, 1985).

TREATMENT FACTORS FACILITATING WEIGHT MAINTENANCE

Continued Care

Perri and colleagues have shown in a series of studies that regular patient-practitioner contact in the year following treatment significantly improves the maintenance of weight loss (Perri, 1992; Perri et al., 1988). Continued care can be as simple as patients' mailing weekly to their practitioner postcards on which they record their weight, calorie intake, physical activity, and related information. The practitioner can respond to this information with a phone call or a return postcard (Perri, McAdoo, Spevak, & Newlin, 1984; Perri, Shapiro, Ludwig, Twentyman, & McAdoo, 1984).

Alternatively, patients can attend bi-weekly group maintenance sessions at which they review their diet and exercise diaries and discuss problems that they have encountered. Patients who received such therapy for 1 year maintained 13.0 kg of their 13.2 kg end-of-treatment loss, whereas those who did not receive it maintained only 5.7 kg of a 10.8 loss (Perri et al., 1988). Taken together, Perri's (1992) studies indicate that continued patient-practitioner contact, by itself, is as effective in maintaining weight loss as are more elaborate interventions that combine continued contact with relapse prevention training, aerobic exercise, or social support.

Mechanisms of Action

The mechanisms by which maintenance therapy improves long-term outcome are poorly understood. Most likely, continued care sustains adherence to diet and exercise modification by providing social support and by increasing patient accountability through regularly scheduled weigh-ins. It should be noted, however, that adherence declined significantly in Perri et al.'s (1988) study as the frequency of visits decreased from weekly to bi-weekly when treatment changed from weight loss to weight maintenance.

Two other points are noteworthy, the first of which is that maintenance therapy appears only to delay rather than to prevent weight regain. Patients treated by Perri et al. (1988) regained an average of 3 kg in the 6 months following completion of the maintenance program, a finding that reveals the need for life-long care, as provided persons with hypertension and diabetes. Bjorvell and Rossner found that intermittent, longer-term care was associated with excellent maintenance of weight loss over a 10-year period (Bjorvell & Rossner, 1985, 1992).

The second point is that maintenance therapy does not appear to be as effective following a very-low-calorie diet as it is following a 1200 kcal/d diet, as used by Perri (1992). Wadden, Foster, and Letizia (1994) found that patients who lost 21.5 kg on a 420 kcal/d liquid diet maintained only a 10.9 kg loss 1 year later, despite their being provided 39 maintenance sessions during this time. By contrast, persons who received a 1200 kcal/d diet lost only 11.9 kg during treatment but maintained a loss of 12.2 kg a year later. We do not know whether the poor results following the VLCD were attributable to the severity of caloric restriction, the greater weight loss induced by this approach, or both. Regardless, we obtained similarly discouraging results in a second investigation of this approach (Wadden, Bartlett, et al., 1994).

Exercise

Several randomized trials have shown that exercise is consistently associated with improved maintenance of weight loss, whether it is combined with a conventional 1200 kcal/d diet (Dahlkoetter, Callahan, & Linton, 1979; Hill et al., 1989) or a VLCD (Pavlou, Krey, & Steffee, 1989; Sikand, Kondo, Foreyt, Jones, & Gotto, 1988). The most promising findings were reported by Pavlou et al. (1989) who observed excellent weight losses 3 years after treatment in mildly obese men who originally received aerobic exercise combined with either a 1200 kcal/d diet or a VLCD. More recently, Skender et al. (1994) reported that treatment by exercise alone produced significantly better weight losses at 2 years follow-up than diet alone or diet plus exercise.

In addition to burning calories, exercise has been hypothesized to facilitate weight maintenance by minimizing the reductions in fat-free mass (Hill et al., 1989) and resting metabolic rate (Mole, Stern, Schultz, Bernauer, & Holcomb, 1989) that normally accompany weight loss. It may also improve mood and self-esteem which, in turn, could facilitate adherence to weight control behaviors (Grilo, Brownell, & Stunkard, 1993). The data concerning preservation of fat-free mass are relatively strong (Saris, 1993), whereas findings for resting metabolic rate are marginal (Saris, 1993), and those for the effects of exercise on mood and adherence are derived almost entirely from studies of non-obese individuals (Kuehnel et al., 1994). Thus, from a clinical standpoint, we know that exercise works, but we still poorly understand the mechanisms by which it facilitates weight control.

Summary

In summary, obese individuals who seek long-term care, as well as programs that emphasize exercise training, are likely to achieve the best maintenance of weight loss. Further research is needed to identify the personal characteristics of these individuals who would appear to be a highly motivated and possibly atypical group.

SUBJECT FACTORS ASSOCIATED WITH WEIGHT MAINTENANCE

Controlled Clinical Trials

When conducting clinical trials, investigators frequently collect baseline information about patients' psychological status, eating and exercise habits, and other factors. They also may collect, during weight reduction and follow-up, process measures that include treatment attendance, adherence to diet and exercise, and assessment of changes in psychological function. All of these variables may then be correlated with short- and long-term changes in weight.

The primary findings of such studies are that persons who, during weight loss, regularly attended treatment sessions and faithfully practiced behavioral weight control skills achieved the largest long-term weight losses (Jeffery et al., 1984; Kramer et al., 1989; Wadden et al., 1992). Continued practice of these skills, after losing weight, was similarly associated with the best long-term results. The most important behaviors included: 1) weighing daily; 2) exercising regularly; 3) recording food intake; 4) and eating low-fat foods (Gormally, Rardin, & Black, 1980; Hartman, Stroud, Sweet, & Saxon, 1993; Jeffery et al. 1984; Katahn, Pleas, Thackery, & Wallston, 1982; Kramer et al., 1989). Although not reported as frequently, several studies found that self-efficacy was positively related to weight maintenance and life stress negatively so (Dubbert & Wilson, 1984; Gormally et al., 1980; Jeffery et al., 1984).

None of the above findings, with the possible exception of weighing daily, is surprising, as they are habits stressed in behavioral weight loss programs. In fact, their correlation with long-term weight maintenance provides indirect support for the assumptions underlying behavioral treatment.

Cause versus correlation. Thus, clinicians cannot go wrong in recommending these behaviors to their overweight patients. Researchers, however, cannot be certain that the behaviors themselves are responsible for the favorable outcome. First, taken together, the behaviors rarely account for more than 25% of the variance in long-term weight change. Other factors, including biological mechanisms, are likely to exert a significant influence (Wadden & Letizia, 1992). Second, the practice of weight control behaviors may be a consequence (or only a correlate) of long-term success rather than a cause. Patients frequently report that they are most likely to exercise and record their food intake when they are "doing well" but are discouraged from following these behaviors when their weight increases (perhaps for reasons unrelated to their behavior).

The author has observed that some individuals fail to maintain their weight loss even when they report strict adherence to diet and exercise modification. The validity of their self-reports can certainly be challenged (Lichtman et al., 1992), but it also appears that behavior modification is simply inadequate, in some cases, to counteract weight regain that may result from a low metabolic rate (Ravussin et al., 1988), genetic influences (Stunkard, Harris, Pedersen, & McClearn, 1990), or other factors (Kern, Ong, Saffari, & Carty, 1990; Wilson, 1993). The model proposed in Figure 1 suggests that the interaction of behavioral and biological factors will yield a variety of "maintenance" outcomes following weight loss. Persons who during treatment adopt appropriate eating and exercise behaviors, and who are relatively free of a biological predisposition to obesity, are likely to achieve the most favorable long-term results. Such an individual might have maintained an appropriate weight all of her life until a recent illness or psychological trauma. With weight loss, she returns to her "normal" weight.

Adherence to the same eating and exercise behaviors, however, would probably be associated with a less favorable outcome in persons predisposed to obesity. Such an individual might walk 12 miles a week and consume a low-fat diet, and yet still struggle with her weight, as she has since childhood (when she first became obese). Persons who failed to modify problem eating and exercise habits (i.e., a sedentary binge eating) during weight loss would also be expected to have an unsatisfactory long-term outcome, even in the absence of clear biological pressures to regain weight. The worst long-term results would be anticipated in persons who failed to correct their eating and exercise habits and who had a strong biological predisposition toward obesity (as suggested by early onset and a family history of obesity).

This model underscores the need to account for biological factors when assessing the contributions of psychological and behavioral factors to long-term weight control. The effects of eating and exercise behaviors, for example, could be compared in individuals with high versus

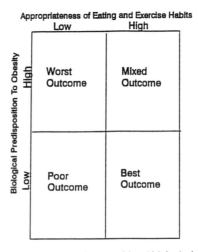

Figure 1. Prediction of maintenance of weight loss based upon subjects' biological predisposition to obesity and the extent to which they adopt appropriate eating and exercise habits.

low daily energy expenditure, as determined by doubly labeled water (Schoeller, 1990). Persons with low energy expenditure might be found to regain weight despite adopting a program of lifestyle modification, a frustrating outcome that could lead them eventually to abandon their efforts at weight control. Such studies should also provide a clearer understanding of whether behaviors such as binge eating (Spitzer et al., 1993; Yanovski, 1993) or weight cycling (Wing, 1992) are predictive of a poor long-term outcome, as often claimed though not demonstrated.

SUBJECT FACTORS ASSOCIATED WITH WEIGHT MAINTENANCE

Uncontrolled Studies

Characteristics of weight loss maintainers identified in uncontrolled studies are generally similar to those identified in controlled investigations with one important difference: Persons in the uncontrolled studies tended to lose weight on their own without professional assistance. Thus, these individuals may differ significantly from those in controlled investigations, perhaps in weighing less and having a milder history of obesity. Unfortunately, most case studies do not describe subjects sufficiently to allow comparison with controlled investigations.

Average weight losses in these uncontrolled studies were reported to be as great as 25 kg and were achieved gradually over 6 to 12 months (Colvin & Olson, 1983). Commonalities observed across studies in the characteristics of successful individuals included their: 1) eating a low-fat diet tailored to their specific food preferences; 2) exercising regularly; 3) monitoring weight and food intake regularly; 4) coping with stress by the use of problem-solving skills; and 5) taking control of and responsibility for their lives (Colvin & Olson, 1983, 1984; Kayman, Bruvold, & Stern, 1990; Marston & Criss, 1984; Schacter, 1983). This last point is particularly salient, as described by Colvin and Olson (1983):

"While a few women are strong advocates of therapeutic systems, it is the absence of the use of such programs which underscores the characteristic that the investigators found most ubiquitous: these women have become autonomous. Listening to their life stories, it is hard to imagine many of them scoring high on a scale of internality before their weight loss. Yet, as if some maturational or developmental landmark had been reached, they recognized their own responsibility for their body size. They felt a strong need to take charge of their own weight loss plan. They developed their own eating and exercise habits to maintain their losses. They moved out of the home into the outside world. They describe themselves as more confident and self-assured (p. 294)."

Further research is needed to illuminate a possible developmental process that occurs in some individuals who have struggled with their weight for years but eventually resolve the psychosocial conflicts that appear to have contributed to it. Clinical experience suggests that these individuals embrace change in their eating and exercise habits as part of a broader change in their psychosocial functioning. This contrasts with the experience that many patients report of having change imposed upon them by their health care provider, despite their having originally initiated weight reduction efforts. Differences between these two groups appear to be more complex than those revealed by simply classifying patients according to their current position on a stages of change continuum (Prochaska & DiClemente, 1985).

Goal weight. Research is also needed to test the hypothesis that attainment of goal weight facilitates maintenance of weight loss (Colvin & Olson, 1983; Wolfe, 1992). Persons who achieve goal weight, as compared with those who do not, are thought to experience greater weight-related self-efficacy and to be willing to work harder to maintain a weight with which they are happy. Those who reduce but fail to reach desirable weight are thought to abandon efforts because their weight losses are not personally satisfying (Wolfe, 1992).

Table 1. Comparison of Behaviors and Reinforcement Associated with Losing Weight.

Weight versus Maintaining a Weight Loss

Weight Loss	Maintenance of weight loss
The goal of treatment is to lose a large amount of weight, after a prolonged period of weight gain.	The goal of treatment is to lose small amounts of weight, as small increases in weight occur.
The dieter's principal strategy is to *avoid* eating all of the foods that have caused the weight problem.	The dieter's principal task is to learn to eat troublesome foods in a controlled fashion (mastery) and to eat new foods, low in fat and calories.
Treatment is time-limited, usually 15 to 25 weeks.	Treatment is on-going and life-long.
The dieter receives support from the diet program and from family and friends.	The dieter receives little or no support from professionals or family members.
Weight loss is highly reinforcing; it is very noticeable and pleasing to dieters and their families.	Maintenance of weight loss is not reinforcing; dieters forget about their accomplishments, as do their family members.
Dieters do not have to exercise to lose weight.	Exercise appears to be critical to maintenance of weight loss.

Belief in the importance of goal weight may well result from a sampling bias in which only those persons who have met goal weight and maintained it are invited to participate in a study (Colvin & Olson, 1983; Marston & Criss, 1984) or are willing to participate (Wolfe, 1992). Many dieters may reach goal weigh, only to regain. The goal-weight hypothesis, however, is an intriguing one that could easily be tested by randomly assigning equivalently obese subjects to treatments designed to have them attain or not attain goal weight. Subjects could be followed for several years thereafter.

CONCLUSIONS AND RECOMMENDATIONS

This review has shown that the individuals who are most likely to maintain their weight loss: 1) exercise regularly; 2) consume a low-fat diet; 3) monitor their weight and food intake frequently; 4) and cope effectively with stress by the use of problem solving skills. Controlled studies indicate that long-term patient-practitioner contact facilitates weight maintenance, probably by sustaining adherence to these behaviors. Uncontrolled investigations, by contrast, suggest that weight maintainers are successful as a result of a maturational change that enables them to recognize their personal needs and to take better care of their physical and emotional health.

The above findings are useful in that they tell patients (and their practitioners) what they should do to maintain their weight loss. Many overweight individuals, however, report that they already know what they should do; the trouble is doing it.

Some of the factors that make "doing it" so difficult are outlined in Table 1, which shows key behavioral differences between losing weight and maintaining a weight loss. These include differences in the goals of these two treatment, the behavioral strategies required, and the reinforcement associated with each set of behaviors. A key difference involves that between avoiding problem foods, as typically occurs during weight loss, and learning to consume such foods in a controlled manner, as well as to eat a varied and low-fat diet, as is required for weight maintenance. Dieters typically find it easier to suppress inappropriate eating habits than to develop new food preferences (such as substituting broiled fish for fried chicken). For every comparison shown in Table 1, weight loss requires less true behavior change but yields far greater immediate rewards than does weight maintenance.

Process of change.

Although this review identified the behaviors practiced by successful weight maintainers, it failed to identify how they adopted them. In short, what allows some persons but not most to use the professional advice that they receive. Thus, future studies of weight maintenance should focus on the process of behavior change. Specifically, what cognitions, behavioral strategies, and affective reactions appear to facilitate patients' exercising regularly and adhering to other weight control behaviors? Do these cognitions and behavioral strategies change over time as patients move from weight loss to initial and then long-term weight maintenance? Moreover, what cognitive and emotional changes occur in individuals who, after repeated cycles of weight loss and regain, finally gain control of their weight and behavior?

Similar study is needed of the opposite side of the coin --the process by which overweight individuals lapse and eventually relapse. We know that most overweight persons regain their lost weight but researchers have only begun to explore the external precipitants, as well as the cognitive, behavioral and affective factors, associated with relapse (Brownell, Marlatt, Lichtenstein, & Wilson, 1986; Grilo, Shiffman, & Wing, 1989). Illumination of these factors should assist clinicians and researchers in developing new strategies to help patients cope with relapse.

In all of this work, it will be important to study the possible contribution of biological factors to weight regain. Some individuals, as a result of a family history of obesity, a low resting metabolic rate or other factors, appear more vulnerable than others to regaining their lost weight. Practitioners must take special care with such individuals to help them understand the causes of their weight problem and to help them cope with their emotional distress. The goal of treatment may change, in such cases, from maintenance of weight loss to promotion of a healthy lifestyle and maintenance of the individual's self-esteem.

ACKNOWLEDGEMENTS

Completion of this article was supported, in part, by a grant from the NIMH (RO 1 MH49451-02).

REFERENCES

Bjorvell, H., & Rossner, S. (1985). Long-term treatment of severe obesity: four year follow up of results of combined behavioural modification programme. British Medical Journal. 291, 379-382.

Bjorvell, H., & Rossner, S. (1992). A ten year follow-up of weight change in severely obese subjects treated in a behavioural modification programme. International Journal of Obesity, 16, 623-625.

Brownell, K.D., Marlatt, G.A., Lichtenstein, E., & Wilson, G.T. (1986). Understanding and preventing relapse. American Psychologist, 41, 765-782.

Colvin, R.H., & Olson, S.B. (1983). A descriptive analysis of men and women who have lost significant weight and are highly successful at maintaining the loss. Addictive Behaviors, 8, 287-295.

Colvin, R.H., & Olson, S.B. (1984). Winners revisited: An 18-month follow-up of our successful weight losers. Addictive Behaviors, 9, 305-306.

Dahlkoetter, J., Callahan, E.J., & Linton, J. (1979). Obesity and the unbalanced energy equation: Exercise versus eating habit change. Journal of Consulting and Clinical Psychology, 47, 898-905.

Dubbert, M., & Wilson, G.T. (1984). Goal-setting and spouse involvement in the treatment of obesity. Behavior Research and Therapy, 22, 227-242.

Gormally, J., Rardin, D., & Black, S. (1980). Correlates of successful response to a behavioral weight control clinic. Journal of Counseling Psychology, 27, 179-191.

Grilo, C.M., Brownell, K.D., & Stunkard, A.J. (1993) The metabolic and psychological importance of exercise in weight control. In A.J. Stunkard & T.A. Wadden (eds) Obesity: Theory and therapy (pp.253-274), New York: Raven Press.

Grilo, C.M., Shiffman, S., & Wing, R.R. (1989). Relapse crises and coping among dieters. Journal of Consulting and Clinical Psychology, 57, 488-495.

Hartman, W.M., Stroud, M., Sweet, D.M., Saxton, J. (1993). Long-term maintenance of weight loss following supplemented fasting. International Journal of Eating Disorders, 14, 87-93.

Hill, J.O., Schlundt, D.G., Sbrocco, T., Sharp, T., Pope-Cordle, J., Stetson, B., Kaler, M., & Heim, C. (1989). Evaluation of an alternating-calorie diet with and without exercise in the treatment of obesity. American Journal of Clinical Nutrition, 50, 248-254.

Jeffery, R.W., Bjornson-Benson, W.M., Rosenthal, B.S., Lindquist, R.A., Kurth, C.L., & Johnson, S.L. (1984). Correlates of weight loss and its maintenance over two years of follow-up among middle-aged men. Preventive Medicine, 13, 155-168.

Katahn, M., Pleas, J., Thackery, M., Wallston, K.A. (1982). Relationship of eating and activity self-reports to follow-up weight maintenance in the massively obese. Behavior Therapy, 13, 521-528.

Kayman, S. Bruvold, W., & Stern, J.S. (1990). Maintenance and relapse after weight loss in women: Behavioral aspects. American Journal of Clinical Nutrition, 52, 800-807.

Kern, P.A., Ong, J.M., Saffari, B., & Carty, J. (1990). The effects of weight loss on the activity and expression of adipose-tissue lipoprotein lipase in very obese humans. New England Journal of Medicine, 322, 1053-1059.

Keuhnel, R.A., Wadden, T.A., Bartlett, S.J., Andersen, R.E., Buckenmyer, P., & Vogt, R. (1994). Effects of exercise on mood, adherence, and short-term weight loss in obese women: A controlled investigation. Manuscript submitted for publication.

Kramer, F.M., Jeffery R.W., Forster, J.L. & Snell, M.K. (1989). Long-term follow-up of behavioral treatment for obesity: Patterns of weight regain in men and women. International Journal of Obesity, 13, 123-136.

Lichtman, S.W., Pisarka, K., Berman, E.R., et al. (1992) Discrepancy between self-reported and actual caloric intake and exercise in obese subjects. New England Journal of Medicine, 327, 1893-1898.

Marston, A.R., & Criss, J. (1984) Maintenance of successful weight loss: Incidence and prediction. International Journal of Obesity, 8, 435-439.

Mole, P.A., Stern, J.S., Schultz, C.L., Bernbauer, E.M., & Holcom, B.J. (1989). Exercise reverses depressed metabolic rate produced by severe caloric restriction. Medicine and Science in Sports and Exercise, 21, 29-33.

Pavlou, K.N., Krey, S., & Steffee, W.P. (1989). Exercise as an adjunct to weight loss and maintenance in moderately obese subjects. American Journal of Clinical Nutrition, 49, 1115-1123.

Perri, M.G. (1992). Improving maintenance of weight loss following treatment by diet and lifestyle modification. In T.A. Wadden & T.B. VanItallie (Eds.), Treatment of the seriously obese patient (pp. 456-477). New York: Guilford Press.

Perri, M.G., McAdoo, W.G., Spevak, P.A., & Newlin, D.B. (1984). Effect of a multicomponent maintenance program on long-term weight loss. Journal of Consulting and Clinical Psychology, 52, 480-481.

Perri, M.G., Shapiro, R.M., Ludwig, W.W., Twentyman, C.T., & McAdoo, W.G. (1984). maintenance strategies for the treatment of obesity: An evaluation of relapse prevention training and posttreatment contact by mail and telephone. Journal of Consulting and Clinical Psychology, 52, 404-413.

Perri, M.G., McAllister, D.A., Gange, J.J., Jordan, R.C., McAdoo, W.G., & Nezu, A.M. (1988). Effects of four maintenance programs on long-term management of obesity. Journal of Consulting and Clinical Psychology, 56, 529-534.

Prochaska, J.O., & DiClemente, C.C. (1985). Common processes of change in smoking, weight control, and psychological distress. In S. Shiffman & T. Willis (Eds.), Coping and substance abuse (pp. 345-364). New York: Academic Press.

Ravussin, E., Lillioja, S., Knowler, W.C., Christin L., Freymond, D., Abbott, W.G., Boyce, V., Howard, B.V., & Bogardus, C. (1988). Reduced rate of energy expenditure as a risk factor for body-weight gain. New England Journal of Medicine, 318, 467-472.

Saris, W. The role of exercise in the dietary treatment of obesity. (1993). International Journal of Obesity, 17, S17-S21.

Schacter, S. (1982). Recidivism and self-cure of smoking and obesity. American Psychologist, 37, 436-444.

Schoeller, D.A. (1990). How accurate is self-reported dietary energy intake? Nutrition Reviews, 48, 373-379.

Sikand, G., Kondo, A., Foreyt, J.P., Jones, P.H., & Grotto, A.M. (1988). Two year follow-up of patients treated with very low calorie dieting and exercise testing. Journal of the American Dietetic Association, 88, 487-488.

Skender, M.L., Goodrick, G.K., Foreyt, J.P., Reeves, R.S., del Junco, D.J., & Gotto, A.M. (1994). Behavioral treatments of obesity: 2-year follow-up of eating, exercise, and combination interventions. Manuscript submitted for publication.

Spitzer, R.L., Yanovski, S., Wadden, T., Wing, R., Marcus, M., Stunkard, A.J., Devlin, M., Mitchell, J., Hasin, D., Horne, R.L. (1993) Binge eating disorder: Its further validation in a multisite study. International Journal of Eating Disorders, 13, 137-153.

Stunkard, A.J., Harris, J.R., Pedersen, N.L., Mc Clearn, G.E. (1990). The body mass index of twins who have been reared apart. New England Journal of Medicine, 322, 1483-1487.

Wadden, T.A., Bartlett, S.J., Foster, G.D., Greenstein, R.A., Wingate, B.J., Stunkard, A.J., & Letizia, K.A. (1994). Pharmacotherapy for weight maintenance following treatment by a very-low-calorie diet. Manuscript submitted for publication.

Wadden, T.A., Foster, G.D., Letizia, K.A. (in press). One-year behavioral treatment of obesity: Comparison of moderate and severe restriction and the effects of weight maintenance therapy. Journal of Consulting and Clinical Psychology.

Wadden, T.A., Foster, G.D., Wang, J., Pierson, R.N., Yang, M., Moreland, K., Stunkard, A.J., & Van Itallie, T.B. (1992). Clinical correlates of short- and long-term weight loss. American Journal of Clinical Nutrition, 56, 271S-274S.

Wadden, T.A., & Letizia, K.A. (1992). Predictors of attrition and weight loss in patients treated by moderate and severe caloric restriction. In T.A. Wadden & T.B. VanItallie (Eds.), Treatment of the seriously obese patient (pp. 283-410). New York: Guilford Press.

Wadden, T.A., Sternberg, J.A., Letizia, K.A., Stunkard, A.J., & Foster, G.D. (1989). Treatment of obesity by very low calorie diet, behavior therapy and their combination: A five-year perspective. International Journal of Obesity, 13, 39-46.

Wilson, G.T. (1985). Psychological prognostic factors in the treatment of obesity. In J. Hirsch & T.B. Van Itallie (Eds.), Recent advances in obesity research: IV. Proceedings of the Fourth International Congress on Obesity (pp.301-311). London: John Libbey.

Wilson, G.T. (1993). Behavioral treatment of obesity: Thirty years and counting. Advances in Behaviour Research and Therapy, 16, 31-75.

Wing, R.R. (1992). Weight cycling in humans: a review of the literature. Annals of Behavioral Medicine, 14, 113-119.

Wolfe, B.L. (1992). Long-term maintenance of weight loss following attainment of goals weight: A preliminary investigation. Addictive Behaviors, 17, 469-477.

Yanovski, S.Z. (1993) Binge eating disorder: Current knowledge and future directions. Obesity Research, 1, 306-324.

APPLICATION OF BEHAVIORAL ECONOMIC PRINCIPLES TO TREATMENT OF CHILDHOOD OBESITY

Leonard H. Epstein

Department of Psychology
State University of New York at Buffalo
235 Park Hall
Buffalo, NY 14260

Obesity is a prevalent problem in childhood (Gortmaker, Dietz, Sobol, & Wehler, 1987), which increases the risk of adult obesity (Stark, Atkins, Wolff, & Douglas, 1981; Abraham, Collins, & Nordsieck, 1971), as well as adult morbidity and mortality (Must, Jacques, Dallal, Bajema, & Dietz, 1992;Nieto, Szklo, & Comstock, 1992). Behavioral treatment procedures have been used with considerable success in treating childhood obesity. Behavioral procedures have been shown to be superior to both no treatment (Epstein, Wing, Koeske, & Valoski, 1984; Israel, Stolmaker, Sharp, Silverman, & Simon, 1984; Kirschenbaum, Harris, & Tomarken, 1984) and attention placebo (Epstein, Wing, Steranchak, Dickson, & Michelson, 1980; Epstein, Wing, Woodall, Penner, Kress, & Koeske, 1985) controls for short term weight control, and behavioral treatments have been successful in maintaining treatment effects over five and then year intervals (Epstein, Valoski, Wing, & McCurley, 1990; Epstein, Valoski, Wing, & McCurley, 1993).

The first generation of treatments we developed were associated with in-treatment (from baseline to six month) percent overweight changes of approximately -15%, with significant differences in maintained weight control over ten years of the same magnitude for families in which both the parents and children were targeted and reinforced for weight loss (Epstein, Valoski, Wing, & McCurley, 1990) and for families in which the parents and children were provided lifestyle or aerobic exercise programs in contrast to those provided a placebo calisthenics control (Epstein, Valoski, Wing, & McCurley, 1993). Over ten years approximately 30% of the children were non-obese, and a similar percentage showed maintained changes of at least a decrease in percent overweight of -20%. These results are among the only in the obesity literature to document successful long-term effects (Epstein, & Wing, 1987), but additional research is needed to improve the in-treatment effects and maintenance of these effects.

One of the most persistent problems in obesity research is the failure to maintain weight loss that is produced by intensive treatments. Newer innovations in treatment such as lengthening treatment (Perri, Nezu, Patti, & McCann, 1989), VLCD (Wadden, Stunkard, &

Obesity Treatment, Edited by D.B. Allison
and F.X. Pi-Sunyer, Plenum Press, New York, 1995

Smoller, 1986) or pharmacotherapy (Craighead, Stunkard, & O'Brien, 1981), are associated with better weight loss than previous methods, but these improved weight losses are not maintained. For this reason research has begun to focus more explicitly on maintenance, and a variety of techniques have been attempted (Perri, Nezu, & Viegener, 1992). In the most comprehensive research program to date on maintenance of treatment effects for adult obesity, Perri and colleagues have evaluated a variety of treatment approaches, including relapse prevention, continued direct therapist contact, use of phone and mail to maintain contact, exercise, new coping skills development and scheduling of maintenance visits (Ibid). In reviewing research on maintenance Perri suggests that current procedures do not enhance maintenance if therapist contact is removed, and recommends continuation of extended treatment using a continued care model (Ibid).

Behavioral treatments for obesity are based on the assumption that the positive energy balance that causes obesity is due in part to eating and exercise behaviors, and that by changing these behaviors weight change can be induced. There is a substantial empirical basis for the fact that excess caloric consumption beyond energy needs causes obesity, and the production of negative energy balance by reducing caloric and fat consumption and increasing exercise expenditure produces weight loss. What was surprising to investigators was that these changes were so hard to maintain, particularly given the fact that some individuals lose substantial amounts of weight, and show important changes in health risk, which have typically been the reasons that investigators presume to be important for weight loss. One possibility worth pursuing is that the improved health that is presumed to motivate a person to lose weight is incorrect, and other factors, such as appearance, improving social life, having more friends, etc. are more important, and these goals may not be met simply by weight loss. The idea that improved quality of life is an important variable that motivates behavior change has been advanced for other problems (Epstein, 1992; Kaplan, 1990), and may be particularly relevant for obesity treatment.

The fact that subjects change behavior during treatment but return to old behavior patterns after the cessation of treatment suggests two important points about the newly acquired behaviors. First, these behaviors are very context specific, and do not easily generalize beyond the constraints placed on the behaviors by treatment. While it is common to assume that the new behaviors have taken the place of the old behaviors, it may be more consistent with the facts to conclude that new eating and exercise behaviors acquired during treatment become associated with numerous components relevant to the context of treatment, such as coming to meetings, meeting with therapists, having weight measured by others, and the support of the therapist. When the context shifts, behaviors associated with the pre-treatment context are reinstated. There is an extensive animal literature on this phenomena, which has been reviewed recently by Bouton and Swartzentruber (Bouton, & Swartzentruber, 1991). These investigators indicate that when a behavior is not engaged in during treatment, either because the behavior has been extinguished or another behavior has been reinforced to take it's place, the behavior is not "destroyed", but the memory of the behavior remains, along with the memory of the new behavior associated with the new context. The performance of the old or new behaviors depend on which context is retrieved. For example, one of the best ways to remove an old behavior is to reinforce new alternative behaviors (Leitenberg, Rawson, & Bath, 1970; Leitenberg, Rawson, & Mulick, 1975). However, reinforcing a new behavior does not erase the original learning, rather it provides a context for the new behaviors. Thus, when the reinforcement for the alternative behaviors is removed, the rate of the original behavior increases (21,22).

The concept of alternate behavior may be critical to maintenance. Before an obese person begins treatment they have a history of excess intake and decreased activity that is maintained by an extensive set of stimulus and reinforcing conditions. The goal of treatment is usually stated as decreasing caloric intake and increasing exercise. It is also reasonable to assume that these obese persons find food very reinforcing, and do not find exercise very reinforcing. Thus, we are asking these subjects to remove a powerful reinforcer and replace it with an aversive stimulus. Under these conditions it is no wonder they go back to their old behaviors. These old behaviors are more reinforcing. Subjects who are reinforced for eating low-fat rather than higher fat foods do not rate low-fat foods as more palatable (Epstein, Wing, Valoski, & Penner, 1987), and subjects who are reinforced for being active do not rate active behaviors as more pleasant than sedentary options (Epstein, Valoski, Vara, McCurley, Wisniewski, Kalarchian, Klein, & Shrager, 1993). More important than their subjective ratings, treated obese persons are given equal opportunity to eat high-fat versus low-fat foods, or be sedentary versus exercising obese persons choose the old behaviors.

A conceptual model for understanding how people make choices among alternatives is behavioral economics, or behavioral theories of choice (Rachlin, 1989). The most direct method for testing the reinforcing value of an event is to vary the accessibility to the event using schedules of reinforcement, and then assess how hard the subject will work for the event. The harder they will work, the more reinforcing the event. When assessing the relative reinforcing effects of a drug, subjects are provided two alternatives, with accessibility varied, and the relative reinforcing value can be derived based on the differential response pattern to the alternatives. The fact that it is hard to change eating or exercise habits should not be surprising when one considers that food is a very powerful reinforcer in comparison to the available alternatives. When food is provided as one alternative in a choice situation, it is invariably the more powerful reinforcer, even when compared with biological (as electrical brain stimulation) or pharmacological (as heroin) reinforcers (Hursh, & Natelson, 1981; Elsmore, Fletcher, Conrad, & Sodetz, 1980). For example, when heroin dependent monkeys were provided access to both food or heroin, and both were easy to obtain, they allocated their responses to maintain access to both food and heroin. However, when the cost for obtaining food and heroin were increased, subjects allocated their responses for food, not heroin (Elsmore, Fletcher, Conrad, & Sodetz, 1980).

The majority of behavioral research in animals has been conducted using food as a reinforcer, and it is easy to also document that food is also a reinforcer for humans (Lappalainen, & Epstein, 1990; Smith, & Epstein, 1991). To address the area of factors that influence the reinforcing effects of preferred food, we have initiated research on the behavioral economics of intake. In the first study (Lappalainen, & Epstein, 1990), normal weight male college subjects were provided access to sandwiches they liked (high preference) versus ones they reported moderate preference for. The reinforcing value of these alternatives were compared by providing access to the lower preferred food at one point per response (FR1) versus the high preference food at schedules varying from FR1 to VR 32. Subjects worked harder to obtain the preferred sandwich up to the FR1/VR2 comparison, showed no difference at VR4/FR1, and responded more to obtain the lower preference at VR8 through VR32. In the second study (Lappalainen, & Epstein, 1990) normal weight male college subjects were provided a choice between preferred breakfast foods versus money during either deprived or non-deprived (just eaten breakfast) conditions. The reinforcing value of each was compared initially at FR1/FR1, and then with access to money kept at VR2 and access to food varied through VR32. As expected, non-deprived subjects chose to work for money at all comparisons. Deprived subjects only chose to work for food when the schedules were equal. When subjects had to work harder to obtain food than money, even at VR2/VR4, they did not show behavioral preference for food. In the third study (Smith, & Epstein, 1991) we used the same behavioral economic methods in non-dieting obese children, who were provided access to highly or less preferred snack foods. Subjects worked to obtain the preferred food when the comparisons were VR2/VR2-VR4, but switched when the access was more limited using VR8-VR32 schedules. These studies suggest that these laboratory methods can be used to assess the reinforcing value of food, and that alternative reinforcers can compete with food, dependent on deprivation and constraints on access to food.

Children who are attempting to change eating patterns are also faced with a number of choices based on the food and non-food alternatives available. The goal of obesity treatment is to reduce the amount of food consumed, as well as modify the type (high-fat) of foods. However, making long term changes in eating habits has proven to be quite difficult. This situation is likely due in part to the greater reinforcing value of eating high-fat than low-fat foods, the increased availability of high-fat convenience foods, and the failure of non-food activities to be as reinforcing as food in eating situations for obese children. The goal for modifying eating behavior depends in part on the specific situation in which eating occurs. For example, at a meal it is desirable for children to consume different types of foods than they usually consumed, reducing caloric and fat intake. In other situations (snack times, between meal eating, etc) it may also be desirable for the child also to eat a different type of food, such as substituting an apple for a bag of potato chips, or to substitute a non-food activity instead of eating. There are three implications from research on behavioral economics that can be directly tried for modifying intake. First, treatments should attempt to reduce access to reinforcing alternatives, making choice of the less reinforcing alternative more likely (Hursh, & Bauman, 1987). It is likely that as long as more reinforcing alternatives are present in the subjects' immediate environment, and access to more reinforcing alternatives is equivalent, subjects will choose the more reinforcing alternative. Second, alternative behaviors that can compete with the reinforcing effects of eating high-fat foods should be identified, just as a major effort in behavioral pharmacology of drug intake is to identify powerful non-drug alternatives to drug taking (Hursh, 1991). Third, methods for reducing the reinforcing efficacy of high fat foods should be evaluated. One interesting method may be derived from research on sensory-specific satiety (Rolls, Rolls, Rowe, & Sweeney, 1981). There is an extensive literature in humans on the influence of food variety on intake within a meal (Ibid), and a smaller but consistent body of research on the effects of variety on intake across meals (Siegel, & Pilgram, 1958). Satiation is one method for reducing reinforcing value, and reduction in the variety of food may reduce the reinforcing value of the remaining choices, thereby changing the relative value of the alternatives.

We have also been studying the behavioral economics of activity choice in children. Obese children are inactive, and the degree of inactivity, as assessed by television watching, is related cross-sectionally and prospectively to changes in obesity (Dietz, & Gortmaker, 1985). It is not surprising that when given the opportunity obese children will choose sedentary versus active alternatives (Epstein, Smith, Vara, & Rodefer, 1991). This may be in part due to the lack of reinforcing value of active behaviors to obese children, but it is also likely due to the powerful reinforcing value of such sedentary alternatives as television, VCR's and computer games. We have completed three laboratory studies on behavioral economics of activity. The first experiment 1 (Ibid) assessed the influence of child percent overweight (<20, 20-80, >80% overweight) on choice of a moderately liked vigorous activity versus a highly-liked sedentary behavior. The active alternative was available on a VR2 schedule, with the schedule for the sedentary alternative varying from VR2, VR4, VR8, VR16, to VR32. As predicted, all children chose the sedentary alternative when access for the two activities was equal (VR2/VR2). As subjects had to allocate more effort to obtain the sedentary alternative, lean and moderately obese children switched to the vigorous activity. Lean children shifted on VR2/VR4, and moderately obese children shifted on VR2/VR8. Very obese children continued to choose the sedentary activity, and did not shift to the active alternative when the schedules were changed. These results suggest that sedentary activities are more reinforcing than active alternatives; that for most children reducing access to sedentary behaviors results in the choice to be active; and the reinforcing value of being sedentary depends in part on the degree of obesity.

Experiment 2 (Ibid) tested in moderately obese children whether preference (high or low) for vigorous activities would influence the point of switching from sedentary to activity alternatives. When the reinforcement schedules were equal, children again chose the sedentary alternative. Children switched from the sedentary to the vigorous activity when the schedules were changed, with no differences as a function of high or low preference for vigorous activities (Ibid). These results suggest that changes in access to the sedentary behaviors were more important than preference in determining choice of sedentary versus active alternatives.

In a third study (Vara, & Epstein, in press) non-exercising female college students women were studied to assess the influence of control over active or sedentary behavior options. Subjects were studied in four sessions, with the sessions varying whether subjects had control over active or sedentary alternatives. Results showed that when the choice was between active alternatives with or without control, subjects reliably allocated more time for the alternative that provided control. Thus, providing options and control over activities increased the reinforcing value of being active, consistent with our research (Epstein, Wing, Koeske, Ossip, & Beck, 1982) and other clinical studies (Thompson, & Wankel, 1980; Martin, Dubbert, Kattell, Thompson, Raczynski, Lake, Smith Webster, Sikora, & Cohen, 1984).

Based on this laboratory research, we initiated a clinical study (Epstein, Valoski, Vara, McCurley, Wisniewski, Kalarchian, Klein, & Shrager, 1993) assessing the benefits of reinforcing a reduced access to sedentary behaviors versus reinforcing subjects for being more active. Body composition, fitness and subjective liking of activity data each showed that reducing access to sedentary behaviors was associated with better treatment effects than reinforcing children for being more active.

In summary, in this brief paper I have attempted to outline the way that contemporary basic behavioral research on variables that regulate intake or activity choice can be incorporated into behavioral treatment programs (Epstein, 1990). It is hoped that a better understanding of behavioral factors that influence choice of the weight regulatory behaviors and resistance to change of these behaviors will improve long-term maintenance of weight control.

ACKNOWLEDGEMENTS

Supported in part by grants (HD25997, HD20829, and HD23713)

REFERENCES

Abraham, S., Collins, G., & Nordsieck, M. (1971). Relationship of childhood weight status to morbidity in adults. Public Health Records, 85, 273-284.

Bouton, M., & Swartzentruber, D. (1991). Sources of relapse after extinction in Pavlovian and instrumental learning. Clinical Psychology Review, 11, 123-140.

Craighead, L. W., Stunkard, A. J., & O'Brien, R. (1981). Behavior therapy and pharmacotherapy for obesity. Archives of General Psychiatry, 38, 763-768.

Dietz, W. H., & Gortmaker, S. L. (1985). Do we fatten our children at the television set? Obesity and television viewing in children and adolexcents. Pediatrics, 75, 807-812.

Elsmore, T. F., Fletcher, G. V., Conrad, D. G., & Sodetz, F. J. (1980). Reduction of heroin intake in baboons by an economic constraint. Pharmacology, Biochemistry and Behavior, 13, 729-731.

Epstein, L. H. (1990). Behavioral treatment of obesity. In E. M. Stricker (ed.), Handbook of Behavioral Neurobiology Volume 10 Neurobiology of Food and Fluid Intake (pp. 61-73). New York: Plenum Press.

Epstein, L. H. (1992). Role of behavior theory in behavioral medicine. Journal of Consulting and Clinical Psychology, 60, 493-498.

Epstein, L. H., Smith, J. A., Vara, L. S., & Rodefer, J. S. (1991). Behavioral economic analysis choice in obese children. Health Psychology, 10, 311-316.

Epstein, L. H., Valoski, A., Vara, L. S., McCurley, J., Wisniewski, L., Kalarchian, M. A., Klein, K. R., & Shrager, L. (1993). Comparative effects of decreasing sedentary behavior and increasing activity on weight change in obese children and their parents. Manuscript submitted for publication.

Epstein, L. H., Valoski, A., Wing, R. R., & McCurley, J. (1990). Ten-year follow-up of behavioral, family-based treatment for obese children. JAMA, 264, 2519-1523.

Epstein, L. H., Valoski, A., Wing, R. R., & McCurley, J. (1993). Ten-year outcomes of behavioral family-based treatment for childhood obesity. Manuscript submitted for publication.

Epstein, L. H., & Wing, R. R. (1987). Behavioral treatment of childhood obesity. Psychological Bulletin, 101, 331-342.

Epstein, L. H., Wing, R. R., Koeske, R., Ossip, D. J., & Beck, S. (1982). A comparison of lifestyle change and programmed aerobic exercise on weight and fitness changes in obese children. Behavior Therapy, 13, 651-665.

Epstein, L. H., Wing, R. R., Koeske, R., & Valoski, A. (1984). The effects of diet plus exercise on weight change in parents and children. Journal of Consulting and Clinical Psychology, 52, 429-437.

Epstein, L. H., Wing, R. R., Steranchak, L., Dickson, B., & Michelson, J. (1980). Comparison of family-based behavior modification and nutrition education for childhood obesity. Journal of Pediatric Psychology, 5, 25-36.

Epstein, L. H., Wing, R. R., Woodall, K., Penner, B. C., Kress, M. J., & Koeske, R. (1985). Effects of family based behavioral treatment on obese 5-8 year old children. Behavior Therapy, 16, 205-212.

Epstein, L. H., Wing, R. R., Valoski, A., & Penner, B. (1987). Stability of food preferences in 8-12 year old children and their parents during weight control. Behavior Modification, 11, 87-101.

Gortmaker, S. L., Dietz, . H., Sobol, A. M., & Wehler, C. A. (1987). Incresing pediatric obesity in the United States. American Journal of Diseases in Children, 141, 535-540.

Hursh, S. R. (1991). Behavioral economics of drug self-administration and drug abuse policy. Journal of the Experimental Analysis of Behavior, 56, 377-393.

Hurch, S. R., & Bauman, R. A. (1987). A behavioral analysis of demand. In L. Green, J. H. Kagel, (Eds.), Advances in behavioral economics: Volume 1 (pp. 117-165). Norwood, NJ: Ablex.

Hursh, S. R., & Natelson, B. H. (1981). Electrical brain stimulation and food reinforcement dissociated by demand elasticity. Physiology and Behavior, 26, 509-515.

Israel, A. C., Stolmaker, L., Sharp, J. P., Silverman, W. K., & Simon, L. G. (1984). An evaluation of two methods of parental involvement in treating obese children. Behavior Therapy, 15, 266-272.

Kaplan, R. M. (1990). Behavior as the central outcome in health care. American Psychologist, 45, 1211-1220.

Kirschenbaum, D. S., Harris, E. S., & Tomarken, A. J. (1984). Effects of parental involvement in behavioral weight loss therapy for preadolescents. Behavior Therapy, 15, 485-500.

Lappaleainen, R., & Epstein, L. H. (1990). A behavioral economics analysis of food choice in humans. Appetite, 14, 81-93.

Leitenberg, H., Rawson, R. A., & Bath, K. (1970). Reinforcement of competing behavior during extinction. Science, 169, 301-303.

Leitenberg, H., Rawson, R. A., & Mulick, J. A. (1975). Extinction and reinforcement of alternative behavior. Journal of Comparative and Physiological Psychology, 88, 640-652.

Martin, J. E., Dubbert, P. M., Kattell, A. D., Thompson, J. K., Raczynski, J. R., Lake, M., Smith, P. O., Webster, J. S., Sikora, T., & Cohen, R. E. (1984). Behavioral control of exercise in sedentary adults. Studies 1 through 6. Journal of Consulting and Clinical Psychology, 52, 795-811.

Must, A., Jacques, P. F., Dallal, G. E., Bajema, C. J., & Dietz, W. H. (1992). Long-term morbidity and mortality of overweight adolescents: A follow-up of the Harvard Growth Study of 1922 to 1935. New England Journal of Medicine, 327, 1350-1355.

Nieto, F. J., Szklo, M., & Comstock, G. W. (1992). Childhood weight and growth rate as predictors of adult mortality. American Journal of Epidemiology, 136, 201-213.

Perri, M. G., Nezu, A. M., Patti, E. T. & McCann, K. L. (1989). Effect of length of treatment on weight loss. Journal of Consulting and Clinical Psychology, 57, 450-452.

Perri, M. G., Nezu, A. M., & Viegener, B. J. (1992). Improving the long-term management of obesity: Theory, research, and clinical guidelines. New York: John Wiley & Sons.

Rahlin, H. (1989). Judgement, decision, and choice: A cognitve/behavioral synthesis. New York: W. H. Freeman.

Rolls, B. J., Rolls, E. ., Rowe, E. A., & Sweeny, K. (1981). Sensory specific satiety in man. Physiology & Behavior, 27, 137-142.

Siegel, P. S., & Pilgram, F. J. (1958). The effect of monotony on the acceptance of food. American Journal of Psychology, 71, 756-759.

Smith, J. A., & Esten, L. H. (1991). Behavioral economic analysis of food choice in obese children. Appetite, 17, 91-95.

Stark, O, Atkins, E., Wolff, O. H., & Douglas, J. W. B. (1981). Longitudinal study of obesity in the National Survey of Health and Development. British Medical Journal, 283, 13-17.

Thompson, C. E., & Wankel, L. M. (1980). The effects of perceived activity choice upon frequency of exercise behavior. Journal of Applied Social Psychology, 10, 436-443.

Vara, L. S., & Epstein, L. H. (in press). Laboratory assessment of choice between exercise or sedentary behaviors. Research Quarterly for Exercise and Sport.

Wadden, T. A., Stunkard, A. J., & Smoller, J. W. (1986). Three-year follow-up of the reatment of obesity by very low calorie diet, behavior therapy, and their combination. Journal of Consulting and Clinical Psychology, 56, 925-928.

PSYCHOSOCIAL PREDICTORS OF OBESITY: IMPLICATIONS FOR PREVENTION

Thorkild I.A. Sørensen

Institute of Preventive Medicine
Copenhagen Municipal Hospital
Copenhage, Denmark

The psychosocial predictors of obesity pertaining to development of obesity may be applicable also to recurrence of obesity in formerly obese patients. The study of psychosocial predictors therefore may be of relevance for both primary and secondary prevention, which should be an integrated part of treatment programmes for obesity.

MEASURES OF PSYCHOSOCIAL FACTORS AND OF OBESITY

Many different measures of psychosocial factors have been employed in previous studies: for example occupation, education, responsibility level, number of employees, income, fortune, housing, living area, social attitudes and norms, self-esteem, body image, and intelligence. Obesity usually has been assessed by degree of overweight, often based on BMI as a continuous variable, or prevalence of overweight using various cutoff levels of BMI or weight-for-height, or percentile values. Few studies have used skinfold thickness as measure of obesity and few have included measures of body fat distribution. These differences in measures of psychosocial factors as well as of obesity may have contributed to the heterogeneity of the results of the studies and make it difficult to extract common conclusions. It remains to be seen whether the relationship between psychosocial factors and obesity is based on some common underlying psychosocial factors or characteristics.

MEANING OF PREDICTION

Prediction of obesity may have three different purposes, all of which are pertinent to prevention: 1) identification or localization of the obesity problem; 2) forecasting of where and in whom obesity will arise; 3) contribution to the evidence of causal relationship between the predictors and obesity. Numerous cross-sectional studies with assessment of the psychosocial factors and obesity at the same time have been carried out. They may serve the first purpose,

Obesity Treatment, Edited by D.B. Allison
and F.X. Pi-Sunyer, Plenum Press, New York, 1995

but can contribute only suggestive evidence for the second and third purposes. Thus, absence of associations in cross-sectional studies makes forecasting and causality less plausible.

REVIEW OF PREVIOUS CROSS-SECTIONAL STUDIES

In a review of 144 published studies, Sobal and Stunkard (Sobal, & Stunkard, 1989) found a strong inverse relationship between socioeconomic status and obesity among women in the developed societies, both in United States and in Europe. Inconsistent results were obtained in studies of men and children. In the developing countries, there were a uniform direct relationship among women, men and children. They concluded that 'a tempting explanation of this paradox is that similar forces - relatively abundant food with few normative constraints about body weight - promote obesity in upper SES women in developing societies and in lower SES women in developed societies'. In the developing societies, low prevalence of obesity in low SES groups is attributed to lack of food, and in the developed societes low prevalence in high SES groups is ascribed to social pressure against obesity. Barring weaker social pressure, Sobal and Stunkard had no explanation of the inconsistent results among men and children in the developed societies. One reason for the inconsistent results might be that the analyses have not taken into account possible non-linear associations in these groups with the inverse relationship becoming apparent only in the obese end of the distribution (Teasdale, Sorensen, & Stunkard, 1992). The remainder of the present paper will exclusively address the inverse relationship between psychosocial factors and obesity.

DIRECTIONALITY OF EFFECTS

The evidence from the cross-sectional studies raise questions about directionality of the prediction: 1) is obesity a predictor of psychosocial status or problems; 2) are psychosocial factors predictors of obesity; 3) is there a bidirectional relationship with both obesity and psychosocial factors predicting each other; or 4) is there an underlying common factor predicting both obesity and the psychosocial status? Prospective studies separating the assessment of obesity and the psychosocial factors in time may address the questions whether risk of development of obesity in the future is related to the current state of the psychosocial factors, or whether the risk of development of certain states (or problems) of the psychosocial factors in the future is related to the current state of obesity. It is essential in this study design that the outcome variable is assessed both at the start of the study and at follow-up. Since changes in body weight and in some psychosocial factors may be a slow process, it will be a great advantage to apply the historical long-term prospective design, in which the development already has taken place. The distinction between bidirectional relationships or common underlying factors influencing both psychosocial status and obesity requires that the underlying factors can be either measured or included as latent factors in models for design and analysis of longitudinal studies (at least two measures over time in each subject).

EFFECTS OF OBESITY ON PSYCHOSOCIAL FACTORS

Although the present topic is the psychosocial predictors of obesity, the interpretation of the available studies becomes less ambigious if question about obesity as a predictor of psychosocial factors or problems is settled. There is abundance of evidence for the negative attitude toward obesity in the developed societies (Sobal, & Stunkard, 1989; Wadden, Stunkard, 1985). One would therefore expect a great influence of obesity on the psychosocial factors. However, there is only little evidence available from few prospective studies.

The classical paper published in 1965 by Goldblatt et al. (Goldblatt, Moore, & Stunkard, 1965), which presented an analysis based on the Midtown Manhatten Study, has frequently been used as evidence for the effect of obesity on psychosocial factors. It was a cross-sectional survey which included data on current obesity status, current social class, and social class of origin, the latter two being used to define social mobility. It showed that obesity was inversely related to upward social mobility. However, since there were no data on earlier obesity status, a distinction between effects of obesity on social mobility and effects of social mobility on obesity cannot be made. In a follow-up study of obese Danish draftees and a comparable control group of non-obese draftees, it was shown that irrespective of parental occupation, intelligence, and educational level at the draft board examination, the obese attained a lower social class (ascertained by their occupation) than the controls (Sonne-Holm, & Sorensen, 1986). Thus, it seems likely that presence of obesity does have an influence on future psychosocial status.

EFFECTS OF PSYCHOSOCIAL FACTORS ON OBESITY

The evidence for effects of psychosocial factors on obesity comes from two sources: 1) cross-sectional studies of the relationship between current obesity and parental social class, and 2) prospective studies where the current psychosocial status is related to the subsequent development of obesity.

There are many studies of the association between obesity in childhood and parental social class, which, however, as mentioned, have given inconsistent results. Few studies address the association between parental social class and obesity in adults, and they all support the inverse relationship. Although the data are collected in a cross-sectional design, the studies are prospective in nature since obesity in the offspring barely affects the social class of the parents. However, since obesity is a familial trait, parental obesity may be a serious confounder of the association of parental social class and obesity in the offspring: parental obesity may influence their own social class as well as obesity in the offspring and thereby create an indirect relationship between parental social class and obesity in the offspring. Other types of relationships between the three variables may exists and be worth exploring. Unfortunately, there are no prospective studies available, in which the relationship between parental social class and obesity in the offspring is examined with control of parental obesity. Indirect support of an independent influence of parental social class has been obtained in the Danish Adoption Study (Teasdale, Sorensen, & Stunkard, 1990) where the social class of the adoptive parents was inversely related to BMI of the adult adoptees despite no relationship in BMI between adoptive parents and adoptees (Stunkard, Sorensen, & Hanis, 1986)

The evidence from the few truly prospective studies where obesity is assessed both at the beginning of the study and at follow-up supports that psychosocial factors have an influence on future obesity. Some of the studies start in childhood Braddon, Rodgers, Wadsworth, & Davies, 1986, Power, & Moynihan, 1988; Lissau-Lund-Sorensen, & Sorensen, 1992; Lissau, & Sorensen, 1993; Lissau-Lund-Sorensen, & Sorensen, 1992), some start in adulthood (Rissanen, Heliovaara, Knekt, Reunanen, & Aromaa, 1991). One of the studies deserves a particular attention because of the surprisingly strong effect (Lissau-Lund-Sorensen, 1992). School children who received no support by their parents according to questionnaire responses from the teachers and children who appeared dirty when examined by the school health nurses showed a greatly increased risk of being obese in young adulthood, also when controlling for BMI in school and parents education and occupation, and the quality of housing in the living area. These findings suggest that parental neglect may be a core components in the psychosocial factors influencing the risk of future development of obesity.

Even these prospective studies may not validly establish the directionality of the relationship between psychosocial factors and obesity for two reasons. First, parental obesity may still play an important role as confounder: the development of obesity between the start and the follow-up in the prospective studies may be influenced by parental obesity, which also may influence the psychosocial factors assessed at the start of the study. Second, development of obesity between the two time points are more likely to occur among those who have been obese earlier than among those who have been normal weight. This allows a relation between state of the psychosocial factors at the start of the study and development of obesity to be a result of previous obesity.

MEDIATORS OF EFFECTS OF PSYCHOSOCIAL FACTORS ON OBESITY

Assuming that there is a causal relationship between the psychosocial factors and obesity, the question arises how this relationship is mediated. Two sets of possible mechanisms may be operative. First, the energy balance may be affected directly either through increased energy intake or decreased energy expenditure, resulting in a positive energy balance and subsequent passive storage of energy as fat. Second, the process of fat storage may be directly influenced, either through increased uptake or decreased fat release from the adipocytes.

Mediation through the energy balance could be put into effect through behavioral changes such as overeating, increased fat intake, increased alcohol consumption, reduced smoking, decreased physical activity. Psycho-neuro-endocrine mechanisms affecting the energy balance through reduced energy expenditure are also conceivable.

There are two problems with the hypothesis about mediating mechanisms primarily affecting the energy balance. One is the necessary assumption of inadequacy of energy balance homeostasis due to changes in the buffering system or to alterations of the energy balance beyond its buffering capacity. The change in the system should be compatible with the very small net positive energy balance that usually is occurring during development of obesity, usually less than 2% of the total energy turnover. Furthermore, taken individually, the suggested mediating mechanisms each exhibit much weaker relationship with development of obesity than the psychosocial factors, and for most of them prospective evidence is scarce. It is, of course, possible that several of the mediating mechanisms are operating at the same time in an additive or synergistic way.

Mediation by direct changes in the fat storage process may be assumed to lead to a positive energy balance corresponding to the energy value of stored fat, and therefore does not assume concomitant inadequacy of energy balance homeostatic mechanims as long as they are not based on amount of fat stored. A number of possible mechanism are available following psycho-neuro-endocrine pathways, but their quantitative role in the fat storage process is still hypothetical.

GENETIC EFFECTS IN THE PSYCHOSOCIAL FACTORS - OBESITY RELATIONSHIP

In both set of possible mediating mechanisms, genetic effects as well as gene-environment interaction could be involved. There is strong evidence for genetic effects on obesity (Stunkard, & Sorensen, 1986; Sorensen, Holst, Stunkard, & Skovgaard, 1992). In the Danish Adoption Study, a preliminary analysis of the possible gene-environment interaction was performed by comparing the correlations in BMI between the adoptee and the biological 1st degree relatives at high and low social class assessed by occupational rating (Sorensen, Holst, & Stunkard, 1992). No clear evidence for gene-environment interaction was found, but further analysis is required.

Rather than a direct causal relationship between psychosocial factors and obesity, there may be common underlying factors. Findings in the Danish Adoption Study suggests that common genetic factors may be in play. It was found that the social class of the biological fathers of the adoptees correlated with the BMI of the adoptees independently of the social class of the adoptee (Teasdale, Sorensen, & Stunkard, 1990). Though small, the correlation was stronger than a correlation that possibly could be explained by the presumed relationship between BMI and social class of the biological fathers of the adoptees. An underlying genetic effect would create an apparently indepedent bidirectional relationship between psychosocial factors and obesity. The genetic effect could theoretically come about by cross-assortative phenotypic mating (mating of of obese persons with persons with the predictive psychosocial factors), by pleiotropic effects (several phenotypes influenced by the same genes), or by epistatic effects (genes influencing psychosocial factors interacts with genes influencing development of obesity).

IMPLICATIONS FOR PREVENTION

On this background the question arises whether the presumed effect of psychosocial factors on obesity can be used in the prevention of obesity despite insufficient evidence and lacking understanding of the mechanisms. The principle of identification of high risk groups by their psychosocial profile and implementation of special preventive programmes for the high risk group may be possible. However, it is necessary to view this suggestion in the general framework of screening (sensitivity, specificity, feasibility, etc), preventive programmes (effectiveness, efficiency, compliance, side-effects, etc), and costs.

There may be specific problems with the use of the relationship between psychosocial factors and obesity reducing the ultimate benefit of preventive programmes. Thus, the psychosocial profile of the high risk group may exhibit greater non-response rates, less motivation, less education, learning difficulties, fewer personal ressources, and lower compliance. Furthermore, the intervention directed at the psychosocial factors as such assuming their causal role is not likely to be successful until we know more about the nature of their relation to obesity.

I conclude that there is not yet a sound basis for using the psychosocial factors in the prevention of obesity.

FUTURE RESEARCH GOALS

This review of the current state of evidence suggests the following goals and strategies for future research in this area:

* Refinement of concepts and measurements of psychosocial factors, perhaps with special emphasis on the effect of parental neglect.
* Improvement of field methods for assessment of body composition and fat distribution.
* Analysis of non-linear relationships between psychosocial factors and obesity, especially in men and children.
* More prospective studies (but no more cross-sectional studies) of the relationship between psychosocial factors and obesity in both directions.
* Comprehensive, two-generational longitudinal studies of psychosocial factors and obesity.
* Prospective studies of mediators of the effects of the psychosocial factors on obesity,

both mediators acting on energy balance and on fat storage.
* Studies of genetic effects in the relationship between psychosocial factors and obesity.

Assuming that in the future evidence supporting the relationship between psychosocial factors and development of obesity will accumulate, the implications for research in prevention may be the following:

* Development of intervention programmes for the high risk groups defined by the psychosocial factors.
* Development of programmes of intervention against the psychosocial factors assuming their causal role.
* Evaluation of the preventive programmes using the highly developed methodology in public health research.

REFERENCES

Braddon, F. E. M., Rodgers, B. Wadsworth, M. E. J., & Davies, J. M. C. (1986). Onset of obesity in a 36 year birth cohort study. British Medical Journal, 293, 299-303.

Goldblatt, P. B. , Moore, M. E..& Stunkard, A.J. (1965). Social factors in obesity. JAMA, 152, 1039-1042.

Lissau-Lund-Sorensen, I., & Sorensen. T. I. A. (1991). The effects of parents' care on risk of becoming overweight in adulthood [Abstract]. International Journal of Obesity, 16(suppl 1), 244.

Lissau-Lund-Sorensen, I., & Sorensen, T. I. A. (1992). Prospective study of the influence of social factors in childhood on risk of overweight in young adulthood. International Journal of Obesity, 16, 169-175.

Lissau, I. & Sorensen, T. I. A. (1993). School difficulties in chldhood and risk of overweight and obesity in young adulthood: A ten year prospective population study. International Journal of Obesity, 17, 169-175.

Power, C. & Moynihan, C. (1988). Social class and changes in weight-for-eight between childhood and early adulthood. International Journal of Obesity, 12, 445-453.

Rissanen, A. M., Heliovaara, M., Knekt, P., eunanen, A., & Aromaa, A. (1991). Determinants of weight gain and overweight in adult Finns. European Journal of Clinical Nutrition, 45, 419-430.

Sobal, J., & Stunkard, A. J. (1989). Socioeconomic status and obesity: A review of the literature. Psychological Bulletin, 105, 260-275.

Sonne-Holm, S., & Sorensen, T. I. A. (1986). Prospective study of attainment of social class of severely obese subjects in relationto parental social class, intelligence, and education. British Medical Journal, 292, 586-589.

Sorensen, T. I. A., Holst, C., & Stunkard, A. J. (1992). Social and familial modification of the genetic influenceson body-mass index of adult adoptees? [Abstract] International Journal of Obesity, 16(suppl. 1), 21.

Sorensen, T. I. A., Holst, C., Stunkard, A. J., & Skovgaard, L. T. (1992). Correlations of body mass index of adult adoptees and their biological and adoptive relatives. International Journal of Obesity, 16, 227-236.

Stunkard, A. J., Sorensen, T. I. A., Hanis, C., et al. (1986). An adoption study of human obesity. New England Journal of Medicine, 314, 193-198.

Teasdale, T. W., Sorensen, T. I. A., & Stunkard, A. J. (1990). Genetic and early environmental components in sociodemographic influenceson adult body fatness. British Medical Journal, 300, 1615-1618.

Teasdale, T. W., Sorensen, T. I. A., & Stunkard, A. J. (1992). Intelligence and educational level in relation to body mas index of adult males. Human Biology, 64, 99-106.

Wadden, T. A., & Stunkard, A. J. (1985). Social and psychologicla consequences of obesity. Annals of Internal Medicine, 103, 1062-1067.

THE ROLE OF EXERCISE IN WEIGHT MAINTENANCE

James O. Hill

University of Colorado Health Sciences Center
Center for Human Nutrition
4200 E. Ninth Avenue-Box C225
Denver, CO 80262

It is not universally accepted by the scientific community that exercise plays an important role in maintenance of a desirable body weight. This uncertainly stems from a substantial number of short-term studies in which the effects of exercise on one or more components of energy balance have been inconsistent. It is important to realize the limitations of many of these acute studies and to design long-term studies more clearly identify the effects of exercise on energy balance.

The intent of this discussion is to critically examine the hypothesis that there is a direct relationship between level of body fatness and level of chronic physical activity. The hypothesis implies that changes in the level of chronic physical activity should lead to changes in body fatness. The extent of such changes depends on characteristics of the subjects and characteristics of the exercise program used.

PHYSICAL ACTIVITY AND BODY WEIGHT MAINTENANCE: THEORETICAL CONSIDERATIONS

It is important to begin by estimating the magnitude of the effect that exercise could have on daily energy balance. For example, when a sedentary person begins regular exercise, the energy deficit is equal to the net increase in daily energy expenditure minus the increase in energy intake.

Energy Expenditure

Energy expenditure is clearly increased during exercise (Astrand, & Rodahl, 1986; Sharp, Reed, Sun, Abumrad, & Hill, 1992) and there is no data to suggest that increases in planned exercise led to decreases in spontaneous physical activity. Whether or not exercise has effects on resting energy expenditure is controversial. Energy expenditure remains elevated for a period of time after exercise, but the magnitude of this effect appears to be minor in untrained or obese subjects engaging in moderate exercise (Bahr, & Haehlum, 1986). Another controversy concerns whether resting metabolic rate (RMR), the largest component of daily energy expenditure, varies with chronic physical activity. Some have suggested that RMR varies directly with maximum aerobic capacity (VO$_2$ max), which is a measure of aerobic fitness (Poehlman, 1989). However, others have found that VO$_2$ max does not affect RMR independently of body composition (Schulz, Nyomba, Alger, Anderson, & Ravussin, 1991; Sharp, Reed, Sun, Abumrad, & Hill, 1992). Finally, many investigators have examined the effects of exercise and chronic physical activity level on the thermic effect of food (TEF) with no consistent results (Hill, 1992).

Exercise also impacts upon daily fat and carbohydrate oxidation rates. The exact effects depend on characteristics of the exercise program. In particular, aerobic exercise and aerobic exercise training are associate with increased fat oxidation.

Energy Intake

When the chronic level of physical activity increases, an energy deficit will result and will lead to body weight loss unless caloric intake is altered to account for the extra energy expended in physical activity. There is surprisingly little data available about factors which determine the effects that changes in exercise will have on food intake. Woo et al. (Woo, Garrow, & Pi-Sunyer, 1982; Woo, & Pi-Sunyer, 1985) found that normal weight subjects showed a greater increase in food intake when given moderate or intense exercise than did obese women. Keim et al. (Keim, Barbieri, & Belko, 1990) found that moderately obese women on a metabolic ward did not alter energy intake significantly when exercised. In further studies (Keim, Canty, & Horn, 1992), they administered the Three Factor Eating Inventory to female subject. It was found that those most likely to increase food intake in response to exercise had higher disinhibition and hunger scores than those least likely to increase food intake.

It is also important to realize that even if the increase in energy intake exactly equals the energy expended in exercise, body weight and body composition could be affected if the composition of the increased energy intake differs (e.g. lower in fat) from the composition of the energy expended. Although such an effect would be small, over time it could contribute to body fatness. Clearly, understanding how changes in exercise affect food intake should be a high priority.

Net Effects of Exercise on Energy Balance

Increasing physical activity clearly increases daily energy expenditure, but the effect is most likely seen only during the exercise. This means that the increase in daily energy expenditure will vary directly with the dose of exercise and will be relatively small in sedentary or obese subjects adding moderate exercise. For example, a sedentary woman who adds 5 hours/week of brisk walking will create an energy deficit of approximately 1400 kcal per week. If there is no caloric compensation this would be expected to produce a loss of about 2 kg of fat in 12 weeks. In a year, such a program would be expected to produce a loss of approximately 8 kg.

If, however, there is caloric compensation for 25% of the energy expended in exercise, the loss of body fat in 12 weeks would be expected to be about 1 kg and in a year, about 6 kg. Overall, it must be realized that the caloric deficit produced by exercise is small and the effects of exercise on body weight and body composition cannot be fairly evaluated in studies of short duration.

PHYSICAL ACTIVITY AND BODY WEIGHT MAINTENANCE: EPIDEMIOLOGICAL STUDIES

If exercise is related to body weight, this should be evident in epidemiological studies. While body weight and body mass index (BMI) are relatively easy variables to measure, it is difficult to accurately estimate the amount of a person's usual physical activity. Epidemiological studies suffer from limited techniques (usually some form of self-report) to assess usual level of physical activity. Despite this limitation, many such studies show an inverse relationship between amount of physical activity and BMI (Romieu, Willett, Stampfer, Colditz, Sampson, Rosner, Hennekens, & Speizer, 1988; Williamson, Serdula, Anda, Levy, & Byers, 1992). Similarly, Lee et al. (Lee, Paffenbarger, & Hsiech, 1992) found in the Harvard Alumni Study that those with the greatest increase in physical activity had the greatest weight loss.

PHYSICAL ACTIVITY AND BODY WEIGHT MAINTENANCE: PROSPECTIVE STUDIES

Despite a strong theoretical reason why exercise might be related to body fatness and despite an association between physical activity and body mass index, prospective studies have not clearly shown that changes in physical activity produce systematic changes in body fatness. Few studies exist in which body weight and body composition changes in response to exercise alone have been studied. Wilmore (Wilmore, 1983) and Ballor and Keesey (Ballor, Keesey, 1991) have reported that the change in body weight and body composition produced by increasing exercise alone is small. This is consistent with the small energy deficit that moderate changes in exercise are likely to have. The majority of such studies have been less than 20 weeks in duration, and the expected change in body weight in this time period would be small. Bouchard et al. (Bouchard, Tremblay, Nadeau, Dussault, Despres, Theriault, Lupien, Serresse, Boulay, & Fourniet, 1990) exercised male subjects for 100 days on a constant food intake. They reported an average loss of body weight of 8 kg and an average loss of body fat of 7 kg. Gwinup (Gwinup, 1987) had sedentary, overweight subjects participate in an exercise program for 6 months. Weight losses of 7-9 kg were reported. It should be noted that the drop-out rate was high and that it was unclear how food intake was altered.

There are many studies in which the effects of exercise during caloric restriction have been compared to caloric restriction alone. These studies have been reviewed in detail by others (Donnelly, Jakicic, & Gunderson, 1980; Epstein, & Wing, 1980; Hill, 1992). In general, results are mixed with some but not all studies showing greater weight loss, greater fat loss, greater fat-free mass preservation, and a lesser reduction in RMR when subjects exercised. In general, such studies have shown a relationship between dose of exercise and amount of weight loss (Epstein, & Wing, 1980). Few of these studies have been longer than 20 weeks in duration and most have been outpatient studies. The variation in true food intake in many such studies is likely to be as large as the increased energy expended in exercise. It appears that the majority of studies evaluating exercise alone or exercise plus food restriction as a treatment for obesity have not been sufficiently long.

The small impact of exercise as compared to caloric restriction on energy balance emphasizes that while caloric restriction is an effective acute means of modifying body weight and body composition, exercise is not. If exercise has a role in maintaining body weight, it is a chronic, not an acute role. Consistent with this hypothesis, the best marker of long-term success in weight maintenance after weight loss is exercise (Kayman, Bruvold, & Stern, 1990). The reason why exercise is a marker of success in weight maintenance after weight loss is not clear. It may simply be a marker of overall compliance, so that exercisers are also maintaining a low caloric intake as compared to pre weight loss. It is clear that daily energy expenditure declines after weight reduction (Hill, Drougas, & Peters, 1993). It appears that the decline in daily fat oxidation is proportionally greater than the decline in protein or carbohydrate oxidation (Schutz, Tremblay, Weinsier, & Nelson, 1992). To maintain a weight loss, total caloric intake and specifically fat intake could be reduced to match the new requirements. Alternatively, exercise, which increases both total energy expenditure and fat oxidation, may be particularly useful. There is no way to maintain a weight reduction without a permanent change in behavior. This can be a change in amount and composition of food eaten, a change in exercise, or both. Exercise is a particularly attractive behavior to change since both total energy expenditure and daily fat oxidation are increased with exercise.

Exercise should be an effective means of preventing weight gain, but again, sufficient long-term data do not exist to demonstrate such an effect. In light of the general failure of efforts for weight reduction, greater emphasis is shifting to prevention. Exercise is a likely prevention intervention, but its effects will be most evident only over long periods of time. As the impact of exercise in obesity prevention is assessed, it is critical that studies be of sufficient duration for exercise to impact upon energy balance.

EXERCISE AND BODY WEIGHT REGULATION-FUTURE DIRECTION

There is a need for long-term prospective studies to examine the relationship between chronic level of physical activity and body fatness. Specifically this would include studies to see if chronic increases in physical activity are associated with chronic reductions in body fat in obese individuals and studies to see if increases in physical activity prevents obesity development in at-risk populations. Such studies will require that subjects remain in exercise programs for periods of several months, if not years, and will be expensive. This may best be done in multi-center trials. Thus, it is important that such trial be undertaken in the most appropriate subject population and using the most appropriate exercise program. Studies to determine how the relationship between physical activity and body fatness is affected by characteristics of the subjects (i.e. age, gender, body fat distribution, body fat percentage, etc.) and of the exercise program (type, intensity, etc.).

Such studies could relative short in duration and could determine if it is possible to identify subjects that may be particularly responsive to exercise. For example, this may be subjects who are least likely to show caloric compensation following increases in exercise. Similarly, different types of exercise have different effects on substrate oxidation (Astrand, & Rodahl, 1986). In general, aerobic exercise of low intensity, long duration is associated with the greatest proportion of fat oxidized (Ibid). Alternatively, resistance training is associated with an increase in FFM (Ibid), which in turn would suggest a greater energy expenditure via RMR. There is a need to examine how different types of exercise affect total daily energy expenditure, total daily fat oxidation, and amount and composition of caloric compensation. It is possible that different types of exercise have different effects in different populations. For example, some data suggest that obese individuals have more Type IIb skeletal muscle fibers, which have a high glycolytic capacity as compared to lean individuals (Wade, Marbut, & Round, 1990). It is possible that the effects of a specific exercise on daily energy expenditure and substrate oxidation vary with differences in skeletal muscle morphology/metabolism.

Although there is strong reason to propose increases in physical activity as a treatment/prevention for obesity, it remains difficult to produce such changes. Most obese subjects who enter exercise programs do not stay in them. There is a great need for behavioral strategies to get people to make permanent changes in their level of physical activity. Difficulties in adherence make it difficult to perform studies of sufficient duration to adequately assess the impact of physical activity on body fatness.

SUMMARY

There is strong theoretical reason to hypothesis a relationship between chronic level of physical activity and body fatness. This is supported by epidemiological data which suggests that high levels of physical activity are associated with low BMI and that changes in physical activity leads to expected changes in BMI. The prospective studies in the literature do not provide strong support for this hypothesis. However, the majority of such studies have used an intervention period which was not sufficiently long to be able to see effects of exercise. In particular, few of these studies choose a sample size and duration based on the expected impact of exercise on overall energy balance. If increases in physical activity lead to reductions in body fatness, this would only occur over periods of time longer than almost all of the existing prospective studies. In light of the general failure of caloric restriction as a chronic treatment for obesity, it may be reasonable to stringently examine whether permanent increases in physical activity can be produced and to determine if these are associated with reductions in body fatness.

REFERENCES

Astrand, P., Rodahl, K. (1986). Textbook of Work Physiology. New York: McGraw-Hill.

Bahr, R. and S. (1986). Maehlum. Excess post-exercise oxygen consumption: A short review. Acta Physiologica Scandinavica 128 Supplement, 556, 99-104.

Ballor, D.L. and R.E. Keesey. (1991). A meta-analysis of the factors affecting exercise-induced changes in body mass, fat mass and fat-free mass in males and females. International Journal of Obesity, 15, 717-726.

Bouchard, C., A. Tremblay, A. Nadeau, J. Dussault, J.-P. Després, G. Theriault, P.J. Lupien, O. Serresse, M.R. Boulay and G. Fourniet. (1990). Long-term exercise training with constant energy intake. 1: Effect on body composition and selected metabolic variables. International Journal of Obesity, 14, 57-73.

Donnelly, J.E., J. Jakicic and S. Gunderson. (1991). Diet and Body Composition Effect of Very Low Calorie Diets and Exercise. Sports Medicine, 12, 237-249.

Epstein, L.H. and R.R. Wing. (1980). Aerobic exercise and weight. Addictive Behaviors, 5, 371-388.

Gwinup, G. (1987). Weight loss without dietary restriction: efficacy of different forms of aerobic exercise. American Journal of Sports Medicine, 15, 275-279.

Hill, J.O. (1992). Exercise, energy expenditure and fat oxidation. In: The Science of Food Regulation, ed. G.A. Bray and D.H. Ryan. Baton Rouge: LSU Press, 67.

Hill, J.O, Drougas, H. and Peters, J.C. (in press, 1993). Obesity treatment: can diet composition play a role? Annals of Internal Medicine.

Kayman, S., W. Bruvold and J.S. Stern. (1990). Maintenance and relapse after weight loss in women: Behavioral aspects. American Journal of Clinical Nutrition, 52, 800-807.

Keim, N.L., T.F. Barbieri and A.Z. Belko. (1990). The effect of exercise on energy intake and body composition in overweight women. International Journal of Obesity, 14, 335-346.

Keim, N.L., Canty, D.J. and Horn, W.F. (1992). Physical activity and food intake. Proceedings of NIH Workshop on Physical Activity and Body Weight, Bethesda, MD.

Lee, I.-M., R.S. Paffenbarger,Jr. and C.-C. Hsieh. (1992). Time trends in physical activity among college alumni, 1962- 1988. American Journal of Epidemiology, 135, 915-925.

Poehlman, E.T. (1989). A review: Exercise and its influence on resting energy metabolism in man. Medicine and Science in Sports and Exercise, 21, 515-525.

Romieu, I., W.C. Willett, M.J. Stampfer, G.A. Colditz, L. Sampson, B. Rosner, C.H. Hennekens and F.E. Speizer. (1988). Energy intake and other determinants of relative weight. American Journal of Clinical Nutrition, 47, 406-412, 1988.

Schulz, L.O., Nyomba, B.L., Alger, S., Anderson, T.E. and Ravussin, E. (1991). Effect of endurance training on sedentary energy expenditure measured in a respiratory chamber. American Journal of Physiology, 260, E257.

Schutz, Y., A. Tremblay, R.L. Weinsier and K.M. Nelson. (1992). Role of fat oxidation in the long-term stabilization of body weight in obese women. American Journal of Clinical Nutrition, 55, 670-674.

Sharp, T.A., G.W. Reed, M. Sun, N.N. Abumrad and J.O. Hill. (1992). Relationship between aerobic fitness level and daily energy expenditure in weight-stable humans. American Journal of Physiology, 263, E121-E128.

Wade, A.J., M.M. Marbut and J.M. Round. (1990). Muscle fibre type and aetiology of obesity. Lancet, 335, 805-808.

Williamson, D.F., M.K. Serdula, R.F. Anda, A. Levy and T. Byers. (1992). Weight loss attempts in adults: Goals, duration, and rate of weight loss. <u>American Journal of Public Health</u> , <u>82</u>, 1251-1257.

Wilmore, J.H. (1983). Body composition in sport and exercise: directions for future research. <u>Medicine and Science in Sports and Exercise</u>, <u>15</u>, 21-31.

Woo, R., J.S. Garrow and F.X. Pi-Sunyer. (1982). Effect of exercise on spontaneous calorie intake in obesity. <u>American Journal of Clinical Nutrition</u>, <u>36</u>, 470-477.

Woo, R. and F.X. Pi-Sunyer. (1985). Effect of increased physical activity on voluntary intake in lean women. <u>Metabolism</u>, <u>34</u>, 836-841.

DIET, PALATABILITY, AND DIETARY IMPLICATIONS OF LONG-TERM WEIGHT MAINTENANCE

Barbara J. Rolls

Program in Biobehavioral Health
The Pennsylvania State University
104 Benedict House
University Park, PA 16802-2311

INTRODUCTION

Palatability relates to stimulus qualities of food which determine its acceptability. Since palatability must be assessed in terms of acceptance, palatability is generally used to refer to the hedonic response of an organism to a food which depends on its taste, smell, flavor, texture and appearance. Palatability can be influenced by a number of factors including learned associations of foods, social, cultural, and economic factors, and the internal physiological state of an organism.

In this review I will consider the role of palatability in the development and maintenance of obesity. Specifically, I will consider how variety in the diet, sweetness, and dietary fat affect food intake and whether changes in these aspects of the diet will aid weight control.

SENSORY-SPECIFIC SATIETY AND VARIETY IN THE DIET

It has been suggested that obese and normal weight individuals differ in the cues which control their eating behavior (Schachter, 1971). In particular overweight individuals appear to be more responsive to the taste of food than normal weight individuals (Spiegel et al., 1989), and they eat more of foods that they find palatable. An important influence on the palatability of a meal is the variety of foods presented. This is related to the fact that as a food is consumed the pleasantness of its sensory properties and the desire to consume it decline, whereas the palatability of foods not yet eaten remains unchanged. This changing hedonic response to a food or "sensory-specific satiety" promotes consumption of a variety of foods and increases the amount eaten in a meal (Rolls, 1986). It is possible that obese individuals might be particularly susceptible to the prolonged palatability provided by a varied meal. However, Pliner et al. (1980) did not find any effect of body weight when they examined the effects of a choice of foods on intake compared to consumption of a single food. Nor do individuals with high dietary restraint (i.e., individuals who are concerned with eating and body weight) differ in the sensory-specific satiety they show following test meals (Tepper, 1992). We (Hetherington & Rolls, 1989) also found that a group of overweight restrained women showed sensory-specific satiety, but the magnitude was not as great as in normal weight unrestrained women in some of the tests.

There have not been studies looking at sensory-specific satiety in overweight binge eaters. Several investigations indicate that such a study could show that this group has impaired sensory-specific satiety which could be important in sustaining their bingeing behavior. We have found (Rolls et al., 1992a) that individuals with bulimia nervosa fail to show sensory-specific satiety after consuming high energy foods. Another recent study suggests that systematic overconsumption of particular foods weakens sensory-specific satiety and this in turn may contribute to overnutrition. Specifically, Hetherington (1993, in press) found that in laboratory tests individuals who described themselves as chocolate addicts ate more chocolate than normal chocolate consumers but showed a smaller decline in the pleasantness of the taste of the chocolate.

Body weight maintentance may depend to some extent on the availability of a varied and palatable diet. In studies of the effects of consumption of a monotonous liquid diet, it was found that both obese and normal-weight individuals voluntarily restricted intake and lost weight (Cabanac & Rabe, 1976). There is also some evidence that if freely available diets are varied and palatable there may be excessive weight gain. In studies of caloric regulation in obese and normal-weight subjects confined to the hospital, a plentiful and varied supply of food led to overeating and weight gain over 3- to 6-day periods (Porikos et al., 1977, 1982). It is difficult to conduct long-term controlled studies of the effects of variety on intake and body weight in humans. Studies in rats (Rolls et al., 1983) indicate that when the palatability and energy density of the available foods are matched, the availability of a variety of foods was associated with excessive weight gain and adiposity over a 7 week period.

Thus the effect of variety on food intake can extend beyond a single meal and can contribute to the development of obesity. It seems likely that in affluent societies where there is continual appetite stimulation by variety within and between meals, there will be little opportunity to compensate for overeating due to variety without conscious limitations of intake. Future studies are needed to determine the influence of variety in the diet on weight maintenance. Clearly there must be a proper balance between the variety in the diet required to keep it palatable and satisfying and that which induces overconsumption.

SUGAR, INTENSE SWEETENERS AND OBESITY

Many people believe that sugar and other carbohydrates contribute to overeating and obesity. Despite this popular belief, there is little direct evidence that obese individuals eat excessive quantities of sweet foods. Indeed , a number of studies show an inverse relationship between reported sugar consumption and degree of overweight (Drewnowski, 1987). Although the literature is contradictory, probably because of the diversity of the obese populations studied and large individual variation in the preference for sweet, there is no strong evidence that obese individuals have an enhanced preference for sweet foods (Drewnowski, 1987). Although there is little evidence that sugar is associated with obesity, sugar is often associated with a high-fat content in foods and serves to increase the palatability of fat and as we shall see in the next section, fat is associated with obesity.

The wide availability of acceptable no-calorie sugar substitutes has meant that a reduction in sugar intake is a relatively easy strategy to employ when dieting to lose weight. Recently, there has been intense debate about the effectiveness of intense sweeteners as an adjunct to weight control. This debate was started by reports suggesting that the sweet taste can increase appetite. The issues related to intense sweeteners have been reviewed in detail (Rolls, 1991), so I will just summarize them here. I will just discuss data related to aspartame use, but it should be borne in mind that different intense sweeteners could have different effects.

Although there have been reports of increases in ratings of hunger associated with aspartame consumption, most investigators have found that aspartame is associated with decreased or unchanged ratings of hunger (see Rolls, 1991). Even if aspartame increases ratings of hunger in some situations, there is no evidence that it has any impact on the controls of food intake and body weight. Aspartame has not been found to increase food intake; indeed several studies showed that consumption of aspartame-sweetened foods or drinks was associated with either no change or a reduction in food intake (Rolls, 1991).

Data from long-term studies are very limited. Laboratory-based studies in which aspartame replaced sugar indicate that if the calorie reduction is substantial, compensation will be incomplete (Porikos et al., 1977, 1983). Thus, there will be some reduction in daily energy intake, but substitution of only a few foods may not result in a reduction in daily energy intake. The caveat here is that most of the studies were conducted in normal-weight, nondieting subjects who were unaware of the manipulation. If an individual voluntarily substitutes a reduced-calorie product for one higher in calories, the effect on caloric intake will probably depend on the subject's motivation. If the individual uses the consumption of a low-calorie food as an excuse to eat more of that food or a high-calorie food, or if the individual is not actively trying to restrict intake, daily energy intake may remain unchanged. However, if intense sweeteners are part of a weight-control program, they could aid calorie control by providing palatable foods with reduced energy (Kanders et al., 1988, 1990). It should be emphasized that there are no data showing that the use of intense sweeteners is associated with elevated food intake or weight gain.

Future studies should determine how long-term sweetener use affects food intake patterns and body weight both in normal weight and obese individuals. Such studies should attempt to assess the motivation of the consumer in choosing a sugar substitute, i.e. are they actively trying to reduce total energy intake and lose weight or are they simply trying to reduce their sugar consumption. Although long-term studies are needed it must be stressed that they are inherently difficult because of problems with ensuring compliance to dietary regimens and in assessing intake. Ideally both field studies and laboratory studies should be run in parallel to determine whether they lead to similar conclusions.

DIETARY FAT AND FAT SUBSTITUTES

Overconsumption of Fat and Obesity

Dietary fat currently comprises approximately 37% of the energy content of the American diet; the guidelines of a number of Federal, professional, and health organizations recommend that this be reduced to 30% (Cronin & Shaw, 1988; U.S. Department of Health and Human Services, 1988). What these guidelines do not take into account, however, is that eating habits are extremely difficult to change. Taste is the primary determinant of food selection and fats endow foods with many textural and sensory characteristics. Fats contribute to the richness of food flavor, and stongly influence the palatability of the diet (Drewnowski, 1988; Mela, 1990). Low-fat diets are often reported to be bland and monotonous, and even highly motivated individuals such as cardiac patients find it difficult to maintain long-term compliance (Drewnowski, 1990).

Although it is presumed that sensory qualities of fat in foods promote overconsumption, only a few studies related to this issue have been conducted. Drewnowski and colleagues (1985, 1991) found that obese and formerly obese individuals preferred higher levels of fat in mixtures of dairy products and sugar than did lean individuals. Mela and Sacchetti (1991) also found a positive relationship between sensory preferences for fat in a variety of foods and percent body fat in normal weight subjects. It has also been shown that as body fat increases, the percent of calories in the diet derived from fat increases (Miller et al., 1990, Strain et al., 1992). Preferences for fat could also be important in the development and maintenance of obesity; in a recent 3 year longitudinal study, high weight gain was associated with high fat intake in both men and women (Klesges et al., 1992).

Additional research is needed to understand how the sensory qualities of fat, and individual differences in preferences for dietary fat, influence human food intake and body composition. Despite the paucity of information, it seems clear that fat enhances the palatability of a wide range of foods. However, it is unlikely that the preference for fat is innate (Mela, 1990). It appears that from an early age high-fat, energy-dense foods become preferred because they are associated with a greater reduction in hunger than foods of lower energy density (Johnson et al., 1991, Birch, 1992). Future studies should examine ways to avoid the early development of a preference for high-fat foods.

Dietary Fat and Satiety

It is commonly believed that meals low in fat may not be very satiating and hunger may return sooner after low-fat meals. However, until recently there was little experimental evidence addressing this issue. A key question is whether fat and carbohydrate have similar effects on hunger and satiety since if the proportion of fat in the diet is reduced, the proportion of carbohydrate will increase.

One way to test the hypothesis that fat has a different satiety value than other macronutrients involves giving fixed amounts of nutrients or foods varying in composition (preloads) and determining the effect on subsequent hunger, satiety and food intake. The amount of fat is varied either by replacing it with other nutrients or by incorporating a non-caloric fat substitute. Preloads must be matched for volume and for sensory characteristics, since these factors could influence food intake.

Two recent studies meeting these criteria employed yogurt preloads varying in carbohydrate and fat levels, with similar sensory properties and energy densities, so that differences in the response to the yogurts would depend on the physiological effects of the nutrients. In the first study it was found that when lean unrestrained (i.e., individuals who were not concerned with their body weight as assessed by the cognitive restraint dimension of the Eating Inventory (Stunkard & Messick, 1985)) males and females consumed preloads 30, 90 or 180 minutes before a self-selected lunch there were no differences related to the level of carbohydrate or fat in the preloads on hunger, fullness, energy intake, or the types of foods or macronutrients consumed (Rolls et al., 1991). The fact that no differences were seen between fat or carbohydrate at either 30 or 180 minutes is important; at 30 minutes it is likely that the main influences on intake would be preabsorptive, whereas by 180 minutes postabsorptive factors would be expected to exert their control (Smith & Gibbs, 1988).

A point that has not yet been emphasized is that individuals may vary markedly in their responses to fat manipulations. Individuals who are obese or who have a tendency to become obese may differ from lean individuals not only in their preference for high-fat foods, but also in their ability to adjust subsequent intake to compensate for consumption of high-fat, high-calorie foods. Such potential individual differences were assessed by testing normal-weight and obese females who were either restrained or unrestrained, in addition to normal weight restrained males. Subjects consumed yogurts with three different energy densities, which also varied in fat and carbohydrate composition, thirty minutes before a lunch meal in a repeated-measures dose-response design. The ability of fat and carbohydrate to reduce lunch intake did not differ in normal-weight unrestrained males and females, confirming the findings of the previous study (Rolls et al., 1991). However, in the restrained or obese groups there was a tendency for fat to be less satiating than carbohydrate. Thus, this preliminary finding suggests that individuals that are concerned with regulation of body weight may be relatively insensitive to the satiety value of fat. This finding requires further investigation since it suggests that alterations in the regulation of fat intake could contribute to the development or maintainance of obesity.

The fat manipulation in the studies discussed thus far was achieved by using commercially available products and involved substituting carbohydrate for fat. Another approach is to replace fat with a non-absorbable fat substitute such as olestra which contributes no calories to the diet. The availability of a fat substitute whose physical and orosensory properties closely duplicate regular fat provides a unique opportunity to examine the effects of a pure fat manipulation on food intake and selection. Fat-derived energy can be varied while preserving identical bulk, appearance, texture and sensory characteristics of food.

In a recent study (Rolls et al., 1992c) in lean, non-dieting men, olestra was used to covertly replace 0, 20, or 36g of fat at breakfast and food intake and ratings of hunger over the following 24 hr were measured. The data showed that consumption of olestra did not affect daily energy intake. However, substitution of fat with olestra led to a dose-dependent reduction in fat intake and a reciprocal increase in carbohydrate intake. There was no "fat specific" compensation for the olestra. There were also no systematic differences in ratings of hunger and fullness between conditions. Another study (Birch et al., in press) was conducted in 2 to 5 year olds over a two day period. Approximately 120 kcal of fat was replaced by olestra over the first part of day 1 and intake was recorded until the end of the second day. Overall, as in the adults, olestra was not associated with a decline in total energy intake, but there was a significant reduction in fat intake. Thus, the replacement of fat with olestra reduced fat intake, but not energy intake in children and in normal weight, non-dieting young men. The implication is that the availability of palatable low-fat foods is likely to aid in the reduction of fat intake if such items are chosen instead of the full fat versions of the same foods.

In all of these studies in which the fat content of the diet was altered covertly, normal weight, unrestrained subjects showed an ability to adjust subsequent intake to compensate for the energy content of the preloads. Caloric compensation was accurate regardless of whether the nutrient composition of foods was changed by substituting carbohydrate for fat or by replacing fat with olestra. In the studies in which the manipulations of fat or carbohydrate were compared directly, there was little indication that the satiety value of the nutrients differed in normal weight individuals. However, the finding that obese individuals or those who are concerned with body weight regulation may not find fat as satiating as carbohydrate requires further study; a reduction in the satiety value of dietary fat could be part of the explanation of why it is overeaten by obese individuals.

Reduced-Fat Diets and Energy Intake

Researchers at Cornell (Kendall et al., 1991) have suggested "that the use of palatable low-fat diets may be an effective means of achieving weight reduction even when no limitations are placed on the quantity consumed." This statement is based on two studies in which they fed subjects foods with a reduced fat content and compared intakes to those when the subjects were consuming foods with the usual fat content (Lissner et al., 1987; Kendall et al., 1991). In both studies subjects could eat as much as they liked of the reduced-fat foods, yet they failed to compensate completely for the reduction in energy in the foods and they lost weight.

While these studies appear to suggest that habitual, unrestricted consumption of low-fat diets may be an effective approach to weight control, this conclusion must be accepted with caution since the subjects in these studies only had access to a limited range of foods and all were low in fat. In studies that we conducted (Foltin et al., 1990, 1992) in which the fat content of the diet was manipulated by up to 1673 kcal, subjects kept daily energy intakes within 15% of baseline. In those studies, subjects had access to a wide range of both high- and low-energy foods. The key issue is how compliance to low-fat diets can be maintained when individuals are surrounded by highly palatable high-fat foods. It seems likely that as the range of palatable low-fat foods broadens through the use of fat substitutes or technological innovations, compliance will become easier (Drewnowski, 1990). It also appears likely from the results of these studies that if individuals consume a high proportion of their diet as low-energy density foods, daily energy intake and the proportion of fat in the diet will be reduced.

Efficacy of Interventions to Reduce Fat Intake

Although conclusive data from long-term clinical trials is not available, it is thought that the best dietary approach to long-term weight maintenance is to permanently change eating habits away from a preference for high-fat foods. Although subjects in long-term experimental protocols (Klesges, et al., 1992, Kristal, et al., 1990) have been able to change their eating habits and adhere to low-fat diets for extended periods of time, most individuals find fat reduction extremely difficult. Since people are often unwilling to change eating habits and to choose foods in which there is a loss of palatability, one strategy for achieving fat reduction is to produce foods with a reduced fat content that taste as good as their high-fat counterparts. A variety of recently introduced fat substitutes and fat mimetics, which retain fatty flavors in food, have provided new tools for reducing fat intake (Schlicker & Regan, 1990). This endeavor has been encouraged by the Department of Health and Human Services which has set an objective for the year 2000 that at least 5000 brand items with reduced fat, saturated fat and cholesterol should be available (U.S. Department of Health and Human Services, 1990).

A critical question is whether individuals will learn with repeat consumption that reduced-fat foods do not satisfy hunger as effectively as the full fat versions of the foods. This is important because it may mean that the palatability of reduced-fat foods will fall so that they are no longer selected; alternatively it could mean that more of these foods or other foods in a meal will be consumed in order to satisfy hunger. A recent pilot study (Lyle et al., 1993) examined this issue by measuring the consumption of clearly labelled fat-free or full-fat versions of condiments (pourable salad dressings or mayonnaise) or frozen yogurt by women in a cafeteria setting. It was found that similar amounts of the condiments were chosen but those who selected the low-fat dessert consumed 8.7% more per serving. These findings must be regarded as preliminary since a single meal was observed, intra-subject comparisons were not made, and little is known about the dieting status of the subjects.

When considering the effects of low-fat foods on food intake and selection, it must be borne in mind that the perception of the fat content may have an effect in addition to the actual fat content. In a recent study (Rolls et al., 1992b) the perception of the fat content of the test food was manipulated. Normal-weight women who received yogurt labelled as "low-fat" consumed more calories during a subsequent lunch than after an equicaloric yogurt labelled as "high-fat". Many commercially available foods that are labelled "low-fat" are high in calories and this conflicting information may disrupt intake regulatory systems. In particular it will be important to assess the responses of obese individuals to disparities between actual and perceived energy content of foods.

A concern about the use of fat substitutes is that they may reinforce the liking for the fatty taste. Ideally, the most effective strategy for fat reduction would be to decrease the preference for dietary fat. Mattes (1993) has looked at the effects of two different reduced-fat diets, one which allowed the use of fat mimetics and one which did not, on the preference for some fatty foods. The results indicated that the group which did not experience fatty flavors showed a decrease in the preferred level of fat in foods, whereas the group using fat mimetics showed no such shift. Mattes (1993) concludes that the preference for fat in foods is governed more by exposure to fatty flavors than by the level of fat in foods. This research is important because it suggests that the preference for fat can be lowered. It also suggests that the best strategy for lowering fat preference is to avoid fat mimetics and fat substitutes. However, this study should be replicated with more controls over the experimental setting. The study was based on instructions to subjects and assessments of diet records with few checks for compliance. Shifts in preference were assessed for only 4 foods and found only for milk and soup. Despite the shift in preference the subjects returned to the high-fat versions of the foods as soon as the low-fat regimen ended.

The few controlled laboratory experiments that have been conducted with low-fat foods indicate that they will help to reduce fat intake. However, more information on population-based consumption is needed to assess the impact low-fat foods will have on reaching the goal of 30% of calories from fat. As population-based data from actual reported intakes of low-fat diets or newly introduced fat substitutes and fat mimetics are not yet available, several recent reports have examined theoretical ways of reducing dietary fat intake. Lyle and colleagues (1992) used historical food and nutrient intakes (derived from menu census surveys) to calculate the potential impact of substituting selected nonfat products for foods currently consumed in comparable food categories. In their study, food categories included cottage, cream, and process cheese, salad dressings, sour cream, frozen desserts, and sweet baked goods. Results of their analyses suggest that diets can be modified to approach dietary recommendations when fat-free products are substituted for current comparable food choices. In this regard, fat-free products offer opportunities for significant reductions in fat intake without altering usual eating habits, and may even influence the perceptions people have about high-fat foods. A recent study (Foreyt & Goodrick, 1992), suggests that use of the fat substitute olestra can provide a means for reducing feelings of "deprivation" associated with low-fat diets, as well as reducing the number of high-fat foods that are considered "tempting".

To assess factors associated with the intake of low-fat diets, Kristal and colleagues (1990) examined correlations of nutrition knowledge and attitudes about diet with consumption of low-fat diets. The authors found that practical knowledge about how to select a low-fat diet was most strongly associated with consumption of a low-fat diet. This finding points to the importance of educating the consumer about effective ways to implement dietary change, i.e. providing strategies for the reduction of dietary fat. To further examine the effects of long-term consumption of low-fat diets, Kristal (1992) studied women who had participated in the "Women's Health Trial", and who had maintained fat intake at $\leq 20\%$ for 1-2 years. In examining strategies used by these subjects for fat reduction, Kristal found that maintenance of substitution (use of low-fat foods or fat substitutes) and modification (trimming the fat from meat or broiling instead of frying) habits was quite good; however, strategies requiring a change in usual food habits or selection (avoiding fat as a flavor, or replacing high-fat foods with fruits and vegetables) were less well maintained. Interestingly, many participants said they had developed a dislike for fat and felt physically uncomfortable after eating high-fat foods. However, it is probably inaccurate to describe this phenomenon in terms of "fat aversion", as these individuals were still consuming substantial amounts of fat.

Implications of Studies on Dietary Fat

Several implications of these studies are of interest in relation to maintaining or reducing body weight. First, varying the fat content of food had little effect on the satiety value of the foods in normal weight individuals. There was, however, an indication that obese individuals or those concerned with body weight regulation may be relatively insensitive to the satiety value of dietary fat and this could be part of the explanation of why they overeat fat. More studies are needed to confirm this and to determine whether their are differences in satiety mechanisms in obesity.

A second implication of the studies is that decreasing the fat content of just some of the available foods may be of little benefit in reducing daily energy intake in non-dieting individuals. When subjects in studies had access to a wide variety of foods, they compensated for the covert caloric manipulation. I emphasize covert because the situation could be different if an individual knowingly chooses to substitute a low-fat food for a high-fat food. Although it is difficult to draw firm conclusions because most of the studies have used covert caloric manipulations, it seems likely that if an individual voluntarily substitutes a low-fat food for one higher in fat, the impact on daily energy intake will probably depend on the individual's motivation. The situation is similar to that in which consumers are using sugar substitutes in that if the individual uses the consumption of a reduced-fat food as an excuse to eat other high-fat foods, or if the individual is not actively trying to restrict energy intake, daily energy intake may remain unchanged. However, if reduced-fat foods are part of a weight-control program, they could aid calorie control by providing substitutes for high-fat foods which could reduce feelings deprivation associated with avoiding a number of foods. It should be stressed that most of the studies reviewed were conducted in normal-weight, non-dieting individuals, and the results may be different in dieting and overweight people.

Finally it appears that consumption of low-fat foods is likely to be of benefit in reducing the daily percentage of calories from fat. In no study was there any indication that a fat-specific appetite developed following consumption of low-fat foods. It seems likely that the reduction in fat intake will be the most important and reliable health benefit associated with low-fat foods. More studies are needed to determine whether a reduction in the proportion of fat in the diet will be associated with weight loss if daily energy intake remains unchanged.

ACKNOWLEDGEMENTS

The author is supported by NIH grants DK39177 and DK40968.

REFERENCES

Birch, L.L., Johnson, S.J., Jones, M.B., Peters, J.C. (1993). Effects of olestra, a non-caloric fat substitute, on children's energy and macronutrient intake. American Journal of Clinical Nutrition, in press.

Birch, L.L. (1992). Children's preferences for high-fat foods. Nutrition Reviews, 50, 249-255.

Cabanac, M. & Rabe, E.F. (1976). Influence of a monotonous diet on body weight regulation in humans. Physiology & Behavior, 17, 675-678.

Cronin, F.J. & Shaw, A.M. (1988). Summary of dietary recommendations for healthy Americans. Nutrition Today, November/December, 26-34.

Drewnowski, A. (1987). Sweetness and obesity. In Sweetness, J. Dobbing (Ed.), pp. 177-192. Berlin: Springer-Verlag.

Drewnowski, A. (1988). Fats and food acceptance: sensory, hedonic and attitudinal aspects. In J Solms, DA Booth, RM Pangborn & et al (Eds.), Food acceptance and nutrition (pp. 189-204). New York: Academic Press.

Drewnowski, A. (1990). The new fat replacements: a strategy for reducing fat consumption. Postgraduate Medicine, 87(6), 111-121.

Drewnowski, A., Brunzell, J.D., Sande, K., Iverius, P.H., Greenwood, M.R.C. (1985). Sweet tooth reconsidered: taste responsiveness in human obesity. Physiology & Behavior, 35, 617-622.

Drewnowski, A., Kurth, C.L. & Rahaim, J.E. (1991). Taste preferences in human obesity: environmental and familial factors. American Journal of Clinical Nutrition, 54, 635-641.

Foltin, R.W., Fischman, M.W., Moran, T.H., Rolls, B.J. & Kelly, T.H. (1990). Caloric compensation for lunches varying in fat and carbohydrate content by humans in a residential laboratory. American Journal of Clinical Nutrition, 52, 969-980.

Foltin, R.W., Rolls, B.J., Moran, T.H., Kelly, T.H., McNelis, A.L. & Fischman, M.W. (1992). Caloric, but not macronutrient, compensation by humans for required-eating occasions with meals and snack varying in fat and carbohydrate. American Journal of Clinical Nutrition, 55, 331-342.

Foreyt, J.P. & Goodrick, G.K. (1992). Potential impact of sugar and fat substitutes in the American diet. Journal of the National Cancer Institute (Monograph), 12, 99-103.

Hetherington, M.M. and Macdiarmid, J.I. (1993) "Chocolate Addiction": a preliminary description and report of its relationship to problem eating. Appetite, in press.

Hetherington, M. & Rolls, B.J. (1989). Sensory-specific satiety in anorexia and bulimia nervosa. In: The psychology of human eating disorders: preclinical and clinical perspectives, L. Schneider, S. Cooper & K.A. Halmi (Eds.), pp. 387-397. New York: New York Academy of Sciences.

Johnson, S.L., McPhee, L. & Birch, L.L. (1991). Conditioned preferences: young children prefer flavors associated with high dietary fat. Physiology and Behavior, 50, 1245-1251.

Kanders, B.S., Lavin, P.T., Kowalchuk, M. & Blackburn, G.L. (1990). Do aspartame (APM)-sweetened foods and beverages aid in long-term control of body weight? American Journal of Clinical Nutrition, 51, 515.

Kanders, B.S., Lavin, P.T., Kowalchuk, M.B., Greenberg, I. & Blackburn, G.L. (1988). An evaluation of the effect of aspartame on weight loss. Appetite, 11, Supplement, 73-84.

Kendall, A., Levitsky, D.A., Strupp, B.J. & Lissner, L. (1991). Weight loss on a low-fat diet: consequence of the imprecision of the control of food intake in humans. American Journal of Clinical Nutrition, 53, 1124-1129.

Klesges, R.C., Klesges, L.M., Haddock, C.K. & Eck, L.H. (1992). A longitudinal analysis of the impact of dietary intake and physical activity on weight change in adults. American Journal of Clinical Nutrition, 55, 818-822.

Kristal, A.R., Bowen, D.J., Curry, S.J., Shattuck, A.L. & Henry, H.J. (1990). Nutrition knowledge, attitudes and perceived norms as correlates of selecting low-fat diets. Health Education Research, 5, 467-477.

Kristal, A.R. (1992). Public health applications of biobehavioral models. In: Promoting dietary change in communities: applying existing models of dietary change to population-based interventions, K.K. DeRoos (Ed.),(pp. 126-132). Seattle, WA: Fred Hutchinson Cancer Research Center.

Lissner, L., Levitsky, D.A., Strupp, B.J., Kalkwarf, H.J. & Roe, D.A. (1987). Dietary fat and the regulation of energy intake in human subjects. American Journal of Clinical Nutrition, 46, 886-892.

Lyle, B.J., McMahon, K.E. & Kreutler, P.A. (1992). Assessing the potential dietary impact of replacing dietary fat with other macronutrients. Journal of Nutrition, 122, 211-216.

Lyle, B.J., McVey, R. & Andrade, J. (1993). Comparing portion sizes of fat free and full fat foods as consumed by women. Federation of American Societies for Experimental Biology Journal, 7, A294.

Mattes, R.D. (1993). Fat preference and adherence to a reduced-fat diet. American Journal of Clinical Nutrition, 57, 373-381.

Mela, D.J. (1990). The basis of dietary fat preferences. Trends in Food Science & Technology, 1(3), 71-73.

Mela, D.J. & Sacchetti, D.A. (1991). Sensory preferences for fats: relationships with diet and body composition. American Journal of Clinical Nutrition, 53, 908-915.

Miller, W.C., Lindeman, A.K., Wallace, J. & Niederpruem, M. (1990). Diet composition, energy intake, and exercise in relation to body fat in men and women. American Journal of Clinical Nutrition, 52, 426-430.

Pliner, P., Polivy, J., Herman, C.P. & Zakalusky, I. (1980). Short-term intake of overweight individuals and normal weight dieters and non-dieters with and without choice among a variety of foods. Appetite, 1, 203-213.

Porikos, K.P., Booth, G. & Van Itallie, T.B. (1977). Effect of covert nutritive dilution on the spontaneous intake of obese individuals: a pilot study. American Journal of Clinical Nutrition, 30, 1638-1644.

Porikos, K.P., Heshka, S., Xavier Pi-Sunyer, F. & Van Itallie, T.B. (1983). Effects of caloric dilution with sucrose polyester on the spontaneous food intake of obese men. Fourth International Congress on Obesity, New York. 79A.(Abstract)

Rolls, B.J. (1991). Effects of intense sweeteners on hunger, food intake and body weight: a review. American Journal of Clinical Nutrition, 53, 872-878.

Rolls, B.J. (1986). Sensory-specific satiety. Nutrition Reviews, 44, 93-101.

Rolls, B.J., Andersen, A.E., Moran, T.H., McNelis, A.L., Baier, H.C. & Fedoroff, I.C. (1992a). Food intake, hunger, and satiety after preloads in women with eating disorders. American Journal of Clinical Nutrition, 55, 1093-1103.

Rolls, B.J., Kim, S., McNelis, A.L., Fischman, M.W., Foltin, R.W. & Moran, T.H. (1991). Time course of effects of preloads high in fat or carbohydrate on food intake and hunger ratings in humans. American Journal of Physiology, 260, R756-R763.

Rolls, B.J., Pirraglia, P.A., Jones, M.B., Peters, J.C. (1992b). Effects of olestra, a non-caloric fat substitute, on daily energy and macronutrient intake. American Journal of Clinical Nutrition, 56, 84-92.

Rolls, B.J., Shide, D.J., Hoeymans, N., Jas, P., Nichols, A. (1992c). Information about the fat content of preloads influences energy intake in women. Appetite, 19, 213.

Schachter, S. (1971). Some extraordinary facts about obese humans and rats. American Psychologist, 26, 129-144.

Schlicker, S.A. & Regan, C. (1990). Innovations in reduced-calorie foods: a review of fat and sugar replacement technologies. Topics in Clinical Nutrition, 6, 50-60.

Smith, G.P. & Gibbs, J. (1988). The satiating effect of cholecystokinin. In M. Winick (Ed.), Control of Appetite (pp. 35-40). New York: John Wiley & Sons.

Spiegel, T.A., Shrager, E.E. & Stellar, E. (1989). Responses of lean and obese subjects to preloads, deprivation, and palatability. Appetite, 13, 45-69.

Strain, G., Hershcopf, R.J. & Zumoff, B. (1992). Food intake of very obese persons: Quantitative and qualitative aspects. Journal of the American Dietetic Association, 92, 199-203.

Stunkard, A.J. & Messick, S. (1985). The three-factor eating questionnaire to measure dietary restraint, disinhibition, and hunger. Journal of Psychosomatic Research, 29, 71-83.

Tepper, B.J. (1992). Dietary restraint and responsiveness to sensory-based food cues as measured by food cues as measured by cephalic phase salivatin and sensory specific satiety. Physiology and Behavior, 52, 305-311.

U.S. Department of Health and Human Services. (1988). The Surgeon General's Report on Health and Nutrition. Washington, DC: US Department of Health and Human Services.

U.S. Department of Health and Human Services, (1990). Healthy people 2000:national health promotion and disease prevention objectives. Washington, D. C.: US Department of Health and Human Services.

INFLUENCE OF THE DIET'S MACRONUTRIENT COMPOSITION ON WEIGHT MAINTENANCE

J.P. Flatt

Department of Biochemistry and Molecular Biology
University of Massachusetts Medical School
Amherst, MA 01002

Changes in nutritional and life-style conditions have led to a progressive rise in the incidence of obesity during this century, first in affluent and now in less industrialized societies as well. The development of an increasingly sedentary life-style, the multiplication of the variety of foods offered and their increased availability throughout the day (Sclafani, 1993; Rolls et al., 1981) as well as the increased proportion of dietary energy provided by fat and sugar (Danforth, 1985) are generally thought to be major factors in contributing to the obesity epidemic. Guidelines for improving health and for limiting excessive weight gain indeed emphasize recommendations to increase physical activity, to reduce the amounts of fat in the diet, as well as to replace sugar-containing products by foods providing complex carbohydrates along with more dietary fiber. A high fat content can contribute to excessive weight gain by increasing the energy-density of foods and by enhancing their hedonic characteristics (Drewnowski et al., 1991; Rolls and Shide, 1992), particularly because the body does not regulate the fat balance with nearly the same accuracy as it does the protein and carbohydrate balances (Flatt, 1987; Abbott et al., 1988; SchŸtz et al., 1989). Yet fat, as well as protein and carbohydrate, must be oxidized in amounts commensurate with those provided by the diet, if body composition and body weight are to be maintained. The main purpose of the discussion presented here is to assess the impact of variations in dietary fat content on the achievement of macronutrient balances and on weight maintenance. It will become apparent, however, that the phenomena which need to be considered to understand this issue also help to understand how other factors, such as food palatability and availability, as well as exercise and hormonal changes affect body weight regulation.

The composition of the fuel mix oxidized is controlled primarily by changes in circulating substrate and hormone levels. These are influenced by nutrient intake, particularly during the post-prandial periods, by physical exertion, and, between meals, by the size of the body's protein pools, the degree of repletion of its glycogen reserves, and the size of the adipose tissue mass. Errors in substrate balances lead to changes in the size of these 'compartments', until the particular body 'configuration' is reached which happens to complement endocrine, enzyme and metabolic regulation in such a way that the composition of the fuel mix oxidized

Obesity Treatment, Edited by D.B. Allison
and F.X. Pi-Sunyer, Plenum Press, New York, 1995

matches, on average, the macronutrient distribution in the diet (Flatt, 1988). The body composition for which this occurs varies greatly among individuals, depending on the interactions between multiple genetic and circumstantial factors. The latter are susceptible to be modified by altering lifestyle parameters, such as exercise, food selection and eating habits. Because a particular body configuration has to be reached to achieve macronutrient balance, body composition, and hence adiposity, are linked to these genetic and circumstantial factors, among which the macronutrient composition of the diet is one.

DIETARY FAT CONTENT AND BODY COMPOSITION

Positive correlations between adiposity and dietary fat content, but not with dietary carbohydrate content, have been established in epidemiological data (Dreon et al., 1988; Romieu et al., 1988; George et al., 1990; Tucker and Kano, 1992). The fact that the impact of differences in dietary fat content appears to be rather small in these studies is due to some extent to the well known uncertainties encountered in assessing nutrient intakes from dietary records, to the fact that in most of the population surveyed dietary fat content varies over a relatively narrow range, and to the influence of numerous other parameters on the interindividual variability in body fat content. The impact of dietary fat content on body fat content under *ad libitum* food intake conditions can be more readily evaluated in animals, because extensive shifts in the *'carbohydrate-to-fat ratio'* can be imposed in such studies. Furthermore, physiological components involved in the regulation of food intake can be studied without the confounding impacts of social interactions and/or conscious restrictions on food consumption, which play considerable roles in man. In *ad libitum* fed mice, gradual increments in dietary fat content, from 4 to 76% of total dietary energy (i.e. a shift in the carbohydrate-to-fat ratio from 20:1 to 1:20, while protein content is kept constant at 18%) lead to a progressive rise in the animals' average body fat content (Fig. 1), which is similar in male and female mice when body fat content is expressed as % of body weight (Salmon & Flatt, 1985; Flatt, 1991). The aberration in the dose-response relationship which is apparent in Figure 1 for the diets with the lowest fat contents is due to the high rates of *de novo* lipogenesis induced by such diets.

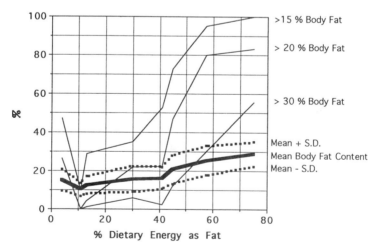

Figure 1. Effect of dietary fat content on % body fat and incidence of obesity in ad libitum fed CD1 mice. Progressive increases in body fat content and in the indicidence of obesity among ad libitum fed male or female CD1 mice elicited by raising the fat content of the diet to male or female CD1 mice. The diets contained 18% of metabolizable energy as protein, the percentage of energy as fat shown on the abscissa, and the balance as starch plus sucrose (1:1). Body fat content was determined by chemical carcass analysis (Salmon and Flatt, 1985).

This process becomes quantitatively insignificant in comparison to the supply of exogenous fat on diets containing more than 12 to 15 % of dietary energy as fat. In man, conversion of carbohydrate to fat is known to be negligible when mixed diets are consumed (Acheson et al., 1984; Hellerstein et al., 1991).

The wide variability in adiposity between animals should be noted, particularly on diets containing substantial proportions of fat (Fig. 1). Such high variability is seen even in highly inbred strains (Flatt, 1989). Evidently, large variations in adiposity are well tolerated and the leverage exerted by the adipose tissue mass on fuel utilization appears to be rather weak, being readily compensated by operating with higher insulin levels (Bjorntorp et al., 1969; Flatt, 1972). This has an important corollary, namely that large alterations in adiposity are necessary to compensate for even minor individual differences in inherited characteristics and/or in life-style. The wide variations in fatness encountered in human populations who consume mixed diets can thus be more readily understood.

When considered over the entire range of carbohydrate-to-fat ratios studied, the impact of dietary fat content on adiposity is considerable (Fig. 1) causing body fat contents to be about 3 times higher on diets with 76%, as compared to 12% of dietary energy as fat. However, the average % Body Fat does not vary very impressively over the range likely to be affected by common attempts to reduce fat consumption, for example by reducing dietary fat content from 45% to 30% of total energy. It is of particular interest, therefore, that the number of mice that one may qualify as being 'overweight', 'obese', or 'very obese' (e.g. % Body Fat >15%, >20%, or >30%, respectively) nevertheless changes considerably as dietary fat content varies through the range of fat contents typical for 'mixed diets' (Fig. 1). This is consistent with the near doubling in the incidence of obesity in the U.S., as compared to France and England, which occurs even though the average Body Mass Index is only slightly higher in the U.S. (Laurier et al., 1992). This suggests that the benefits of efforts at reducing dietary fat content should not be judged merely by the impact on average adiposity expected on the basis of epidemiological data, particularly since even relatively modest declines in fatness may provide significant health benefits. Furthermore, the effect of changing dietary fat content when studied longitudinally is much more clearly evident, even under conditions of *ad libitum* intake. Substantial reductions in the fat content of the foods consumed lead to a losses of 2 to 4 kg of body fat (Sheppard et al., 1991; Prewitt et al., 1991), even when the palatability of the foods provided is designed to be comparable on the high and low fat diets (Lissner et al., 1987; Kendall et al., 1991).

DIFFERENCE IN THE METABOLIC LEVERAGE OF DIETARY CARBOHYDRATE AND FAT

It is important to understand why the macronutrient distribution in the diet should affect body composition, and, in particular, why fat in the diet is more likely to lead to obesity than dietary carbohydrate, even though the latter generally makes up a larger share of total energy intake. It may be noted, first, that the consumption of foods in amounts meeting individual energy requirements almost always provides more than enough protein to sustain Nitrogen balance, or stable rates of protein accretion during growth. Evidently, the body's metabolism is programmed to effectively adjust amino acid oxidation to protein intake, and it is able to do so irrespective of the carbohydrate-to-fat ratio in the diet. Weight maintenance is thus determined primarily by events pertaining to the metabolism of carbohydrate and fat, which together provide the bulk of the substrates used for energy generation. The body's carbohydrate reserves, mainly as muscle and liver glycogen, are usually maintained in a range between 250 to 500 g in a 70 kg adult (equivalent to 1000-2000 kcal) (Bjšrntorp and Sjšstršm, 1978). They are therefore not much larger than the amount of carbohydrates usually consumed in one day. By contrast, the body's fat stores, typically 10 to 25 kg (equivalent to some 100,000-200,000

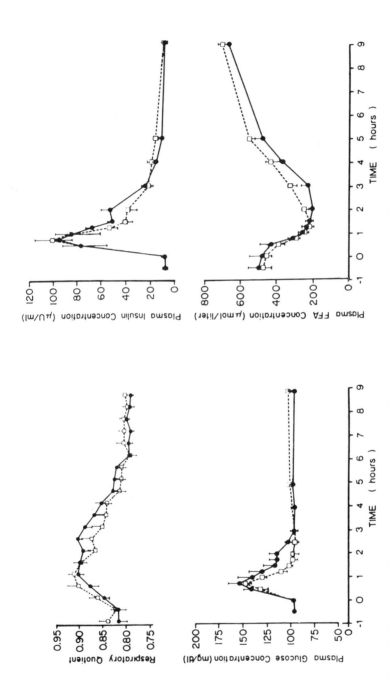

Figure 2. Changes in the Non-Protein Respiratory Quotient, in blood glucose, and in plasma insulin and free fatty acid (FFA) levels observed in 7 young men in response to a low fat breakfast consisting of white bread, jam and dried meat (73 g carbohydrate, 6 g fat and 30 g protein Y------Y), and after consuming the same breakfast on another day with a supplement of 50 g of margarine (41 g of additional fat o------o). Means + SEM. (Adapted with permission from Flatt et al. (1985): Effects of dietary fat on post-prandial substrate oxidation and on carbohydrate and fat balances. J. Clin. Invest. 76: 1019-1024.)

kcal) contain 100 to 200 times more fat than common daily fat intakes. Considering the importance of the body's glycogen stores in maintaining stable blood glucose levels and in assuring muscular responses to sudden increases in physical exertion, biological evolution was compelled to develop regulatory mechanisms and endocrine signals that give a high priority to the adjustment of carbohydrate oxidation to carbohydrate availability (Mayer and Thomas, 1967; Flatt, 1987). When ingestion of food fails to replenish the glycogen reserves, carbohydrate oxidation must be rapidly and effectively restrained. On the other hand, ingestion of a meal containing carbohydrates promptly elicits an increase in carbohydrate (glucose) oxidation, evidenced by the post-prandial increase in the RQ. This response is hardly affected by the presence of fat in the meal, and it occurs even when the proportions of dietary carbohydrate and fat are equal to the relative proportions of glucose and fatty acids being oxidized (Fig. 2). Thus, whereas carbohydrate intake markedly promotescarbohydrate oxidation, fat intake promotes fat oxidation only minimally (Flatt et al., 1985, Griffiths et al., 1993). The goal of maintaining fat balance evidently receives a rather low priority in the regulation of metabolic fuel utilization, a fact that deserves to be recognized as a major factor in permitting excessive fat accumulation (SchŸtz et al., 1989; Thomas et al., 1992; Ravussin & Swinburn, 1992).

To understand the lack of control over the fat balance, one should remember that total substrate oxidation is determined by overall energy expenditure, which itself depends on body size and physical activity. Since metabolic regulation effectively strives to adjust amino acid to protein intake, and glucose oxidation to carbohydrate intake (plus the small amounts of glucose gained by gluconeogenesis from protein and triglyceride-glycerol), fat oxidation cannot also be freely adjusted to fat intake. Fat oxidation is in effect mainly determined by the gap between total energy expenditure and the amounts of protein and carbohydrate energy consumed (Flatt, 1991a). One has to wonder, then, why body fat contents nevertheless tends to remain fairly constant in spite of considerable differences in life-style and while consuming diets containing different proportions of fat. Some adjustment of fat oxidation to fat intake occurs due to a lesser increase in the post-prandial RQ when fats replace carbohydrates in meals. Further changes in fat oxidation rates can be elicited by altering the range within which the body's glycogen stores are maintained. As will be discussed below, operating with lower glycogen levels when consuming diets with a relatively high fat content, allows for a greater use of fat as fuel between meals. But this reduction is frequently insufficient to prevent fat accumulation, particularly when there is unrestricted access to appetizing foods.

INTERACTIONS BETWEEN CARBOHYDRATE AND FAT METABOLISM

Several of the main interactions between carbohydrate and fat metabolism can be illustrated by a model comprizing two reservoirs of very different sizes (Fig. 3) (Flatt, 1989). The small reservoir is meant to represent the body's limited capacity for storing glycogen, whereas the large reservoir stands for its large fat stores. A conduit from the small to the large reservoir represents conversion of carbohydrate into fat, but, as shown by the conduit's position, glycogen levels are usually maintained below the level at which appreciable *de novo* lipogenesis occurs (Acheson et al., 1984; Hellerstein et al., 1991). The small turbine B represents the exclusive use of glucose by the brain under usual conditions, i.e. about 20% of total flux in resting man. The contributions made by the small and by the large reservoirs to the flux through turbine A are assumed to occur in proportion to the *'pressures'* prevailing at the bottom of the two reservoirs. This is analogous to the fact that carbohydrate oxidation remains high for many hours when the body's glycogen reserves have been filled by the consumption of large doses of carbohydrates (Acheson et al., 1984) on one hand, and, on the other hand, to the fact that expansion of the adipose tissue mass enhances fat oxidation by raising circulating free fatty acid

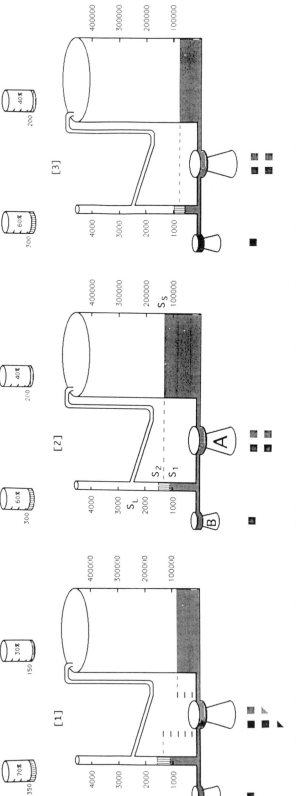

Figure 3. Two-compartment model used as analogy for the body's acquisition, storage and oxidation of carbohydrate (small reservoir) and of fat (large reservoir) (adapted from Flatt, 1989). Units are chosen to correspond to the amounts of glycogen and of triglycerides typically present in the human body, expressed in terms of kcal. Three steady-state situations are illustrated.

(FFA) levels and turnover (Randle et al., 1963; Bjšrntorp et al., 1969). Higher FFA availability reduces the amount of intracellullar CoA available for pyruvate oxidation (Groop et al., 1991) and contributes to induce a state of insulin resistance favoring greater fat oxidation (Felber et al., 1987). Together these phenomena tend to limit further fat accumulation (Flatt, 1988; Swinburn et al., 1991; Seidell et al., 1992).

Replenishment occurs from time to time, in portions illustrated by the contents of the small containers shown above the reservoirs. The fraction of the added total that falls into the large reservoir is analogous to the fat content of the diet. Given its large dimensions, the amount of fuel added to the large reservoir during one 'outflow-replenishment cycle' will cause only an insignificant change in its level. On the other hand, marked changes in the content of the small reservoir occur during each cycle, which are much more likely to be detectable and more suitable for triggering replenishment at appropriate intervals. In the model it is thus assumed that fuel addition is elicited whenever the content of the small reservoir has fallen to a particular minimal level (S_1). The cumulative effect of repeated imbalances between addition and outflow can lead to substantial changes in the content of the large reservoir. Ultimately, it will be filled to the level where the 'pressure' prevailing in it causes its contributrion to the flow through the large reservoir to be equal to the amount of fuel added to it in one cycle. Subsequent replenishments triggered at a frequency appropriate to maintain the content of the small reservoir in its operating range (i.e., between S_1 and S_2) will cause no further accumulation or depletion in the large reservoir. A 'steady-state' is then reached which will tend to perpetuate itself, without there being a sensor to measure its content, nor any mechanism designed to bring the system to some predetermined 'set point' value.

The three panels of Fig. 3 illustrate the changes brought about by increasing the proportion of fuel added to the large reservoir (analogous to increasing a diet's content) from 30% (left panel) to 40% (middle and right panels). The amount added in one 'meal' is '500 kcal', and the outflow in one cycle, assuming that steady-state conditions have become established, is also 500 kcal, as shown by the squares and triangles (representing 100 and 50 kcal, respectively) describing the outflux from each turbine. If the level triggering replenishment (i.e. S_1) remains constant, the steady-state condition for which outflows from the two resevoirs are equal to their inflows will rise, from 3/5 of the average level in the small reservoir (left panel), to the average level (middle panel) prevailing in the small reservoir . However, such an increment in the content of the large reservoir can be prevented by changing the level for which replenishment of the small reservoir is triggered, as seen by examining the right panel, where a change from 30% to 40% in the fraction of the total influx falling into the large reservoir is compensated by keeping the content of the small reservoir in a lower range. Thus, the dietary fat content and the range within which glycogen levels are maintained can both be expected to influence the degree of adiposity for which the steady-state of weight maintenance tends to become established.

Therefore, when foods with relatively high fat contents are consumed, glycogen levels must be maintained at reduced levels to permit the use of fat as fuel to reach an average rate commensurate with the diet's fat content. Often this is not the case, as illustrated by the fact that the relative proportions of fat and carbohydrate in the diet markedly affect average fatness among *ad libitum* fed mice (Fig. 1). However, multiple regression analysis also shows that the mice which had high liver glycogen levels at the time of sacrifice also were fatter, i.e.:

% Body Fat = 6.6 + 0.21 ($\pm$ 0.02) x % Dietary Fat + 1.32 ($\pm$ 0.19) x % Liver Glycogen

($N = 557$; $R^2 = 0.27$; $P < 0.0001$). Differences in the range within which 'habitual glycogen levels' are maintained thus appear to be a factor contributing to inter-individual variations in fatness. This is important because such differences could explain how and why food palatability and availability, and individual responsiveness to these factors, can influence adiposity and the prevalence of obesity, at any given level of dietary fat content.

MECHANISMS OF WEIGHT MAINTENANCE

Energy expenditure and energy intake vary substantially from day to day, and their daily variations are not closely synchronized in man (Edholm and Fletcher, 1955). Although a complex set of physiological responses operates in limiting the size of the daily errors in maintaining energy balance (Foltin et al., 1992), large deviations from energy balance can occur for several days in individuals having unrestricted access to food in spite of such *'diurnal regulation'* of food intake (Rising et al., 1992). Long-term maintenance of stable body composition and body weight thus depends on the operation of compensatory phenomena. Three kinds of *'corrective responses'* are possible, (a) alteration of the composition of the substrate mix used for energy generation, (b) adjustment of food intake, and/or (c) modification of the rate of energy expenditure. As demonstrated by the rise in the RQ after food ingestion, the first of these responses is prompt and powerful. It does not affect the overall energy balance, but serves to adjust glucose oxidation to the amounts of carbohydrate available. Changes in resting energy expenditure can only attenuate, but not reverse errors in the energy balance. Compensation for deviations from the energy balance can therefore only be brought about by appropriate up or down adjustments of food intake.

Changes in daily carbohydrate and fat balances determined with the help of indirect calorimetry (Flatt, 1991b) for many consecutive days in *ad libitum* fed mice show that changes

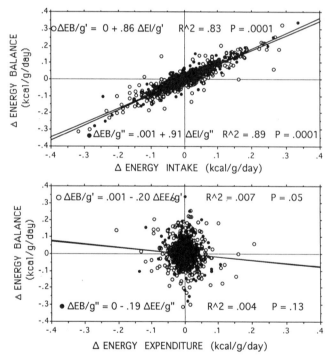

Figure 4. Effect of changes from one day to the next in energy intake and in energy expenditure on energy balances in 5 normal weight (o) (mean body weight = 51.7+3.8 g) and 5 'overweight' (y) (62.3+7.6 g) male CD1 mice maintained ad libitum on diets providing 18% of dietary energy as casein, 13, 30, or 41% of as fat, and the balance as starch plus sucrose (1:1). (Reproduced with permission from Flatt (1991c): Dietary fat content, exercise and body composition.)

in the energy balance from one day to the next are overwhelmingly determined by changes in food intake ($R^2 > 0.8$), rather than by variations in energy expenditure ($R^2 < 0.05$) (Fig. 4) (Flatt, 1991c). Furthermore changes in food intake are influenced twice as much by deviations from the carbohydrate, than from the fat balance (Table 1) (Flatt, 1991). Transfer from a low to a high fat diet induces a positive fat balance during a few days, following which a new steady-state of approximate weight maintenance becomes reestablished (Fig. 5). Transfer from the high to the low fat diet, on the other hand, led to a transiently negative fat balance, followed by weight maintenance at a lower degree of adiposity.

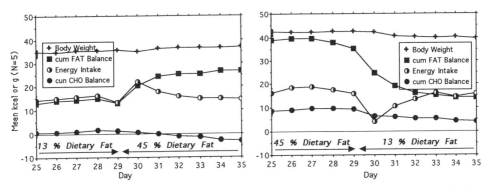

Figure 5. Average body weight (g), cumulative carbohydrate and fat balances (kcal), and daily energy intakes (kcal/day) in two groups of 5 female CD1 mice, during the days preceding and following transfer from a diet containint 13% to one with 45% of dietary energy as fat (left panel) and vice-versa (right panel). Substrate oxidation rates were determined by indirect calorimetry as described in Flatt (1991b).

By contrast, changes in the carbohydrate balances were essentially negligible. The daily food consumption data which are also shown in the figure demonstrate that changes in the adipose tissue mass were a prerequisite for the reestablishment of rates of food intake commensurate with energy expenditure, and that the reestablishment of macronutrient balance and weight maintenance is delayed by the time necessary to gain (left panel) or lose (right panel) a certain amount of fat. Together with the data shown in Fig. 4 and Table 1, this suggests that the establishment of a state of weight maintenance is due to the chronic influence of the adipose tissue mass on the relative rates of glucose and fat oxidation, and that short-term changes in food intake serve primarily the goal of maintaining carbohydrate balance. Such *'modulation of food intake'* elicits adjustments in energy intake that will also lead to long-term energy balance, but only when the body has reached the particular configuration for which it complements the body's metabolic fuel regulation in such a manner that the carbohydrate-to-fat ratio in the fuel mix oxidized matches, on average, the relative proportions of carbohydrate and fat in the diet.

ROLE OF THE FAT MASS IN WEIGHT MAINTENANCE

Provision of sucrose solutions or of a selection of highly palatable foods (*'supermarket'* or *'cafeteria-diets'*) to experimental animals generally causes them to overeat markedly (Sclafani and Springer, 1976), but even under conditions of unrestricted access, food intake diminishes spontaneously after some weight gain has occurred (Rogers and Blundell, 1984). Expansion of the adipose tissue mass (which may or may not be accompanied by changes in glycogen levels) thus appears able to compensate for differences in food palatability, permitting the steady-state of weight maintenance to become reestablished, though at a higher degree of adiposity. It seems quite likely that food availability, palatability, and variety would influence food intake to an even greater extent in man than in *'cafeteria-fed'* animals. A varied selection of appealing dishes will enhance meal size (Rolls et al., 1981), as satiety feelings must reach greater intensity to restrict further food intake than in the face of unappealing foods. (In the model of Fig. 3, this corresponds to raising the S_2 level). This and the inducement to eat between meals, a consequence of the ubiquitous availability of foods (which is analogous to raising S_1 in the model of Fig. 3) have the effect of raising the range within which glycogen levels are habitually maintained. Even in the face of *'terrible'* food selection and eating habits, however, expansion of the fat mass ultimately allows satiation to manifest itself and to restrict food intake enough to limit further weight accumulation in most individuals. This attests to the power of physiological food intake regulation over the long haul, even though the control over daily food intake appears to be rather weak, being often demonstrable only among lean 'unrestrained' subjects (Foltin et al., 1992). The leverage which the size of the adipose tissue mass exerts on the composition of the fuel mix oxidized and the fact that glycogen levels are spontaneously maintained below the level at which *de novo* lipogenesis becomes a significant pathway for the disposal of carbohydrates, thus provide an explanation for the long-term stabilization of body fat contents, and hence of body weights. Although such stability has often been considered to show that the energy balance is regulated, this is quite probably an illusion which can be dispelled by considering the powerful drive to overeat to restore fat losses encurred during periods of food restriction, as well as the spontaneous trend to lose the fat gained during periods of deliberate overeating (Roberts et al., 1990; Diaz et al., 1992; Tremblay et al., 1992).

Fatness thus depends on the amount of body fat necessary to induce a rate of fat oxidation commensurate with fat intake, and on the extent to which genetic factors may alter the impact of circumstantial variables thereon. In this regard, it would seem likely that the impact of abdominal fat accumulation on FFA levels and on intermediary metabolism is greater than that of fat deposition peripherally, just as hepatic glycogen levels would be presumed to influence blood glucose and insulin levels to a greater extent than muscle glycogen. Because adjustment of fat oxidation to fat intake is not achieved by regulatory mechanisms directed at adjusting fat oxidation to fat intake, but rather through the impact of long-term changes in the adipose tissue mass, it is quite natural that diets high in fat should lead to increases in adiposity, until rates of fat oxidation become commensurate with fat intake. This effect of diet composition on body composition tends to be enhanced in affluent situations, as the constant availability of a wide variety of appetizing foods tends to keep glycogen levels well repleted, thereby restricting fat oxidation between meals. Because variations in the size of the adipose

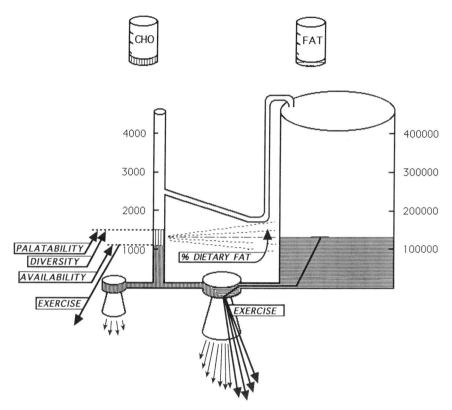

Figure 6. Two-compartment model illustrating the impact of circumstantial and life-style factors on adiposity. The small and the large reservoirs describe the human body's limited capacity for storing glycogen, and its large capacity for fat storage, respectively (as expressed in terms of kcal). The small turbine represents the exclusive use of glucose by the brain. The relative proportions of glucose and of fatty acids used by the large turbine are assumed to be influenced by the levels to which the two reservoirs are filled at a given time. Replenishment of the body's glycogen and fat stores occurs from time to time by consumption of meals (illustrated by the contents of the smal containers shown above the reservoirs). of which the fraction corresponding to the diet's fat content is delivered into the large reservoir. Food consumption is determined by the habitual pattern of meal consumption. complemented by physiological regulatory mechanisms. which assure that glycogen reserves are sufficient to avoid hypoglycemia, while also preventing their build-up to levels at which *de novo* lipogenesis would be induced. (i.e.: the conduit from the small to the large reservoir). Additions of fuel to the large reservoir cause only insignifiant changes in its level, whereas marked changes in the content of the small reservoir occur. This causes the rate of glucose oxidation by the large turbine to adjust itself to glycogen availablity. The interplay between this phenomenon and the factors controlling food intake results in glycogen levels being maintained within a particular operating range. If outflow from the large reservoir (=fat oxidation) is not commensurate with inflow (=fat ihntake), its content (=adipose tissue mass) will change slowly over time, until it is filled to the level that causes its contribution to flow through the large reservoir to be equal on avarage to the amount of fuel added to it, when a 'steady-state' is reached.

The model shows why the size of the fat mass for which weight maintenace tends to become established is influenced by the diet's fat content as well as by the range within which glycogen levels are habitually maintained. The model also illustrates the impact of circumstantial and life-style parameters on adipostiy: food availability, palatability and diversity, because they influence the range within which the glycogen stores are habitually maintained; predilection for, or avoidance of foods,which influence the diet's avarage fat content; exercise, because it increases substrate oxidation in skeletal muscle where fatty acids are readily oxidised and causes greater glycogen depletion between meals (For further explanantion see Fig. 3 and its discussion in the text) tissue depots exert only a relatively weak impact on metabolic fuel regulation (cf. discussion of Fig. 1), large gains or losses of fat must occur before their influence becomes sufficiently manifest, resulting in large inter-individual variations in adiposity. As shown in Fig. 6, the two-compartment model thus allows to envision how rather simple and plausible mechanisms can account for the impact of the food supply on the incidence of adiposity in a manner that indeed leads to the expectation of a high incidence of obesity in affluent societies, particularly among sedentary individuals, as will be seen below.

EFFECTS OF EXERCISE IN THE ESTABLISHMENT OF MACRONUTRIENT BALANCE

Being physically active is generally quite effective in limiting the accumulation of excess weight, or in inducing loss of excess adipose tissue. It is generally not well understood why increments in food intake elicited by exercise are sometimes sufficient to assure weight maintenance (i.e., in a physically active individual), but sometimes not (i.e., when someone initiates a physical training program).

The impact of physical activities on glucose and fatty acid oxidation depends on their intensity and duration. Strenuous effort leads to high RQ's, whereas sustainable exertion, after an initial rise, lead to a progressive decline in the RQ. Furthermore, the impact of physical exertion on the RQ extends into the post-exercise period (Bielinski et al., 1985), in part due to the glycogen depletion that it causes (Flatt, 1987). It is important to realize, in addition, that physical activity lengthens the intervals between meals, if such intervals are judged by the

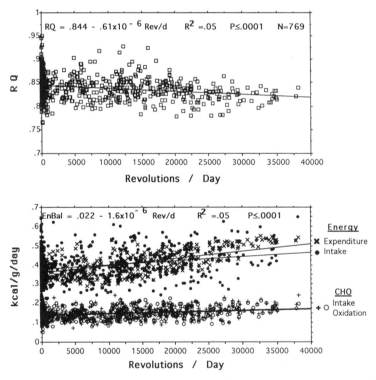

Figure 7. Effects of spontaneous running activity on 24-h RQ and on daily energy and carbohydrate turnover and balances in 10 ad libitum fed female CD1 mice maintained on a diet providing 18% of metabolizable as protein, 45% of dietary energy as fat, and the balance as starch plus sucrose (1:1). (Reproduced with permission from Flatt (1991): The RQ/FQ concept and body weight maintenance. Nestle Foundation, Annual Report, p. 49-71.)

amounts of calories expended, rather than by the time elapsed. This allows glycogen reserves to become more depleted, favoring greater fat oxidation during the periods preceding the next meal. The fact that the steady state of weight maintenance is reached with a lesser expansion of the adipose tissue mass when sustained physical activities are part of the daily routine, implies that the overall effect of exercise is to promote fat oxidation to a greater extent than carbohydrate oxidation. This is indeed directly demonstrable in *ad libitum* fed mice, in whom spontaneous use of a running wheel leads to lower 24-hour RQs (Fig. 7).

Food intake is stimulated by running, but only to the extent needed to maintain carbohydrate balance. Given the decrease in the 24-h RQ, fat and energy balances become negative. Thus one comes to the realization that exercise substitutes for greater adiposity, and greater adiposity substitutes for lack of exercise, in bringing about rates of fat oxidation commensurate with fat intakes. The leverage of exercise on body fatness can be readily explained with the two compartment model (Fig. 6), by its effects in pulling down the lower limit of the range within which habitual glycogen levels are maintained (i.e. an effect opposite

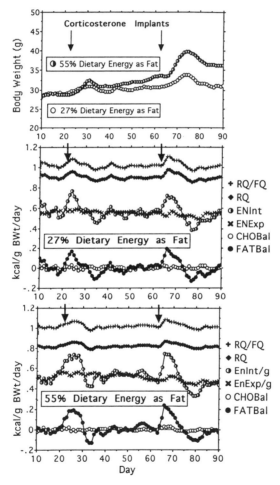

Figure 8. Average bogy weight (g), RQ and RQ/FQ, 24-h energy expenditure, food intake, carbohydrate and fat balances (kcal/g body weight/day) in two groups of 5 female CD1 mice, before and following subcutaneous implantation of corticosterone-releasing pellets (25 mg; Innovative Reserach Inc., Toledo, OH) on days 22 and 64. The points are shown as moving averages over three-day periods. The animals had free access to pelleted diet formulas containing 18 % of energy as casein, 27% or 55% as fat, and 55% or 27% of as sucrose plus starch (1:1). (Reproduced with permisison from Flatt (1993): Dietary fat, carbohydrate balance, and weight maintenance. Ann NY Acad Sci, 683, 122-140).

to the influence exerted by food availability), and because exercise enhances substrate oxidation in muscle, which readily oxidizes fatty acids. Furthermore, increased flux through the large turbine reduces the impact of the exclusively glucose-using small turbine on whole-body carbohydrate and fat oxidation.

GLUCOCORTICOID EFFECTS ON MACRONUTRIENT BALANCE

Administration of corticosterone to *ad libitum* fed mice affects macronutrient balance by increasing carbohydrate and decreasing fat oxidation (Fig. 8). This effect is the opposite of that elicited by exercise, and it causes the energy balance to become positive, rather than negative. Although energy expenditure remained unchanged, the increase in the RQ forced the animals to consume more food to maintain carbohydrate balance, bringing about a period of markedly positive fat balance. This effect was more pronounced on the diet providing 55% of total energy as fat, as compared to the diet with 27% dietary fat, as more total energy has to be consumed to match an increase in carbohydrate oxidation when the proportions of fat to carbohydrate in the diet are 2:1, as compared to 1:2, respectively. This experiment suggests that the obesity-promoting role of glucocorticoid hormones may be due to their effect in enhancing carbohydrate oxidation, or in inhibiting fat oxidation. Considering that these hormones induce insulin resistance, the latter appears to be more likely, possibly because the high insulin levels needed to control blood glucose levels inhibit fat mobilization and/or activate pyruvate dehydrogenase (see below). In a situation like this, where insulin resistance elicits increased insulin secretion to prevent hyperglycemia, insulin resistance promotes the development of obesity. By contrast, when increased insulin secretion is needed to prevent excessive fatty acid release from an enlarged adipose tissue mass (Flatt, 1972), the insulin resistance induced by chronic hyperinsulinemia counteracts further fat accumulation (Flatt, 1988; Swinburn et al., 1991; Seidell et al., 1992). The role of altered insulin sensitivity and changes in insulin levels in the development of obesity can in effect not be judged merely by measuring these changes, since it depends on whether their overall impact tends to raise or to lower the average RQ.

The time course of the changes described in Fig. 8 also shows that the animals spontaneously went into negative energy balance when the corticosterone-releasing pellets became exhausted. This appears to be due to the fact that the 'artificially' enlarged adipose tissue mass caused increased fat oxidation and carbohydrate-sparing, shown by low 24-h RQ values, as well as inhibition of food intake, until the animals body composition had returned to their normal steady-state situations and growth curves.

EXTREME OBESITY: A FAILURE TO ACHIEVE FAT BALANCE

In cases of extreme obesity, accumulation of body fat evidently does not promote fat oxidation effectively enough to induce rates of fat oxidation commensurate with fat intake. This can be described as a failure of excessive fatness to appropriately spare carbohydrate from oxidation. This alternate description conveys an interesting new slant, leading one to focus on the metabolic reaction by which glucose is irreversibly degraded, namely by oxidation of pyruvate to acetyl-CoA by pyruvate dehydrogenase (PDH). PDH is a very complex enzyme whose activity is, among other, enhanced by insulin and inhibited by FFA (Denton et al., 1987; Mandarino, 1989), both of which are raised by increases in the adipose tissue mass. The balance between these opposing effects on the regulation of PDH may vary among different individuals, possibly because adjustments in insulin and FFA levels are influenced by differences in insulin resistance. Pyruvate oxidation is also driven by high pyruvate concentrations (French et al., 1988), which could reinforce the action of high insulin on PDH when glycogen levels are excessively high due to hyperphagia. At any rate, it seems to be of particular interest to examine the notion that the failure of excess body fat accumulation to elicit appropriate inhibition of food intake may be linked to insufficient inhibition of PDH activity.

REDUCTION IN DIETARY FAT INTAKE AND WEIGHT CONTROL

In individuals previously consuming substantial amounts of fat, a marked reduction in fat intake leads to a gradual decline in the adipose tissue mass even in the absence of restrictions on the amounts of food consumed (Kendall et al., 1991), consistent with the expection that low-fat diets allow the steady-state of body weight maintenance to become established at lower degrees of adiposity. In considering this type of dietary intervention, it is important to have reasonable expectations about likely rates of weight changes. For an individual accustomed to a diet providing 45% of total calories as fat, a reduction in fat intake to 30% of total calories, while protein and carbohydrate consumptions remain constant, would create an energy deficit of some 250 to 450 kcalories per day, depending on body size and physical activity on daily energy turnover. This would cause a fat loss of 30 to 50 grams per day, or a weekly reduction of the adipose tissue mass by 1/2 to 1 pound. This is not likely to sustain much enthusiasm in a markedly obese individual who needs to shed much weight, and who therefore may need a more intensive initial intervention. These numbers also serve to illustrate that the admonition to eat carbohydrate freely while cutting fat intake, though perhaps not unreasonable for individuals aiming to maintain weight, is counter-productive for subjects who want to lose weight, as it will attenuate the impact of a reduction in fat intake on the energy balance. To be effective as a measure for weight correction, a reduction in fat intake should thus be complemented by efforts to limit (or at least to not increase) carbohydrate intake. This is facilitated by restricting sugar intake, and selecting preferentially complex carbohydrates (i.e., carbohydrates in the form of starch still accompanied by natural fiber, such as vegetables and whole-grain products), which have a *'low glycemic index'* (Wolever et al., 1991) and are more likely to exert a prolonged satiating influence (Duncan et al., 1983).

There is not enough information as of now to judge to what level the percentage of energy consumed as fat must be reduced to prevent obesity, a limit which is in fact apt to vary among different individuals. It seems likely that the 30% target proposed by current dietary guidelines will not by itself be sufficient to prevent adiposity among individuals prone to developing obesity. However, even if limiting fat intake to 30% does not guarantee or restore ideal body weights, such a dietary measure can be expected to have an impact by altering the dietary habits of obese subjects, who often have a predilection for fatty foods (Drewnowski et al., 1991). It is of course also feasible to further reduce dietary fat intake, restricting it to 25% or even to 20% of total caloric intake. This requires a sustained commitment to an increasingly exclusive selection of food items, differing substantially from the assortment of foods preferred in western societies.

In addition to the metabolic leverage thereby achieved, and to the reduction in caloric density of the allowed food, this has the effect of markedly restricting food choices. This may well prove to be the main advantage for many individuals, as it counteracts the influence of food palatability and variety in raising the range within which glycogen levels are habitually maintained (cf. Fig. 6). One may start to wonder whether the proliferation of low-fat foods may ultimately tend to nullify this advantage.

Finally, in trying to implement such dietary changes, one should be aware of the fact that a recent study revealed that consumption of ethanol selectively reduces fat, but not carbohydrate oxidation (Suter et al., 1992), so that energy consumed in the form of alcohol should be counted with that provided by fat in computing and managing the fat-to-carbohydrate ratio of the diet (Flatt, 1992).

Table 1. Modulation of Food Intake in 10 Male CD1 Mice

		Prev. Day's CHO Bal.†	Prev. Day's FAT Bal.†	R^2
(1) Δ Energy Intake† =	-.002	-1.51	-.46	.5
(2) =	-.004	-1.51	-.45	.34
(3) =	.002	-1.01	-.59	.33
5 Normal Weight Mice (B.Wt. = 51.7 ± 3.8; N=1387)				
(4) =	0	-1.25	-.61	.37
5 Overweight Mice (B.Wt. = 62.3 ± 7.6; N=1386)				
(5) =	-.004	-1.24	-.45	.34

(1) 13% Dietary Fat; N= 634   (2) 30% Dietary Fat; N=480
(3) 41% Dietary Fat; N=1660   (4&5) All diets; N=1387
†(kcal/g B.Wt./day)

CONCLUSIONS

The goal of weight control is in the achievement of fat balance without the need to depend on excessive expansion of the adipose tissue mass to raise fat oxidation. Since the body will spontaneously and effectively maintain protein and carbohydrate balances, but does not (or cannot) regulate the fat balance (and hence the energy balance) nearly as accurately, it makes sense to direct voluntary efforts at this relatively *'soft target'*. Concentrating on the fat balance also has the advantage of providing a more specific goal than one based on controlling overall energy exchanges. Since it is obviously easier to ensure that fat oxidation be at least equal to fat intake when fat intake is small, a key measure is to avoid fatty foods. The overall approach to weight control can thus be summarized by two simple recommendations: *"Do not eat more fat than you oxidize, considering your exercise habits!"* , or *"Exercise enough to burn as much fat as you eat!'*

ACKNOWLEDGEMENTS

The collaboration of K.E. G. Sargent and of D. Demers is gratefully acknowledged. This work was supported by HIH grant DK 33214.

REFERENCES

Abbott, W. G. H., Howard, B. V., Christin, L., et al. (1988): Short-term energy balance: relationship with protein, carbohydrate, and fat balances. American Journal of Physiology, 255, E332-E337.

Acheson, K. J., SchŸtz, Y., Bessard, T., Ravussin, E., Jequier, E. and Flatt, J. P. (1984): Nutritional influences on lipogenesis and thermogenesis after a carbohydrate meal. American Journal of Physiology, 246, E62-E70.

Bielinski, R., SchŸtz, Y. and Jequier, E. (1985): Energy metabolism during the post-exercise recovery in man. American Journal of Clinical Nutrition, 42, 69-82.

Bjšrntorp, P., Bergman, H., Varnauskas, E. and Lindholm, B. (1969): Lipid mobilization in relation to body composition in man. Metabolism, 18, 840-851.

Bjšrntorp, P. and Sjšstršm, L. (1978): Carbohydrate storage in man: speculations and some quantitative considerations. Metabolism, 27, 1853-1865.

Danforth, E., Jr (1985): Diet and obesity. American Journal of Clinical Nutrition, 41, 1132-1145.

Denton, R. M., McCormack, J. G., Midgley, P. J. W. and Rutter, G. A. (1987): Hormonal regulation of fluxes through pyruvate dehydrogenase and the citric acid cycle in mammalian tissues. Biochemical Society Symposia, 54, 127-143.

Diaz, E. O., Prentice, A. M., Goldberg, G. R., Murgatroyd, P. R. and Coward, W. A. (1992): Metabolic response to experimental overfeeding in lean and overweight healthy volunteers. American Journal of Clinical Nutrition, 56, 641-655.

Dreon, D. M., Frey-Hewitt, B., Ellsworth, N., Williams, P. T., Terry, R. B. and Wood, P. D. (1988): Dietary fat: carbohydrate ratio and obesity in middle aged men. American Journal of Clinical Nutrition, 47, 995-1000.

Drewnowski, A., Kurth, C. L. and Rahaim, J. E. (1991): Taste preferences in human obesity: enviromental and familial factors. American Journal of Clinical Nutrition, 54, 635-641.

Duncan, K. H., Bacon, J. A. and Weinsier, R. L. (1983): The effects of high and low energy density diets on satiety, energy intake, and eating time of obese and nonobese subjects. American Journal of Clinical Nutrition, 37, 763-767.

Edholm, O. G. and Fletcher, J. G. (1955): The energy expenditure and food intake of individual men. British Journal of Nutrition, 9, 286-300.

Felber, J., Ferrannini, E., Golay, A., et al. (1987): Role of lipid oxidation in pathogenesis of insulin resistance of obesity and type II diabetes. Diabetes, 36, 1341-1350.

Flatt,J.P. (1972): Role of the increased adipose tissue mass in the apparent insulin insensitivity of obesity. American Journal of Clinical Nutrition, 25:1189-1192.

Flatt, J. P. (1987): Dietary fat, carbohydrate balance, and weight maintenance: effects of exercise. American Journal of Clinical Nutrition, 45, 296-306.

Flatt, J. P. (1988): Importance of nutrient balance in body weight regulation. Diabetes/Met. Rev. 4, 571-581.

Flatt, J. P. (1989): Differences in the regulation of carbohydrate and fat metabolism and their implication for body weight maintenance in: Hormones, thermogenesis and obesity. Lardy, H.A., Stratman, H., eds, Elsevier, New York, p. 3-17

Flatt, J. P. (1991): The RQ/FQ concept and body weight maintenance. Nestle Foundation Annual Report, p. 49-71.

Flatt, J. P. (1991a): Opposite effects of variations in food intake on carbohydrate and fat oxidation in ad libitum fed mice. Journal of Nutritional Biochemistry, 2, 186-192.

Flatt, J. P. (1991b): Assessment of daily and cumulative carbohydrate and fat balances in mice. Journal of Nutritional Biochemistry, 2, 193-202.

Flatt, J. P. (1991c). Dietary fat content, exercise, and body composition. In Obesity: Dietary factors and control, Rousos, D.R., Himms-Hagen, J. and Suzuki, M. eds. Karger, Basel P. 239-250.

Flatt, J. P. (1992): Body weight, fat storage, and alcohol metabolism. Nutrition Reviews, 50, 267-270.

Flatt,J.P. (1993): Dietary fat, carbohydrate balance, and weight maintenance. Annals of the New York Academy of Science, 683, 122-140.

Flatt, J. P., Ravussin, E., Acheson, K. J. and Jequier, E. (1985): Effects of dietary fat on postprandial substrate oxidation and on carbohydrate and fat balances. Journal of Clinical Investigations, 76, 1019-1024.

Foltin, R. W., Rolls, B. J., Moran, T. H., Kelly, T. H., Mcnelis, A. L. and Fischman, M. W. (1992): Caloric, but not macronutrient, compensation by humans for required eating occasions with meals and snack varying in fat and carbohydrate. American Journal of Clinical Nutrition, 55, 331-42.

French, T. J., Goode, A. W., Holness, M. J., MacLennan, P. A. and Sugden, M. C. (1988): The relationship between changes in lipid fuel availability and tissue fructose 2,6-bisphosphate concentrations and pyruvate dehydrogenase complex activities in the fed state. Biochemical Journal, 256, 935-939.

George, V., Tremblay, A., Despres, J. P., LeBlanc, C. and Bouchard, C. (1990): Effect of dietary fat content on total and regional adiposity in men and women. International Journal of Obesity, 14, 1085-1094.

Griffiths, A.J., Humphreys. S.M., Clark, M.L., Fielding, B.A. and Fragn, K.N. (1993): Immediate metabolic availability of dietary fat in combination with carbohydrate. American Journal of Clinical Nutrition, (in press).

Groop, L. C., Bonadonna, R. C., Shank, M., Petrides, A. S. and DeFronza, R. A. (1991): Role of free fatty acids and insulin in determining free fatty acid and lipid oxidation in man. Journal of Clinical Nutrition, 87, 83-89.

Hellerstein, M. K., Christiansen, M., Kaempfer, S., et al. (1991): Measurement of de novo hepatic lipogenesis in humans using stable isotopes. Journal of Clinical Investigations, 87, 1841-1852.

Kendall, A., Levitsky, D. A., Strupp, B. J. and Lissner, L. (1991): Weight loss on a low fat diet: consequence of the imprecision of the control of food intake in humans. American Journal of Clinical Nutrition, 53, 1124-1129.

Laurier, D., Guiguet, M., Chau, N. P., Well, J. A. and Valleron, A. J. (1992): Prevalence of obesity: a comparative survey in France, the United Kingdom, and the United States. International Journal of Obesity, 16, 565-572.

Lissner, L., Levitsky, D. A., Strupp, B. J., Kalkwarf, H. J. and Roe, D. A. (1987): Dietary fat and the regulation of energy intake in human subjects. American Journal of Clinical Nutrition, 46, 886-892.

Mandarino, L. J. (1989): Regulation of skeletal muscle pyruvate dehydrogenase and glycogen synthase in man. Diabetes/Metab Rev, 5, 475-486.

Mayer, J. and Thomas, D. W. (1967): Regulation of food intake and obesity. Science, 156, 328-337.

Prewitt, T. E., Schmeisser, D., Bowen, P. E., et al. (1991): Changes in body weight, body composition, and energy intake in women fed high and low-fat diets. American Journal of Clinical Nutrition, 54, 304-310.

Ravussin,E. and Swinburn,B.A. (1992): Pathophysiology of obesity. Lancet, 340, 404-408.

Ravussin, E., and Swinburn, B.A. (1993): Metabolic predictors of obesity: Cross-sectional versus longitudinal data (In press)

Randle, P.J., Hales, C.N., Garland, P.B. and Newsholme, E.A. (1963): The glucose-fatty acid cycle, its role in insulin sensitivity and the metabolic disturbances of diabetes mellitus. Lancet, i: 785-789.

Rising, R., Alger, S., Boyce, V., et al. (1992): Food intake measured by an automated food selection system: relationship to energy expenditure. American Journal of Clinical Nutrition, 55, 343-349.

Roberts, S. B., Young, V. R., Fuss, P., et al. (1990): Energy expenditure and subsequent nutrient intakes in overfed young men. American Journal of Physiology, 259, R461-R469.

Rogers, P. J. and Blundell, J. E. (1984): Meal patterns and food selection during the development of obesity in rats fed a cafeteria diet. Neuroscience and Biobehavioral Review, 8, 441-453.

Rolls, B. J., Rowe, E. A., Rolls, E. T., Kingston, B., Megson, A. and Gunary, R. (1981): Variety in a meal enhances food intake in man. Physiology & Behavior, 26, 215-221.

Rolls, B. J. and Shide, D. J. (1992): The influence of dietary fat on food intake and body weight. Nutritional Review, 50, 283-290.

Romieu, I., Willett, W. C., Stampfer, M. J., et al. (1988): Energy intake and other determinants of relative weight. American Journal of Clinical Nutrition, 47, 406-412.

Salmon,D.M.W. and Flatt, J.P. (1985): Effects of dietary fat content on the incidence of obesity among ad libitum fed mice. International Journal of Obesity, 9, 443-449.

SchŸtz, Y., Flatt, J. P. and Jequier, E. (1989): Failure of dietary fat intake to promote fat oxidation: A factor favoring the development of obesity. American Journal of Clinical Nutrtion, 50, 307-314.

Sclafani, A. (1993). Dietary Obesity. In: <u>Obesity: Theory and Therapy. 2nd ed.</u>, Stunkard, A.J. and Wadden, T.A. eds. New York, Raven Press, p 125-136.

Sclafani, A. and Springer, D. (1976): Dietary obesity in adult rats: similarities to hypothalamic and human obesity syndromes. <u>Physiological Behavior, 17</u>, 461-471.

Seidell, J. C., Muller, D. C., Sorkin, J. D. and Andres, R. (1992): Fasting respiratory exchange ratio and resting metabolic rate as predictors of weight gain: the Baltimore Longitudinal Study on Aging. <u>International Journal of Obesity, 16</u>, 667-674.

Sheppard, L., Kristal, A. R. and Kushi, L. H. (1991): Weight loss in women participating in a randomized trial of low fat diets. <u>American Journal of Clinical Nutrition, 54</u>, 821-828.

Suter, P. M., SchŸtz, Y. and Jequier, E. (1992): The effect of ethanol on fat storage in healthy subjects. <u>New England Journal of Medicine, 326</u>, 983-987.

Swinburn, B. A., Nyomba, B. L., Saad, M. F., et al. (1991): Insulin resistance associated with lower rates of weight gain in Pima Indians. <u>Journal of Clinical Investigations, 88</u>, 168-173.

Thomas, C. D., Peters, J. C., Reed, G. W., Abumrad, N. N., Sun, M. and Hill, J. O. (1992): Nutrient balance and energy expenditure during *ad libitum* feeding of high fat and high carbohydrate diets in humans. <u>American Journal of Clinical Nutrition, 55</u>, 934-942.

Tremblay, A., Despres, J.P., Theriault, G., Fournier, G., Bouchard, C. (1992): Overfeeding and energy expenditure in humans. <u>American Journal of Clinical Nutrition, 56</u>, 857-862.

Tucker, L. A. and Kano, M. J. (1992): Dietary fat and body fat: a multivariate study of 205 adult females. <u>American Journal of Clinical Nutrition, 56</u>, 616-622.

Wolever, T. M. S., Jenkins, D. J. A., Jenkins, A. L. and Josse, R. G. (1991): The glycemic index: methology and clinical implications. <u>American Journal of Clinical Nutrition, 54</u>, 846-854.

WHAT ARE OUR PSYCHOTHERAPEUTIC OPTIONS?

Rena R. Wing

University of Pittsburgh
Western Psychiatric Institute and Clinic
3811 O'Hara Street
Pittsburgh, PA 15213

Over the past two decades, behavioral treatment programs have become increasingly more effective in producing initial weight loss. The best programs now yield average weight losses of approximately 10 kg at the end of treatment (usually 20-24 weeks). However, long-term results are still modest, averaging about 5 kg (Wadden, & VanItallie, 1992). Therefore,the key problem facing us today is how to improve long-term results.

Several approaches deserve our consideration. First, it seems necessary that <u>longer treatments</u> be developed, and a chronic disease approach to obesity be adopted. It may well be that obese patients need to remain in therapy forever. Evidence supporting the concept of longer treatment interventions comes from a study by Perri, et al (Perri, McAdoo, Spevak, & Newlin, 1984). These investigators found that subjects treated with a standard 20 week behavioral program with no subsequent treatment contact lost weight initially, but maintained a loss of only 3.6 kg at 12 month follow-up. In contrast, subjects given the same initial treatment, but seen biweekly throughout the 12 months of follow-up, maintained weight losses of 8.4 - 13.5 kg. A recent study that we conducted with Type 2 diabetic patients also used a chronic disease model. In this study, where subjects attended treatment every week for 52 weeks, the mean weight loss at the end of the 52 week program was 10.2 kg.

However, one of the major problems in developing such long-term interventions is burn-out. Most patients are unwilling to attend treatments weekly for a year, and attendance in such programs decreases markedly over time. Thus, we need to carefully consider what can be taught in a chronic disease approach to obesity and how we can maintain interest and attendance over time. Using different treatment approaches at different phases of treatment may be helpful, such as starting the program with a focus on diet and adding exercise strategies at 6 months. Techniques to increase group cohesiveness may also be useful.

Moreover, lengthening treatments may be only one component of a more general issue--the need to develop <u>more intensive approaches to behavior change</u>. To date, behavioral treatments have been primarily educational in nature; participants are instructed in techniques for modifying the cues and reinforcers that control eating and exercise behavior, but the burden of implementing these procedures and modifying the home environment is left entirely to the patient. Better results might be obtained by more directly modifying the antecedents and reinforcers in the patients' environment for them. A recent study, using more direct manipulations of the antecedent cues for eating, by actually providing subjects with the foods they should eat, showed positive effects of this approach (Jeffery, Wing, Thorson, Burton, Raether, Harvey, & Mullen, in press). In contrast, a stronger incentive approach, based on paying people to lose weight, had no effect. Further research using stronger approaches to modifying the environment are clearly needed.

Other more intensive approaches to behavior change may also be warranted. The positive results obtained by Ornish (Ornish, Bron, Scherwitz, Billings, Armstrong, Ports, McLanahan, Kirkeeide, Brand, & Gould, 1990) with a very low fat diet and meetings held twice a week are of interest. These results suggest that setting stricter goals (i.e. <10% of calories from fat vs 20-30% as is customary in behavioral programs) may actually be helpful to patients. Similarly, Bjorvell and Rossner (Bjorvell, & osser, 1992) obtained positive results with a treatment program that involved weekly meetings for 4 years. This program started with a 6 week in-hospital program, which included instruction in behavior modification, a low calorie diet (600 kcal/day) and aerobic exercise. Patients were able to return to the hospital for 2 week phases of inpatient therapy as needed over the 4 years. In subsequent studies, it would be interesting to determine whether it is possible to replicate the success of this program and to identify the active ingredients in the intervention. There are several aspects of the treatment that could be related to its success, including the long-term, ongoing contact, the self-initiated return to strict dieting, and the use of periods of in-hospital intervention.

Another option that has received only limited attention is the use of <u>combination therapies</u>. Combining pharmacotherapy and behavioral treatment produced significant long-term weight loss in both a study by Weintraub, where the drugs phentermine and fenfluramine were used in combination with behavior therapy (Weintraub, 1992), and in a study by Marcus et al. (Marcus, Wing, Ewing, Kern, McDermott, & Gooding, 1990), which combined fluoxetine with behavior modification.

The strategies discussed thus far all maintain the current focus on changing diet and exercise behaviors. Another option is to <u>broaden our target</u> and to realize that obese patients may have problems in other psychosocial domains that affect their eating. Targeting these other areas may be more helpful than targeting the eating per se. For example, an individual may be having marital problems, and stressful interactions with the spouse may trigger eating. Perhaps better outcomes would be achieved by intervening on the marital problems, and reducing the source of stress, rather than merely trying to teach patients not to eat in response to the stress. This approach would clearly require more individualized therapy, as the associated psychosocial issues would differ across patients.

We should also consider the range of reinforcers currently available to the subject. For some overweight individuals, food may be one of the few reinforcers in their life. It is unrealistic to expect these individuals to give up food without some type of substitute reinforcer. Stuart emphasized this in his early, successful treatment of obesity (Stuart, 1967). A key part of his treatment was to help subjects cultivate other activities that were reinforcing to them, such as birdwatching or caring for African violets. The development of alternative reinforcers is also a key component of Azrin's community reinforcement approach to the treatment of alcoholism (Hunt, & azrin, 1973).

As we consider broadening the therapeutic targets, we should also consider <u>utilizing other psychotherapeutic approaches</u> in addition to behavior therapy and cognitive behavior therapy. For example, interpersonal therapy has been shown to be effective in the treatment of bulimia nervosa; in one recent study, results with interpersonal therapy were comparable to those achieved with cognitive behavior therapy at long-term follow-up (Fairburn, Jones, Peveler, Hope, & O'Connor, 1993). This is of interest since interpersonal therapy focuses on interpersonal relations and does not specifically address issues related to eating, weight or shape, which are considered central to bulimia nervosa.

Since obesity has proven so difficult to treat, we should consider whether periods of caloric restriction, independent of weight loss, may be helpful in preventing or treating the medical complications of obesity, such as hypertension and diabetes. Several recent studies have shown that one week of caloric restriction can improve cardiovascular risk factors, including insulin and triglycerides (Weisier, James, Darnell, Wooldridge, Birch, Hunter, & Bartolucci, 1992). We have recently demonstrated that 7 days of an 800 kcal/day diet markedly reduces fasting glucose in obese Type II diabetic patients and ameliorates the three abnormalities associated with hyperglycemia in these individuals, namely abnormalities in insulin secretion, insulin sensitivity, and hepatic glucose output (Kelley, Wing, Buonocore, Sturis,Polonsky, & Fitzsimmons, in press). Thus, there may be benefits to using intermittent periods of calorie restriction in the treatment of obese patients with Type II diabetes, rather than focusing on weight loss per se.

Finally it is time that we begin to learn more about those individuals who have succeeded in weight loss. To date, there has been little research on this important group--how numerous are successful weight losers, who are they, and how do they do it? By learning from their success, we may be able to improve our treatment interventions.

REFERENCES

Bjorvell, H., Rossner, S. (1985). Long-erm treatment of severe obesity: Four year follow up of results of combined behavioural modificaiton programme. British Medical Journal, 291, 379-382.

Fairburn, C. G., Jones, R., Peveler, R. C., Hope, R. A., & O'Connor, M. (1993). Psychotherapy and bulimia nervosa: Longer-term effects of interpersonal psychotherapy, behavior therapy, and cognitive behavior therapy. Archives of General Psychiatry, 50, 419-428.

Hunt, G. M., & Azrin, N. H., (1973). A community reinforcement approach to alcoholism. Behaviour Research and Therapy, 11, 91-104.

Jeffery, R. W., Wing, R. R., Thorson, C. Burton, L. R., Raether, C., Harvey, J., & Mullen, M. (in press). Strengthening behvarioral interventions for weight loss: A randomized trial of food provision and monetary incentives. Journal of Consulting and Clinical Psychology.

Kelley, D. E., Wing, R. Buonocore, C., Sturis, J., Polonshiy, K., & Fitzsimmons, S. (in press). Relative effects of calorie restriction and weight loss in non-insulin dependent diabetes mellitus. Journal of Clinical Endocrinology Metabolism.

Marcus, M. D. Wing, R. R>, Ewing, L. Kern, E., McDermott, M. & Gooding, W. (1990). A double-blind, placego-controlled trial or fluoxetine plus behavior modification in the treatment of obese binge-eaters and non-binge eaters. American Journal of Psychiatry, 147, 876-881.

Ornish, D., Brown, S. E., Scherwitz, L. W., Billings, J. H., Armstrong, W. T. Ports, T. A., McLanahan, S. M., Kirkeeide, R. L, Brand, R. J., & Gould, K. L. (1990). Can lifestyle changes reverse coronary heart disease? Lancet, 336, 129-133.

Perri, M. G., McAdoo, W. G., Spevak, P. A., & Newlin, D. B. (1984). Effect of a multicomponent maintenance program on long-term weight loss. Journal of Consulting and Clinical Psychology, 52(3), 480-481.

Stuart, R. B. (1967). Behavioral control of overeating. Behaviour Research and Therapy, 5, 357-365.

Wadden, T. A., & VanItallie, T. B. (1992). Treatment of the Seriously Obese Patient. New York, Guilford Press.

Weinsier, R. L., James, L. D., Darnell, B. E.,Wooldridge, N. H, Birch, R. Hunter, G. R., & Bartolucci, A. A. (1992). Lipid and insuln concentrations in obese postmenopausal women: Separate effects of energy restriction and weight loss. American Journal of Clinical Nutrition, 56, 44-49.

Weintraub, M. (1992). Long-term weight control study. Clinical Pharmacological Therapy, 51, 581-646.

POTENTIAL SIDE COSTS AND SIDE BENEFITS OF PHARMACOLOGICAL TREATMENT OF OBESITY

Teis Andersen

Departments of Medical Gastroenterology and Endocrinology
University of Copenhagen
Copenhagen, Denmark

This paper deals with other effects of obesity drugs than weight loss itself and weight loss related effects. The review does not pretend completeness. Rather will the effects - good and bad - be dealt with from examples putting the stress on experience from human studies of clinical relevance.

NUTRITIONAL CHANGES

A quantitative change in the form of a reduction in food intake, is the essential impact of an anorexic and as such well accepted by the patients treated. When increasing treatment periods, malnutrition secondary to the use of anorexic drugs is a potential side effect that should be looked for, in particular if more potent anorexic drugs come into use.

Qualitative changes include an influence on macronutrient preferences as well as on specific aspects of satiation and satiety.

Whereas amfetamine as well as related drugs are considered to reduce intake of the various macronutrients proportionally (Foltin, Kelly, & Fischman, 1990), other drugs have been claimed to have specific effects on macronutrient selection. For serotonergic drugs the rational is based on the theory that the release from central serotonine containing neurons reflects the plasma ratio between tryptophan and large neutral amino acids. A high carbohydrate meal increases this ratio, which in turn increases brain tryptophan levels and synthesis and release of serotonine. The finding (Wurtman, & Wurtman, 1984) that dexfenfluramine by its central serotonergic effect should be particularly effective in so-called carbohydrate cravers is well known. However, the selective reduction of carbohydrate intake, in particular from snacks, has not been uniformly supported by others (Anderson, Astrup, & Quaade, 1989; Blundell, 1992; Mathus-Vliegen, van de Voorde, Kok, & Res, 1992). Among the probable reasons are differences in patient selection, composition of diet, and duration of treatment.

It may also be questioned whether a reduction of carbohydrate intake is appropriate, as the general nutrition advice calls for a higher carbohydrate intake at the expense of fat consumption. Moreover, recently it has been found that dexfenfluramine is more liable to reduce the intake of non-sweet than sweet carbohydrates (Goodall, Feeney, McGuirk, & Silverstone, 1992).

A selective reduction of fat intake is more in accordance with current nutrition recommendations. No current anorexic offers such effect, but lipid absorption inhibitors may prove clinically to act in this way. A too high lipid intake during treatment with e.g. the inhibitor of gastric and pancreatic lipases, tetrahydrolipstatin (orlistat, Roche) will lead to an unpleasant flatulence, steatorrhea and in some cases even fecal incontinence (Drent, & an der Veen, 1993). Further analysis of ongoing clinical trials will reveal whether these side effects parallel the alcohol-disulfiram reaction utilized in the treatment of alcoholism.

A limitation of fat uptake carries the risk of inadequate supplies af fat soluble vitamins and essensial fatty acids. Careful surveillance is justified during the further testing of lipase inhibitors.

Also certain peptides seem to exhibit a nutrient-specific influence on food intake. Enterostatin is formed by cleavage of the pancreatic peptide procolipase, which is secreted in response to lipid intake. In rats, enterostatin selectively depresses fat intake (Bray, 1992), and human studies are ongoing.

INFLUENCE ON LEAN AND FAT TISSUES

Investigations prompted by the discussions about use of very-low-calorie formula diets have made it clear that dietary treatments without increase in physical activity are typically associated with some loss of lean body mass (LBM) corresponding to the increasing LBM during weight gain. Still, of course, the best possible LBM preservation should be aimed at during weight loss in order to keep up energy expenditure and reduce the risk of weight regain.

During energy restriction the organism defends itself against loss of LBM by a decline in T_3 levels. Decades ago it was demonstrated that attempts to compensate this decline by giving supplements of thyroid hormones lead to a further weight loss almost exclusively consisting of LBM.

An intension to compensate the low-T_3 syndrome and the associated fall in energy expenditure during weight loss has been an important motivation for the development and use of beta adrenergic thermogenic drugs. In animal studies many of the newly developed thermogenic drugs have been found to conserve to some extent the lean tissues, but human data are very limited. A combination of ephedrine and caffeine as adjuvant to a diet has in a small series been found to reduce the LBM reduction by 70% compared to placebo (Astrup, Buemann, Christensen, Toubro, Thorbek, Victor, & Quaade, 1992). Ephedrine alone has also been found to preserve LBM during VLCD (Pasquali, Casimirri, Melchionda, Grossi, Bortoluzzi, Labate, Stefanini, & Raitano, 1992). The concordance of these results with those from animal studies is suggestive. If the findings can be further reproduced, we are dealing with an important effect of an anti-obesity agent.

The serotonergic agent fluoxetine may have the opposite effect on LBM. Thus, it was resently shown (Visser, Seidell, Koppeschaar, & Smits, 1993) that fluoxetine treated patients lost relatively more LBM than did placebo patients. In fact, 40% of the weight loss in the fluoxetine group was LBM, a value considerably above the accepted level.

Thus, in the evaluation of the often relatively small weight losses obtained from drug treatment, a measurement of the composition of lost body mass should be included. Furthermore, keeping in mind the current evidence for a major negative impact on health of the intraabdominal adipose tissue mass, also drug influence on fat distribution should be evaluated. The Dutch study just referred to (Ibid) found by using the MR technique a relatively larger loss of subcutaneous than intraabdominal fat in the fluoxetine group compared to the placebo treated control patients. The alpha-2 antagonist yohimbine have been found to have no effect on fat distribution as estimated by CT scans (Sax, 1991). No substantial data on body composition changes during treatment with beta-adrenergic agonists seem present.

Testosterone and growth hormone are investigated for their ability to improve body composition. In support of the hypothesis that relatively low testosterone levels may be involved in the development of intraabdominal fat accumulation in some populations, it has been shown (Marin, Holmang, Jonsson, Sjostrom, Kvist, Holm, Lindstedt, & Bjorntorp, 1992) in abdominally obese middle-aged men that moderate doses of testosterone cause a statistically significant reduction of intraabdominal adipose tisssue mass and a decline in the associated metabolic variables. However, body weight and BMI are unaffected.

As found in animal studies, also growth hormone supplementation in humans decreases the intaabdominal adipose tissue mass without any net change in body weight (Bengtsson, Eden, Lonn, Kvist, Stokland, Lindstedt, Bosaeus, Tolli, Sjostrom, & Isaksson, 1993). Contrary to the testosterone supplementation results, growth hormone substitution causes an overall increase in LBM at the expense of fat mass (Snyder, Underwook & Clemmons, 1990; Skaggs, & Crist, 1991). Obesity is associated with a lowered 24-h growth hormone secretion and a blunted growth hormone response to a number of stimuli, and growth hormone treatment may also for this reason be of particular interest. Insulin-like growth factor-1 (IGF-1) is also depressed in obesity and it has been found inversely associated with intraabdominal adipose tissue mass (Rasmussen, Frystyk, Andersen, Breum, Christiansen, & Hilsted, 1993). Contrary to growth hormone, IGF-1 influences insulin resistance favourably. This fact makes IGF-1 a candidate for further studies of body composition modulation in obesity.

METABOLIC CHANGES

Glucose metabolism, which plays a key role in the risk- carrying metabolic profile of obesity, is an obvious target for side actions of obesity drugs. Literature is contradictory in the evaluation of a possible beneficial effect of serotonergic drugs on glucose-insulin metabolism. Probably, independent of weight loss a weak improvement of insulin sensitivity results from dexfenfluramine as well as from fluoxetine with according improvements of glucose and insulin levels (Andersen, Richelsen, Bak, Schmitz, Sorensen, Lavielle, & Pedersen, 1993; Potter van Loon, Radder, Frolich, Krans, Zwinderman, & Meinders, 1992).

On their side, the adrenergic agonists do not lead to any significant weight loss independent improvement of the glycaemic control in humans.

Regarding *lipid metabolism*, favourable independent effects of the serotonergic agents are even more uncertain than the effects on glucose metabolism. The adrenergic agonists increase lipid oxidation (Astrup, Buemann, Christensen, Toubro, Thorbek, Victor, & Quaade, 1992) but do not lead to any improvement of the lipid profile (Krieger, Daly, Dulloo, Ransil, Young, & Landsberg, 1990).

It is perhaps more surprising that the lipase inhibitor tetrahydrolipstatin has been found without effect on cholesterol and triglyceride levels (Drent, & van der Veen, 1993). It should be recalled, however, that the patients of this study had near-normal lipid levels, and studies on hyperlipidemics are ongoing.

CARDIOVASCULAR EFFECTS

The positive and negative side effects of obesity drugs have mostly been evaluated from quite simple parameters such as heart rate, blood pressure, ECG's and clinical findings. Of the serotonergic agents, at least dexfenfluramine seems in short term studies (Andersen,

Zimmermann, Hedner, & Bjorntorp, 1991) to have an independent blood pressure lowering effect, pulse rate being unaffected or marginally lowered. The effect on the supine systolic and diastolic blood pressure is in the order of 4 mmHg and is probably due to a reduction in sympathetic outflow.

Contrariwise, the adrenergic agents induce to a varying degree tachycardia and hypertension as could be expected from their nature. These effects have been a limiting factor for clinical use of new thermogenic agents, whereas the problem seems less marked in relation to some of the old adrenergic agonists such as ephedrine and caffeine (Astrup, Breum, Toubro, Hein, & Quaade, 1992). These compounds have a less pronounced hypertensive and chronotropic effect and tolerance to the cardiovascular effects develops within a few weeks whereas the anorectic and the thermogenic effect are more prolonged. Still, the risk of blood pressure increase at the start of the treatment makes these compounds generally unsuitable for weight reduction in hypertensive patients. An exeption seems to be phenylpropranolamine that has been extensively examined, also in hypertensives (Morgan, & Funderburk, 1992). Patients with pre-existing heart disease should be given adreneric drugs only with caution as worsening of angina and arrythmias have been reported (Bradley, Blum, & Scheib, 1974) in such patients treated with Mazindole.

A serious but rare cardiovascular complication to drug treatment of obesity is the pulmonary hypertension reported casuistically in relation to fenfluramine as well as to dexfenfluramine (Atanassoff, Weiss, Schmid, & Tornic, 1992).

CNS EFFECTS

One of the oldest concerns in connection with adrenergic anorectics was the concern about dependency stemming from the abuse potential of amfetamine. The amfetamine derivatives currently marketed for obesity treatment do have, however, a very small abuse potential. This is illustrated by the fact that no abuse was reported in the large long-term National Heart, Lung and Blood Institute study, in which fentermine was administered for hundreds of patient years in combination with fenfluramine (Weintraub, 1992). On the other hand, abuse has been reported casuistically, for example from ephedrine, which can also in very rare cases promote psychoses (Battig, 1993). In relation to combined ephedrine-caffeine treatment tiredness and headache have been reported as withdrawal symptoms (Astrup, Breum, Toubro, Hein, & Quaade, 1992). Taken together the abuse concern should not dominate the discussion about these drugs as long as they are administered as prescription drugs only. The serotinergic drugs and all other drug categories for obesity treatment are considered being without any risk of dependency.

In general, side effects to adrenergic agonists and to serotonergic substances are opposite. The adrenergic drugs very often induce a feeling of excitation, power and energy sometimes turning into restlessness and insomnia. On the other hand, the serotonergic drugs are associated with tiredness and drowsiness. Whereas dl-fenfluramine has been associated with some risk of depression, in particular in relation to abrupt withdrawal, the risk is considerably less pronounced or even absent when using dexfenfluramine. Fluoxetine is even widely registered as an antidepressant.

A great deal of clinical interest has been devoted to the possible effects of sertonergic agents in particular obesity disorders, which have been associated with lowered serotonine levels and a tendency to increased carbohydrate intake. The available data should however be concluded from with caution, especially because the syndromes are difficult to define and because results origin from only a limited number of centers.

Seasonal affective disorder is characterized by mild depressive symptoms and modified eating patterns leading to obesity. Dexfenfluramine has been found to influence the psychiatric as well as food related parameters favourably (McTavish, & Heel, 1992). Similarly, the claimed entity *premenstrual disorder* has been reported to be significantly improved by dexfenfluramine (Ibid).

Smoking cessation is a significant contributor to overweight. Perhaps more importantly, the justified fear of gaining weight is a major obstacle to the success of non-smoking campaigns. Dexfenfluramine as well as fluoxetine have prevented or minimized weight gain in relation to smoking cessation in several trials (Spring, Pingitore, & Kessler, 1992), but comparative studies including drugs from for example the adrenergic agonist group are lacking. It is therefore impossible to tell whether or not the effect observed is specific to the neurophysiologic changes characterizing smoking cessation or rather a general one linked to anorexic medication.

Obesity related to *binge eating* has also been proposed as being particularly sensitive to treatment with serotonergic agents. A controlled study (Marcus, Wing, Ewing, Kern, McDermott, & Gooding, 1990) using fluoxetine has not, however, showed the drug to be superior to behaviour modification.

Fluoxetine has also been tested against *alcohol abuse*, and it was demonstrated to reduce alcohol intake in heavy drinkers by about 16% over a 2 week period (Naranjo, Kadlec, Sanhueza, Woodley-Remus, & Sellers, 1990). Accordingly, dl-fenfluramine in combination with fentermine has been observed to reduce alcohol craving in obese alcoholic patients (Hitzig, 1993).

Finally, fluoxetine has been shown (Kopelman, Elliott, Simonds, Cramer, Ward, & Wedzicha, 1992) to improve respiratory function in obese subjects suffering from *sleep apnoea*. Fluoxetine limited the fall in arterial oxygen saturation, which could be related to a suppression in REM sleep.

FUTURE PROSPECTS

Patients are mostly concerned about the desired weight loss whereas we as professionals are more concerned about the degree to which we can improve the risk profile of our obese patients without notable hazards. As the potency of the drugs are almost equal, the choice between drugs will very much depend upon their side-effects and their potential beneficial side actions as reviewed above.

As the side-benefits, with our current insight, do only persist as long as treatment is maintained, they will typically become clinically significant only if we become prepared in the future to practice long-term or even life-long pharmacological treatment of obesity.

REFERENCES

Andersen, P. H., Richelsen, B., Bak, J., Schmitz, O., Sorensen, N. S., Lavielle, R., & Pedersen, O. (1993). Influence of short-term dexfenfluramine therapy on glucose and lipid metabolism in obese non-diabetic patients. Acta Endocrinologica, 128, 251-258.

Andersen, T., Astrup, A., & Quaade, F. (1989). d-Fenfluramine reduces overweight but does not change food preferences. International Journal of Obesity, 13 (suppl 1), A136.

Andersson, B., Zimmermann, M. E., Hedner, T., & Bjorntorp, P. (1991). Haemodymanic, metabolic and endocrine effects of short-term dexfenfluramine treatment in young, obese women. European Journal of Clinical Pharmacology, 40, 249-254.

Astrup, A., Breum, L., Toubro, S., Hein, P., & Quaade, F. (1992), The effect and safety of an ephedrine/caffeine coumpund compared to ephedrine, caffeine and placebo in obese subjects on an energy restricted diet: A double blind trial. International Journal of Obesity, 16, 269-277.

Astrup, A. Buemann, B., Christensen, N. J., Toubro, S., Thorbek, G., Victor, O. J., & Quaade, F. (1992). The effect of ephedrine/caffeine mixture on energy expenditure and body composition in obese women. Metabolism, 41, 686-688.

Atanassoff, P. G., Weiss, B. M., Scmid, E. R., & Tornic, M. (1992). Pulmonary hypertension and dexfenfluramine. Lancet, 339, 436.

Battig, K. (1993). Acute and chronic cardiovascular and behavioural effects of caffeine, aspirin and ephedrine. International Journal of Obesity, 17(suppl 1), S61-64.

Bengtsson, B-A, Eden, S., Lonn, L., Kvist, H., Stokland, A., Lindstedt, G., Bosaeus, I., Tolli, Sjostrom, L., & Isaksson, O. G. P. (1993). Journal of Clinical Endocrinology and Metabolism, 76, 309-317.

Blundell,, J. E. (1992). Serotonin and the biology of feeding. American Journal of Clinical Nutrition, 55, 155S-159S.

Bradley, M. J., Blum, N. J., & Scheib, R. K. (1974). Mazindol in obesity with known cardiac disease. Journal of International Medical Research, 2, 347-354.

Bray, G. A. (1992). Peptides affect the intake of specific nutrients and the sympathetic nervous system. American Journal of Clinical Nutrition, 55, 265S-271S.

Drent, M. L., & van der Veen, E. A. (1993). Lipase inhibition: A novel concept in the treatment of obesity. International Journal of Obesity, 17, 241-244.

Foltin, R. W., Felly, T. H., & Fischman. M. W. (1990). The effect of d-amphetamine on food intake of humans living in a residential laboratory. Appetite, 15, 33-46.

Goodall, E., Feeney, S., McGuirk, J., & Silverstone, T. (1992). A comparison of the effects of d- and l-fenfluramine and d-amphetamine on energy and macronutrient intake in human subjects. Psychopharmacology, 106, 221-227.

Hitzig, P. (1993). Combined dopamine and serotonin agonists: A synergistic approach to alcoholism and other addictive behaviors. Maryland Medical Journal, 42, 153-156.

Kopelman, P. G., Elliott, M. W., Simonds, A., Cramer, D., Ward, S., & Wedzicha, J. A. (1992). Short-term use of fluoxetine in asymptomatic obese subjects with sleep-related hypoventilation. International Journal of Obesity, 16, 825-830.

Krieger, D. R., Daly, P. A., Dulloo, A. G., Ransil B. J., Young, J. B., & Landsberg, L. (1990). Ephedrine, caffeine andaspirin promote weight loss in obese subjects. Transactions of the Association of American Physicians, 103, 307-312.

Marcus, M. D., Wing, R. R., Ewing, L., Kern, E., McDermott, M., & Gooding, W. (1990) A double-blind, placebo-controlled trial of fluoxetine plus behavior modification in the treatment of obese binge-eaters and non-binge eaters. American Journal of Psychiatry, 147, 876-881.

Marin, P., Holmang, S., Jonsson, L., Sjostrom, l., Kvist, H., Hom, G., Lindstedt, G., & Bjorntorp, P. (1992). The effects of testosterone treatment on body composition and metabolism in middle-aged men. International Journal of Obesity, 16, 991-997.

Mathus-Vliegen, E. M. H., van de Voorde, K., Kok, A. M., & Res, A. M. A. (1992). Dexfenfluramine in the treatment of severe obesity: A placebo-controlled investigation of the effects on weight loss, cardiovascular risk factors, food intake and eating behaviour. Journal of Internal Medicine, 232, 119-127.

McTavish, D., & Heel, R. C. (1992). Dexfenfluramine. A review of its pharmacological properties and therapeutic potential in obesity. Drugs, 43, 713-733.

Morgan, J. P., & Funderburk, F. K. (1992). Phenylpropanolamine and blood pressure: A review of prospective studies. American Journal of Clinical Nutrition, 55, 206S-210S.

Naranjo, C. A., Kadlec, K. E., Sanhueza, P, Woodley-Remus, D., & Sellers, E. M. (1990). Fluoxetine differentially alters alcohol intake and other consummatory behaviors in problem drinkers. Clinical Pharmacology and Therapeutics, 47, 490-498.

Pasquali, R., Casimirri, F., Melchionda, N., Grossi, G. Bortoluzzi, L., Labate, A. M. M., Stefanini, C.,& Raitano, A. (1992). Effects of chronic administration of ephedrine during very low calorie diets on energy expenditure, protein metabolism and hormone levels in obese subjects. Clinical Science, 82, 85-92.

Potter van Loon, B. J., Radder, J. K., Frolich, M., Krans, H. M. J., Azinderman, A., H., & Meinders, A. E. (1992). Fluoxetine increases insulin action in obese nondiabetic and in obese non-insulin-dependent diabetic individuals. International Journal of Obesity, 16, 79-85.

Rasmussen, M. H., Frystyk, J., Andersen, T., Breum, L, Christiansen, J. S., & Hilsted, J. (1993). The impact of obesity, fat distribution and energy restriction on insulin-like growth factor-1 (IGF-1), IGF-binding protein-3, insulin and growth hormone. Metabolism, in press.

Sax, L. (1991). Yohimbine does not affect fat distribution in men. International Journal of Obesity, 15, 561-565.

Skaggs, S. R. & Crist, D. M. (1991). Exogenous human growth hormone reduces body fat in obese women. Hormone Research, 35, 19-24.

Snyder, D. K., Underwood, L. E., & Clemmons, D. R. (1990). Anabolic effects of growth hormone in obese diet-restricted subjects are dose dependent. American Journal of Clinical Nutrition, 52, 431-437.

Spring, B., Pingitore, R., & Kessler, K. (1992). Strategies to minimize weight gain after smoking cessation: Psychological and pharmacological intervention with specific reference to dexfenfluramine. International Journal of Obesity, 16(suppl 3), S19-23.

Visser, M., Seidell, J. C., Koppeschaar, H. P. F., & Smits, P. (1993). The effect of fluoxetine on body weight, body composition and visceral fat accumulation. International Journal of Obesity, 17, 247-253.

Weintraub, M. (1992). Long-term weight control study: Conclusions. Clinical Pharmacology and Therapeutics, 51, 642-646.

Wurtman, J. J. & Wurtman, R. J. (1984). d-Fenfluramine selectively decreases carbohydreate but not protein intake in obese subjects. International Journal of Obesity, 8(suppl 1), 79-84.

DRUG TREATMENT OF OBESITY: THE ARGUMENT IN FAVOR

George A. Bray

Pennington Biomedical Research Center
Baton Rouge, LA 70808-4124

INTRODUCTION

Treatment of obesity has many analogies with treatment of hypertension. Both diseases are defined by arbitrary cut points on a continuous variable. The impact of health of any deviation varies with the degree of deviation, duration of follow-up, gender, age and race. Several mechanisms can cause each disease and hyperinsulimia is characteristic of most patients with either disease. A number of the underlying realities for treatment of this disease (NIH Consensus Developement Conference Statement, 1985) argue for long term treatment.

FEATURES OF OBESITY AS A DISEASE

First, obesity is a chronic disease, which has many causes. Cure is rare, but palliatation is possible. Weight loss is slow and recidivism is common. Weight regain may also be slow but is often rapid. Finally, treatment is often more frustrating than the underlying disease.

Medications do not work if not taken. Because of its chronic nature, the argument for use of drugs might be best accomplished against a background of a desirable pharmacological agent.

FEATURES OF AN IDEAL DRUG

Any should be safe. Secondly, it should produce a dose related reduction in body fat. It should also spare body protein and other body tissues. There should be few, if any, side effects and it should be free of abuse potential. It should be safe and acceptable for chronic administration. At present none of the available drugs meet these criteria, but the future holds promise that one or more drugs will be developed which could be used for the appropriate degree of obesity.

Obesity Treatment, Edited by D.B. Allison
and F.X. Pi-Sunyer, Plenum Press, New York, 1995

HISTORICAL PERSPECTIVE

Drugs were first used to treat obesity in 1893. The first of these was thyroid hormone. It was used because obesity was thought to be due to a low metabolic rate. Two other treatments were also introduced in the pre-World War II period. The first of these was dinitrophenol, a drug which was noted to increase metabolic rate by uncoupling oxidative phosphorylation. This drug was abandoned in 1936 because of undesirable side effects. Dextroamphetamine was originally developed for narcolepsy, but was noted to produce weight loss. When it was shown to produce weight loss by reducing appetite, and a new era of pharmaceutical therapy for obesity opened (Bray, 1976).

APPETITE SUPPRESSING DRUGS

Amphetamine-Like Drugs

Amphetamine has many of the pharmacological properties of the naturally occurring neurotransmitters, norepinephrine and epinephrine. Amphetamine, however, suffers from the serious disadvantage of being a drug with substantial abuse potential (Griffiths, Brady, & Bradford, 1979). Its central excitatory properties led to the search for derivatives which contained the appetite suppressant effects without the potential for drug abuse. Chemical manipulations of the side chain and ring structure of amphetamine produced a group of drugs with markedly reduced risks for abuse and with much reduced stimulation effects on the central nervous system, yet which retain the appetite suppressing effects. All of these drugs with the exception of fenfluramine have a similar spectrum of pharmacologic actions.

In a review of the effectiveness of amphetamine-like drugs, the Food and Drug Administration reanalyzed all of the controlled studies submitted to that agency claiming effectiveness for an anoretic drug up to the early 1970s (Scoville, 1975). There were over 200 such studies which included nearly 10,000 patients in trials lasting 4 - 20 weeks. This project which analyzed 105 new drug applications, found that in more than 90% of the studies, the active drug produced more weight loss than placebo, but the weight loss due to drug was not great nor invariable. In 40% of the 160 trials comparing placebo and active drug, the patient receiving active drug lost significantly more weight than those receiving placebo. Pooling the drug-treated and placebo-treated patients included in studies using two parallel arms, yielded 4,543 patients treated with drug and 3,182 patients treated with placebo. For those who returned after 4 weeks of therapy, the dropout rate for patients on active drug was 24.3% compared to 18.5% for those receiving placebo. Of patients on active drug, 44% were able to loose one pound or more per week compared with 26% of patients receiving placebo. Of patients receiving active drug, 2% lost more than three pounds per week compared to only 1% of those receiving placebo. Average weight loss for patients taking the drug was 0.25 Kg/wk (0.56 lb/wk) more than those receiving placebo at the end of 4 weeks of therapy. Lumping all patients together at their final weights, Scoville (1975) found that patients taking active drug lost approximately 0.25 Kg/wk more than those taking placebo. In his paper Scoville noted that "because drugs do not provide complete cures, however is no reason to reject them out of hand; partial success is clearly better than failure".

Since the work of Scoville (1975) a number of additional trials of appetite suppressing drugs have been published. The most important of these is the study combining fenfluramine and phentermine (Weintraub, Fundaresan, Schuster, Ginsberg, Madan, Stein, et al, 1992). In this 4 year study, drug-treated patients lost an average of 15 Kg during the first double-blind period compared to 4.6 Kg in placebo-treated patients. The drug-treated patients continued to do better than placebo-treated patients throughout the study.

Serotonergic Drugs

A new chapter in pharmacologic therapy of obesity began with the introduction of fenfluramine, a drug which is chemically similar to the amphetamines but pharmacologically very different. Fenfluramine is like a serotonin-agonist. It was found to partially inhibit the re-uptake of serotonin and to release serotonin from nerve endings. A number of different drugs are now available which will enhance extra neuronal serotonin concentration and thus inhibit food intake (Blundell, 1992). The mechanisms of action are diverse ranging from the precursors of serotonin action, to drugs which primarily inhibit serotonin re-uptake into nerve terminals, to drugs which have a major effect on serotonin release as well as serotonin uptake and to drugs which act directly on serotonin receptors. Of these drugs, only dl-fenfluramine in the United States and d-fenfluramine in Europe are available for clinical use. Several long term studies with fenfluramine have been reported (Guy-Grand, Apfelbaum, Crepaldi, Gries, Lefebvre, & Turner, 1989; Finer, Craddock, Lavielle, & Keen, 1988; Weintraub, Fundaresan, Schuster, Ginsberg, Madan, Stein, et al., 1992; Douglas, Munro, itchin, Muir, & Proudfoot, 1981). Among patients who remain in the trials, fenfluramine is clearly more effective than placebo in producing and maintaining weight loss for periods up to one year. In a double-blind crossover study, fenfluramine enhanced the magnitude of weight loss over and above what could be achieved with the best behavior modification, exercise and nutrition program (Weintraub, Fundaresan, Schuster, Ginsberg, Madan, Stein, et al, 1992). The principal drawback to use of fenfluramine is the development of depression when it is withdrawn abruptly and rare reports of pulmonary hypertension (Douglas, Munro, Kitchin, Muir, & Proudfoot, 1981; McMurra, Bloomfield, & Miller, 1986; Pouwels, Smeets, Ceriex, & Wouters, 1990; Atanassoff, Weiss, Schmid, & Tornic, 1992).

Fluoxetine, an inhibitor of serotonin reuptake, is currently marketed as an antidepressant drug. During trials of effectiveness as an antidepressant, fluoxetine-treated patients were noted to lose small amounts of weight. Subsequently, a number of clinical trials for obesity have been published with the drug (Levine, Enas, Thompson, Byyny, Dauer, Kirby, Kreindle, Levy, Lucas, & McIlwain, 1989; Ferguson, & Feighner, 1987; Darga, Carroll-Michals, Botsford, & Lucas, 1991; Gray, Fujioka, Devine, & Bray, 1992). Fluoxetine shows a dose response effect on weight loss over 8 weeks of treatment (Levine, Enas, Thompson, Byyny, Dauer, Kirby, Kreindle, Levy, Lucas, McIlwain, 1989). When patients are treated with the drug for more than 16-20 weeks however, on average they begin to regain weight. The mechanism for this weight regain is unclear, since it does not occur in all patients. Fluoxetine may thus be a useful drug for continued therapy for the subset of patients who do not regain weight.

LIMITATIONS

At the present time, the drugs which are available for treatment of obesity are of relatively limited potency and relatively few long-term trials exist. Because most of the older "noradrenergic" agents derived from amphetamine are no longer protected by patents, there is little incentive to conduct long-term clinical trials with these agents. With the newer agents, dl-fenfluramine, dexfenfluramine and fluoxetine, drug trials of 6 to 44 months have been published and the drugs are clearly more effective than placebo. At the present, there is only one trial known to this reviewer combining a serotonergic and noradrenergic drug

(Weintrab, & Bray, 1989). If one is to learn from the experience of treating hypertensive patients, it is likely that the use of combination therapy will produce a greater effect than any single agent alone. In addition to the lack of patent protection, a number of other barriers exist to use of the current appetite suppressing drugs (Weintraub, & Bray, 1989; Bray, 1991).

First, the public perceives obesity as a disorder of willpower. Second, health professionals also often believe that weight regain after termination of treatment reflects failure of the drug. That is, drugs are expected to cure obesity. Third, regulatory rigidity limits use of existing drugs to "a few weeks". Fourth, state licensing boards are eager to prosecute physicians for alleged misuse of appetite suppressing drugs. Finally, inadequate funding for clinical trials limits the study of the treatment for obesity.

REFERENCES

Arch, J. R. S., Ainsworth, A. T. Cawthorne, M. A., Piercy, V., Sennitt, M. V., Thody, V. E., Wilson, C., & Wilson, S. (1984). Atypical beta-adrenoceptor on brown adipocytes as target for anti-obesity drugs. Nature, 309(5964), 163-165.

Astrup, A., Toubro, S., Christensen, N. J., & Quaade, F. (1992). Pharmacology of thermogenic drugs. American Journal of Clinical Nutrition, 55, 245WS-248S.

Atanassoff, P. G., Weiss, B. M., Schmid, E. R., & Tornic, M. (1992). Pulmonary hypertension and dexfenfluramine. Lancet, 339, 436-437.

Banting, W. (1863). A letter on corpulence addressed to the public. London: harrison and Sons.

Blundell, J. E. (1992). Serotonin and the biology of feeding. American Journal of Clinical Nutrition, 55, 155S-159S.

Bray, G. A. (1991). Barriers to the treatment of obesity: Editorial. Annals of Internal Medicine, 115, 152-153.

Bray, G. A. (1990). Obesity: Historical development of scientific and cultural ideas. International Journal of Obesity, 14, 909-926.

Bray, G. A. (1976). The obese patient. 9th Edition Major Problems in Internal Medicine. W. B. Saunders Co., Philadelphia, 1-450.

Bray, G. A. (1991). Treatment for obesity: A nutrient balance/nutrient partition approach. Nutrition Reviews, 49(2), 33-45.

Bray, G. A., & Gray, D. S. (1988). Treatment of obesity: An overview. Diabetes/Metabolism Reviews, 4(7), 653-679.

Bray, G. A., & Inoue, S. (Ed.) (1992). Pharmacological Treatment of Obesity. American Journal of Clinical Nutrition, 55, 1S-319S.

Darga, L. L., Carroll-Michals, L., Botsford, S. J., & Lucas, C. P. (1991). Fluoxetine's effect on weight loss in obese subjects. American Journal of Clinical Nutrition, 54, 321-325.

Douglas, J. G., Munro, J. F., Kitchin, a. H., Muir, A. L., & Proudfoot, A. T. (1981). Pulmonary hypertension and fenfluramine. British Medical Journal, 283, 881-883.

Ferguson, J. M., & Feighner, U. P. (1987). Fluoxetine-induced weight loss in over-weight non-depressed humans. International Journal of Obesity, 11(suppl 1), 163-170.

Finer, N., Craddock, D., Lavielle, R. & Keen, H. (1988). Effect of 6 months therapy with dexfenfluramine in obese patients: Studies in the United Kingdon. Clinical Neuropharmacology, 11(suppl 1), S179-S186.

Gray, D. S., Fujioka,K. Devine, W., & Bray, G. A. (1992). Fluoxetine treatment of the obese diabetic. International Journal of Obesity, in press.

Griffiths, R. R., Brady, J. V., & Bradford, L. D. (1979). Predicting the abuse liability of drugs with animal drug self-administration prodecures: Psychomotor stimulants and hallucinogens. Advances in Behavioral Pharmacology, 2, 163-208.

Guy-Grand, B. Apfelbaum, M., Crepaldi, G. Gries, A., Lefebvre, P. & Turner, P. (1989). International trial of long-term dexfenfluramine in obesity. Lancet, 2, 1142.

Levine, L. R., Enas, G. G., Thompson, W. L., Byyny, R. L., Dauer, A. D., Kirby, R. W., Kreindle, T. G., Levy, B. Lucas, C. P., & McIlwain, H. H., (1989). Use of fluoxetine, a selective serotonin-uptake inhibitor, in the treatment of obesity-a dose response study. International Journal of Obesity, 13(5), 635-645.

McMurray, J., Bloomsfield, P, & Miller, H. C. (1986). Irreversible pulmonary hypertension after treatment with fenfluramine. British Medical Journal, 292, 239-240.

NIH Consensus Development Conference Statement. (1985). Health implications of obesity. Annals of Internal Medicine, 103, 1973-1077.

Pouwels, H. M., Smeets, J. L., Cheriex, E. C., & Wouters, E. F. (1990). Pulmonary hypertension and fenfluramine. European Respiratory Journal, 3, 606-607.

Scoville, B. A. (1975). Review of amphetamine-like drugs by the Food and Drug Administration: Clinical data and value judgements. In: Obesity in Perspective DHEW Publ No (NIH), Ed. G. A. Bray, Bethesda, Maryland, 75-708, 441-443.

Weintraub, M., & Bray, G. A. (1989). Drug treatment of obesity. Medical Clinics of North America, 73, 237-250.

Weintraub, M., Fundaresan, P. R., Schuster, B., Ginsberg, G., Madan, M. Stein, E., C., et al. (1992). National Heart, Lung and Blood Institute long-term weight control study: I-VII. Clinical Pharmacology and Therapeutics, in press.

PREDICTING TREATMENT OUTCOME, GENETICS, NEUROENDOCRINOLOGY, AND METHODOLOGICAL ISSUES

Stanley Heshka

Obesity Research Center
St. Luke's/Roosevelt Hospital
Columbia University College of
Physicians and Surgeons
New York, NY 10025

There is general agreement that our present obesity treatment methods are, by and large, unsatisfactory. Our aim is to bring together people to identify research questions, the answers to which help us develop better, more effective treatments. Each of us, I hope, will leave this meeting with a somewhat sharper and more focused idea about exactly what kind of research, and in what way our own research, could contribute to resolving the present shortcomings.

When they analyze behavior problems, psychologists like to think in terms of a behavioral equation formulated by Kurt Lewin in the 1940's. He noted that behavior is a joint function of the organism and the environment (Lewin, 1936). Over the past two days we've been looking at various parts of this equation as it relates to obesity treatment. We have looked at the behaviors which are the goals of our change efforts. These behaviors include dietary restraint and increased physical exercise which result in a lower body weight. We have noticed immediately a tremendous shortcoming in what we know and what we can do. If we exclude those people who are massively obese or who have very high BMI's, and those people with co-morbid conditions, then the fact is that we do not know whether we should intervene with these individuals or not. The data are conflicting. It seems that in the short term, there are improvements in health indicators. One would think that a period of time spent with lower serum lipids, lower blood pressure and a lower body weight might produce less wear and tear on the joints and have some long-term beneficial effect.

In fact, the epidemiological studies are not at all clear in confirming this. Some of them show that weight stability or changes of less then a few kilograms have the best long term association with survival (Lissner, Odell, D'Agostino, et al. 1991). Other studies on weight variability seem to suggest that variation in weight is not beneficial (Wing, 1992). Given that our treatment outcomes at the moment are not producing permanent changes, the obvious question in need of an answer is, should we intervene with these people at all, or should we leave them alone and at the very least, do no harm? This is something that I hope those who have access to relevant data or who are in a position to mount a study which would investigate the issue of weight variability, will undertake with great urgency.

Obesity Treatment, Edited by D.B. Allison
and F.X. Pi-Sunyer, Plenum Press, New York, 1995

We have also looked at the other side of the behavioral equation -- the organism in the environment. In regard to the organism, we heard from Dr. Weintraub about a long-term study of a medication which modifies the organism. He was the principle investigator on what has been, to this date, the longest medication study (Weintraub, 1992). As we saw, the results that Dr. Weintraub presented were less then entirely satisfactory. There were a large number of non-responders and, over a long period of time, there was weight regain. We clearly need additional long-term studies on medication and whether or not that is a viable method of producing enduring weight loss.

On the environmental part of the behavioral equation, we have had reports from researchers who do behavior modification, which presumably achieves its effects by modifying the environment and by altering the contingencies between the cues in the environment and the reward structure or consequences of the actions of the organism. It appears that a large part of our efforts in that field have consisted of "harassing" the organism. We have not been able to find clever, effective ways to make permanent changes in the environment which would sustain the dietary practices and physical activity to maintain a lower weight. Clearly, we need ingenious, creative work in that field to find some way to maintain these changes over long periods of time.

Today we are going to continue with our main theme. It is a truism that treatment should be tailored to the patient. In our field it is not clear that we know how to do this. Must we proceed in a stepwise fashion, trying one thing after another until we finally find something that works? Or might we be able to find some way of predicting at the outset who will be successful, or at least relatively successful, and with what mode of treatment? If we can make such predictions, what modes of treatment are availabe? On the other hand, if we cannot predict, why not? Why is it that we have been unsuccessful in finding predictors of success and what can we do about it? Or, is this a problem that can not be solved? After examining this, we will look at two promising lines of research to see what they have to say about maximizing our treatment outcomes and effectiveness. These are the topics of the genetic component of obesity and some recent work in neuroendocrinology. Finally, we will call upon some experts in data analysis to comment and to make suggestions as to how we can take our incomplete data with all of its missing values and error variability and try to draw valid conclusions from it. If the data have tremendous inadequacies suggestions will be made as to how we might collect data differently given the nature of the problems that we are trying to study. Perhaps these individuals will to try to wean us from the canned computer programs and statistical packages which we routinely use, such as the T-tests and the analyses of variance, in favor of something more creative.

REFERENCES

Lewin, K. (1936). A Dynamic Theory of Personality. NY, McGraw Hill.

Lissner, L., Odell, R. M., D'Agostino, R. B., et al. (1991). Variability of body weght and health otcomes in the Framingham population. New England Journal of Medicine, 324, 1839-1844.

Weintraub, M., Fundaresan, P. R., Schuster, B., Ginsberg, G., Madan, M., Stein, E. C., et al. (1992). National Heart, Lung and Blood Institute long-term weight control study: I-VII. Clinical Pharmacological Therapy.

Wing. R. (1992). Weight cycling in humans: A review of the literature. Annals of Behavioral Medicine, 14(2), 113-116.

BEHAVIORAL AND PSYCHOLOGICAL PREDICTORS OF TREATMENT OUTCOME IN OBESITY

G. Terence Wilson

Rutgers University
Busch Campus
PO Box 819
Piscataway, NJ 08855-0819

The identification of predictor variables in the treatment of obese patients can focus on four separate albeit related facets: attrition during treatment; short-term weight loss; long-term weight loss; and changes in maladaptive lifestyle behaviors associated with obesity, such as high fat intake, physical inactivity, and binge eating.

Identifying predictor variables in the treatment of any clinical disorder is predicated on the assumption that there is variability in outcome. In the case of obesity the following revision of the classic Stunkard (1958) edict holds: most patients will stay in treatment. Of those who do, most will lose weight by treatment end. Of treatment responders, roughly two-thirds will maintain weight loss over the next 1 to 2 years. Of those who lose weight, virtually all will regain it within 3 to 5 years. As such, it is useful to search for predictors of attrition during treatment and short-term weight loss. There is hardly any variance in long-term outcome, however. Following even the most comprehensive and sophisticated dietary and behavioral treatments, virtually all obese patients inexorably regain all of the weight they had lost during treatment at three and five year follow-up (Garner & Wooley, 1991; Wadden et al., 1989). In other words, response to dietary and behavioral treatments can be predicted. Irrespective of patient characteristics or treatment processes, the majority of patients fail to show long-term weight loss. With respect to attrition and short-term effects, three classes of variables are potential predictors of treatment outcome: pretreatment patient characteristics; process variables correlated with weight loss and maintenance; and treatment features that produce differential effects.

PRETREATMENT PATIENT CHARACTERISTICS

Behavioral Variables

Weight Cycling. Brownell et al.'s (1986) initial study showed that a cycle of weight loss and regain made it more difficult for rats to lose weight on a second equally restricted diet. Consistent with these data, Blackburn et al. (1989) found that obese patients lost weight more slowly the second time they received the same restricted diet. Other studies have failed to replicate these effects (Wing, 1992). For example, Wadden, Bartlett, et al. (1992) showed that patients who recalled a history of weight cycling fared as well as those who did in a six month combined VLCD and behavioral treatment program. There is no reliable effect of a history of weight cycling.

Dietary Restraint. There is an extensive and complex literature linking patterns of dietary restraint to anomalies in eating behavior in the laboratory, including apparent loss of control over intake which has been viewed as an analogue of binge eating (Polivy & Herman, 1985). One of the problems in this field is that different measures of this concept predict different eating patterns (Lowe, 1993). None has been shown to predict treatment outcome reliably. Herman and Polivy's Restraint Scale is unrelated to treatment outcome (Stuart & Guire, 1978). The data on the predictive value of the cognitive restraint scale of Stunkard and Messick's (1985) Three Factor Eating Questionnaire (TFEQ) are mixed (Wadden & Letizia, 1992). Dietary restraint is not a unitary construct (Lowe, 1993), and Westenhoefer (1991) has subdivided the cognitive restraint scale of the TFEQ into "rigid control" and "flexible control." The latter, but not the former, has been associated with successful weight loss (Pudel & Westenhoefer, 1992).

Binge Eating. Clinical lore has long held that binge eating is a negative prognostic factor in weight control treatment (Wilson, 1976). This view has been put forward as evidence of the predictive validity of the newly proposed DSM-IV diagnosis of binge eating disorder (BED) (Spitzer et al., 1992). Nevertheless, the majority of studies to date have failed to show the purported negative effects of binge eating (Brody et al., 1993; deZwaan et al., 1992; Dubbert & Wilson, 1974; Marcus et al., 1990; Schlundt et al., 1991; Telch & Agras, 1993; Wadden et al., 1992; Yanovski & Sebring, 1994). Marcus et al. (1988) reported greater relapse in obese binge eaters at 6 month follow-up, but not at posttreatment or 12 month follow-up. The only two studies that have shown that binge eating affects posttreatment weight loss had methodological shortcomings (Beliard et al., 1992; Keefe et al., 1984). Therefore, it must be concluded that binge eating has not relably been shown to be a predictor of treatment outcome in obese patients. (Parenthetically, obese binge eaters consistently report a greater history of weight cycling compared with non-bingers. The absence of a reliable difference between the two groups casts still further doubt on the predictive value of weight cycling. The same logic applies to the Disinhibition scale of the TFEQ, on which binge eaters score significantly higher than non-bingers [Yanovski, in press]).

Future research should focus more broadly on different forms of overeating rather than solely on the much-publicized BED criteria (Fairburn et al., 1992). For example, Wadden et al. (in press) found that overeating (without the sense of loss of control that helps define binge eating) but not binge eating was associated with greater drop-out rates. Using cluster analysis of two weeks of self-monitoring of eating habits, Schlundt et al. (1991) identified five different patterns in obese patients: chronic food restriction; alternating patterns of restriction and binge eating; emotional overeating; and unrestricted overeating. Significantly, the chronically restricting cluster had less lean body mass, lower resting metabolic rate, and higher waist-to-hip ratios than the unrestricted overeaters. Consistent with other research (Fitzgibbon & Kirschenbaum, 1991), the alternating dieting-binge eating cluster reported greater emotional distress than the other clusters. Nevertheless, over the course of behavioral treatment the different groups did not differ in drop-out rates, amount of weight lost, or exercise compliance. Underscoring the inconsistency in most of the literature on prediction of weight loss, the finding that emotional overeating cluster did not show greater problems with weight control conflicts with Blair et al.'s (1990) report to the contrary.

Psychological Variables

Personality Tests. Standardized personality measures fail to predict treatment outcome (Wilson, 1985).

Psychopathology. Despite data indicating that distressed patients have more problems in regulating food-related behavior (Fitzgibbon & Kirschenbaum, 1991; Schlundt et al., 1991), psychological distress seems to have no reliable effect on outcome (Cooke & Meyers, 1980). Beliard et al. (1992) found that the presence of a psychiatric diagnosis was unrelated to outcome. It was only when they created a composite psychopathology measure from three questionnaires (the Symptom Checklist, the Borderline Symptom Inventory, and the Binge Scale) that high levels of psychopathology were associated with poorer weight loss. The inconsistency in this literature is further illustrated the finding that pre-existing depression had different effects on weight loss in different studies by the same research group (Wadden & Letizia, 1992). Obese binge eaters have significantly greater psychiatric psychopathology than non-bingers, yet binge eating does not predict outcome. Yanovski (in press) has suggested that only a subgroup of obese binge eaters with a concomitant psychiatric disorder may be non-responders to treatment. This possibility remains to be explored.

Theory-Based Processes of Behavior Change. Speculation about psychological factors linked to understanding obesity has been endless. A more rational approach to finding predictor variables would be to examine the relation between well-established principles of behavior change and weight control treatments. Two examples of theory-based processes that have been shown to predict treatment-induced behavior change in other disorders are self-efficacy theory (Bandura, 1986) and the stages of change model (Prochaska et al., 1992).

In contrast to trait-like personality measures, ratings of self-efficacy reflect people's confidence that they can cope effectively in specific situations (e.g., resist eating [or overeating] when anxious). Patients' efficacy ratings have predicted short-term weight loss in several studies of dietary and behavioral treatments (e.g., Bernier & Avard, 1986; Clark et al., 1991; Edell et al., 1987). The effect is a modest one. Moreover, different studies have yielded variable findings concerning the specific nature of efficacy ratings that predict outcome (Stotland & Zuroff, 1991). In a study comparing several different psychological variables, Prochaska et al. (1992) found that self-efficacy was a less powerful significant predictor than other factors.

The stages of change model describes a series of phases through which people pass in the course of making a lifestyle change. In the precontemplation phase the individual is largely unaware of a problem and has
not considered the possibility of change. In the contemplation phase the individual is aware of a problem, but is ambivalent about addressing it directly. Motivation to do something about it wanes and waxes. The preparation stage marks a serious intention to attempt change. In the action stage efforts are made to change with or without therapeutic assistance. The maintenance stage involves the attempt to sustain behavior change over time. Relapse is an event that terminates the maintenance stage and triggers a recycling through the earlier stages. The model emphasizes that in the process of change, people cycle and recycle through the different stages before achieving a stable outcome. A recent study of the process of smoking cessation illustrates the utility of the model. Stage of change differences in smokers volunteering for a minimal intervention cessation program strongly predicted attempts to quit and cessation success at one and six month follow-ups (DiClemente et al., 1991).

Patients not in the preparation or action stage in the early sessions are likely to drop-out or fail to lose weight in behavioral treatment for obesity (Prochaska, 1993). The finding that the more committed and motivated patients fare better in treatment is neither new or surprising. Compliance with self-monitoring instructions, which marks motivation as noted below, has been a strong predictor of short-term success. This model fails to account for the universal lack of long-term success. Most patients in formal obesity programs complete treatment and lose weight. By definition, they have completed the action stage and should have passed into the maintenance stage. Yet weight is regained inexorably. The explanation is that unlike addictive behaviors such as cigarette smoking to which the model has been successfully applied, obesity is a chronic biological malfunction rather than a behavioral disorder (Wilson, 1993). Specific behaviors such as food intake and physical activity are only loosely related to weight control.

PROCESS VARIABLES CORRELATED WITH WEIGHT LOSS AND MAINTENANCE

Program Attendance

Not surprisingly, attendance at treatment sessions in dietary and behavioral programs is correlated with weight loss (Wadden & Letizia, 1992). No causal inference can be made. Attendance at treatment sessions may simply be a proxy for motivation.

Early Weight Loss

Weight loss in the first few sessions has been consistently and significantly associated with weight loss at the end of different dietary and behavioral treatments (Wadden & Letizia, 1992; Wilson, 1985). Patients who do not lose weight at the outset can be considered very poor risks for continued treatment.

Self-Monitoring

Patients who consistently self-monitor food intake fare better in treatment than those who are less compliant (Perri et al., 1989; Wilson, 1985). Although self-monitoring is arguably as potent a self-regulatory strategy as there is, it also reflects overall patient motivation. As is the case with early weight loss, patients who do not comply with instructions to self-monitor will almost certainly fail to respond to treatment.

Coping Strategies

In general, active problem-solving coping is more adaptive than more passive forms. It is therefore not surprising that successful maintenance of weight loss over two years was associated with the use of problem-focused rather than emotion-focused coping strategies (Kayman et al., 1990). The former entail problem-solving skills aimed at directly resolving challenging situations, whereas the latter involve ways of reducing emotional distress (perhaps by eating). The correlational nature of this study does not permit the inference that people who use specific coping strategies will necessarily maintain weight loss. Patients who maintained weight loss differed from those who did not on several variables, including exercise, the use of social support, and vigilance about eating. Grilo et al. (1992) examined the role of different coping strategies in response to situations linked to relapse. No advantage attached to any particular type of coping. What was significant in preventing relapse was an immediate coping response of some kind. As in other studies of the correlates of short-term maintenance of weight loss, causal connections cannot be made.

Exercise

Although evidence on the effect of exercise on initial weight loss is mixed, the correlation of exercise with maintenance of weight loss is a robust finding (Wadden & Letizia, 1992). The explanation of this positive association remains unknown.

TREATMENT FACTORS AFFECTING WEIGHT LOSS AND MAINTENANCE

Duration of Treatment

Longer behavioral treatment results in greater weight loss (Wadden & Bartlett, 1992). This effect is limited, however. Perri et al. (1989) extended their treatment program to 40 weeks. Subjects lost 9.9 kg during the first 20 weeks, but only an extra 3.6 kg from week 21 to 40 even though they remained clearly obese. Weight loss is not maintained in the long-term in part because it is not sufficiently reinforcing intrinsically to sustain the dietary restraint needed to continue a negative energy balance. External pressure is required, leading to calls for continual or lifelong dietary/behavioral "treatment" (Foreyt & Goodrick, 1991). The feasibility of this prospect is questionable (Wilson, 1993).

Type of Treatment

Differences between alternative treatments can be seen in short-term weight loss. For example, behavioral treatment combined with a VLCD is superior to the VLCD alone (Wadden & Bartlett, 1992). Nevertheless, all dietary and behavioral treatments appear equally ineffective in maintaining long-term weight loss (Garner & Wooley, 1991; Wilson, 1993). Continuous pharmacological treatment (fenfluramine) is the single most promising treatment for sustained long-term weight loss in moderate obesity (Bray, 1992; Guy-Grand, 1992; Weintraub, 1992). Surgery seems recommended for severely obese patients (Kral, 1992).

REFERENCES

Bandura, A. (1986). Social foundations of thought and action: Social cognitive theory. Englewood Cliffs, NJ: Prentice-Hall, Inc.

Beliard, D., Kirschenbaum, D. S., & Fitzgibbon, M. L. (1992). Evaluation of an intensive weight control program using a priori criteria to determine outcome. International Journal of Obesity, 16, 1-13.

Bernier, M., & Avard, J. (1986). Self-efficacy, outcome, and attrition in a weight-reduction program. Cognitive Therapy and Research, 10, 319-338.

Blackburn, G. L., Wilson, G. T., Kanders, B. S. et al. (1989). Weight cycling: The experience of human dieters. American Journal of Clinical Nutrition, 49, 1105-1109.

Blair, A. J., Lewis, V. J., & Booth, D. A. (1990). Does emotion eating interfere with success in attempts at weight control? Appetite, 15, 151-157.

Bray, G. A. (1992). Drug treatment of obesity. American Journal of Clinical Nutrition, 55, 538-544.

Brody, M., Walsh, B.T., & Devlin, M. (1993). Binge eating disorder: Reliability and validity of a new diagnostic category. Unpublished manuscript, Columbia University.

Brownell, K. D., Greenwood, M. R. C., Stellar, E., Shrager, E. E. (1986). The effects of repeated cycles of weight loss and regain in rats. Physiology and Behavior, 38, 459-464.

Clark, M. C., Abrams, D. B., & Niaura, R. S. (1991). Self-efficacy in weight management. Journal of Consulting and Clinical Psychology, 59, 739-744.

Cooke, C. J., & Meyers, A. (1980). Assessment of subject characteristics in the behavioral treatment of obesity. Behavior Assessment, 2, 59-70.

deZwaan, M., Nutzinger, D.O., & Schoenbeck, G. (1992). Binge eating in overweight women. Comprehensive Psychiatry, 33, 256-261.

DiClemente, C. C., Prochaska, J. O., Fairhurst, S. K., Velicer, W. F., Velasquez, M. M., & Rossi, J. S. (1991). The process of smoking cessation: An analysis of precontemplation, contemplation, and preparation stages of change. Journal of Consulting and Clinical Psychology, 59, 295-304.

Dubbert, P.M., & Wilson, G.T. (1984). Goal setting and spouse involvement in the treatment of obesity. Behaviour Research and Therapy, 22, 227-242.

Edell, B. H., Edinton, S., Herd, B., O'Brien, R. M., & Witkin, G. (1987). Self-efficacy and self-weight loss in family-based behavior modification program. Journal of Consulting and Clinical Psychology, 5, 674-685.

Fairburn, C. G., Welch, S. L., & Hay, P. J. (1993). The classification of recurrent overeating: The "Binge Eating Disorder" proposal. International Journal of Eating Disorders, 13, 155-160.

Fitzgibbon, M. L., & Kirschenbaum, D. S. (1991). Distressed binge eaters as a distinct subgroup among obese individuals. Addictive Behaviors, 16, 441-451.

Foreyt, J. P., & Goodrick, G. K. (1991). Factors common to successful therapy for the obese patient. Medicine and Science in Sports and Exercise, 23, 292-297.

Garner, D. M., & Wooley, S. C. (1991). Confronting the failure of behavioral and dietary treatments for obesity. Clinical Psychology Review, 11, 729-780.

Grilo, C.M., Shiffman, S., & Wing, R. (1992). Dieters' strategies for coping with relapse crises. Paper presented at 26th Annual Meeting of the Association for Advancement of Behavior therapy, Boston, November.

Guy-Grand, B., Apfelbaum, M., Crepaldi, G., Gries, A., Lefebvre, P., Turner, P. (1992). International trial of long-term dexfenfluramine in obesity. Lancet, 2, 1142-1144.

Kayman, S., Bruvold, W., & Stern, J. (1990). Maintenance and relapse after weight loss in women: Behavioral aspects. American Journal of Clinical Nutrition, 52, 800-807.

Keefe, P. H., Wyshogrod, D., Weinberger, E., & Agras, W. S. (1984). Binge eating and outcome of behavioral treatment in obesity: A preliminary report. Behaviour Research and Therapy, 22, 319-321.

Kral, J. G. (1992). Surgical treatment of obesity. In T. A. Wadden & T. B. VanItallie (Eds.), Treatment of the seriously obese patient. New York: Guilford Press.

Lowe, M.R. (1993). The effects of dieting on eating behavior: a three-factor model. Psychological Bulletin, 114, 100-121.

Marcus, M.D., Wing, R.R., & Hopkins, J. (1988). Obese binge eaters: Affect, cognitions, and response to behavioral weight control. Journal of Consulting and Clinical Psychology, 56, 433-439.

Marcus, M. D., Wing, R. R., Ewing, L., Kern, E., Gooding, W., & McDermott, M. (1990). Psychiatric disorders among obese binge eaters. International Journal of Eating Disorders, 9, 69-77.

Perri, M. G., Nezu, A. M., Patti, E. T., & McCann, K. L. (1989). Effect of length of treatment on weight loss. Journal of Consulting and Clinical Psychology, 57, 450-454.

Polivy, J., & Herman, C. P. (1985). Dieting and bingeing: A causal analysis. American Psychologist, 40, 193-201.

Prochaska, J.O. (1993). Working in harmony with how people change naturally. The Weight Control Digest, 3, 249-254.

Prochaska, J. O., Norcross, J. C., Fowler, J. L., Follick, J., & Abrams, D. B. (1992). Attendance and outcome in a work site weight control program: Processes and stages of change as process and predictor variables. Addictive Behaviors, 17, 35-45.

Schlundt, D. G., Taylor, D., Hill, J. O., Sbrocco, T., Pope-Cordle, J., Kasser, T., & Arnold D. (1991). A behavioral taxonomy of obese female participants in a weight-loss program. American Journal of Clinical Nutrition, 109.

Spitzer, R. L., Devlin, M., Walsh, B. T., Hasin, D., Wing, R., Marcus, M., Stunkard, A., Wadden, T., Yanovski, S., Agras, S., Mitchell, J., & Nonas, C. (1992). Binge eating disorders: A multi-site field trial of the diagnostic criteria. International Journal of Eating Disorders, 11, 191-203.

Stotland, S., & Zuroff, D. C. (1991). Relations between multiple measures of dieting self-efficacy and weight change in a behavioral weight control program. Behavior Therapy, 22, 47-59.

Stuart, R.B., & Guire, K. (1978). Some correlates of the maintenance of weight loss through behavior modification. International Journal of Obesity, 2, 225-235.

Stunkard, A.J. & Messick, S. (1985). The three-factor eating questionnaire to measure dietary restraint and hunger. Journal of Psychosomatic Research, 29, 71-83.

Telch, C.F., & Agras, W.S. (1993). The effects of a very low calorie diet on binge eating. Behavior Therapy, 24, 177-194.

Wadden, T. A., & Bartlett, S. J. (1992). Very low calorie diets: An overview and appraisal. In T. A. Wadden & T. B. VanItallie (Eds.). Treatment of the seriously obese patient (pp. 44-79). New York: Guilford Press.

Wadden, T. A., Bartlett, S., Letizia, K. A., et al. (1992). Relationship of dieting history to resting metabolic rate, body composition, eating behavior and subsequent weight loss. American Journal of Clinical Nutrition , 56, 2065-2115.

Wadden, T. A., Foster, G. D., & Letizia, K. A. (1992). Response of obese binge eaters to treatment by behavioral therapy combined with very low calorie diet. Journal of Consulting and Clinical Psychology, 60, 808-811.

Wadden, T. A., & Letizia, K. A. (1992). Predictors of attrition and weight loss in patients treated by moderate and severe caloric restriction. In T. A. Wadden & T. B. VanItallie (Eds.). Treatment of the seriously obese patient (pp. 383-410).

Wadden, T. A., Sternberg, J. A., Letizia, K. A., Stunkard, A. J., & Foster, G. D. (1989). Treatment of obesity by very low calorie diet, behavior therapy, and their combination: A five-year perspective. International Journal of Obesity, 13, 39-46

Weintraub, M. (1992). Long-term weight control: The National Heart, Lung, and Blood Institute funded multimodal intervention study. Clinical Pharmacological Therapy, 51, 581-646.

Westenhoefer, J. (1991). Dietary restraint and disinhibition: Is restraint a homogeneous construct? Appetite, 16, 45-55.

Wilson, G.T. (1976). Obesity, binge eating, and behavior therapy: Some clinical observations. Behavior Therapy, 7, 700-701.

Wilson, G.T. (1985). Psychological prognostic factors in the treatment of obesity. In J. Hirsch & T. Van Itallie (Eds.), Recent advances in obesity research, IV. London: John Libbey & Co.

Wilson, G.T. (1993). Behavioral treatment of obesity: Thirty years and counting. Advances in Behaviour Research and Therapy, 16, 31-75.

Wing, R. R. (1992). Weight cycling in humans: A review of the literature. Annals of Behavioral Medicine, 14, 113-119.

Yanovski, S. Z. (in press). Binge eating disorder: Current knowledge and future directions. Obesity Research.

Yanovski, S. Z., & Sebring, N. G. (1994). Recorded food intake of obese women with binge eating disorders before and after weight loss. International Journal of Eating Disorders, 15, 135-150.

PREDICTING TREATMENT OUTCOME:
WHY WE HAVE BEEN SO UNSUCCESSFUL

David B. Allison and Cheryl N. Engel

Obesity Research Center - St. Luke's/Roosevelt Hospital
Columbia University College of Physicians and Surgeons
New York, NY 10025

Following Dr. Wilson's paper (Wilson, this volume), we will discuss a bit more about prediction. From a somewhat more methodological point of view, we will explore some reasons why we have such trouble predicting treatment outcome.

First, why would one want to predict treatment outcome? One reason is to be able to supply treatment to those who will benefit and conversely, not supply it for those who will not benefit. Adequate predictors of treatment outcome might help resolve much of the disagreement between those who advocate weight loss and members of the "antidiet movement." Most would agree that there is no point in directing weight loss efforts at those for whom attempts at weight loss are completely futile, while there is a point concerning those for whom treatment might be successful. Moreover, a good predictor allows one to reduce iatrogenesis by withholding treatment from those who will not benefit. Finally, a good predictor would allow treatment research to focus on the core group of individuals who are most resistant to current treatments, rather than on everyone, as is occurring now.

There are at least three outcomes one can try to predict. They include: 1) staying in treatment, 2) losing weight, and 3) maintaining weight losses. Staying in treatment may be one of the most important outcomes, because longer treatment seems to be more successful (Brownell & Wadden, 1986; Perri, Nezu, Patti, & McCann, 1989; Wadden & Bell, 1990). However, because there is not a great deal of research in either this area or regarding maintaining weight loss, we will focus primarily on losing weight, the area in which we have the most data.

A variety of predictors of treatment outcome have been tried (see Table 1), including demographic variables such as age, gender, and age of onset (Borden, 1974; McReynolds & Lutz, 1974; Stein, Hassanein, & Lukert, 1981), physiological predictors such as weight and glucose tolerance (Yang, 1988), and psychological predictors (Kelly, 1975). The particular types of psychological predictors that are used include measures like the Minnesota Multiphasic Personality Inventory (MMPI) and the Sixteen Personality Factor Questionnaire (16PF) (Johnson, Swenson, & Gastineau, 1976). The MMPI and the 16PF are large personality inventories or psychopathology inventories. In some sense, they are a psychologist's "shotgun,"

Table 1. Some Predictors of Treatment Outcome

Demographic	Physiological	Psychological
Age	Weight	MMPI
Gender	Glucose Tolerance	16PF
Age-at-Onset	Adipocyte Size	Locus-of-Control
Dieting History	Adipocyte Number	Self-efficacy
Marital Status	Adipose Tissue	Eating Behavior
Race	Distribution	Activity Patterns
Family History	Resting Metabolic Rate	Attitudes Toward Fat People

in that they measure a little bit of everything, while not necessarily measuring any one construct in an especially focused manner. This is an important point we will return to later.

PREVIOUS REVIEWS

We will now touch upon some reviews other researchers have presented. An older, very thorough review, Weiss (1977) suggested that "neither demographic, personality or personal weight measures have been shown to possess much predictive validity, with the possible exception of age of onset [later age of onset is associated with better outcomes] and locus of control" (p. 199). Because age of onset and locus of control are interesting to take note of, we will return to them later and discuss why these two measures might work in predicting treatment outcome.

Wilson and Dubbert (1983 and references therein) note that "despite attempts by numerous investigators to demonstrate a relationship between demographic, personality and behavioral variables and success or failure in weight reduction, reviewers are in agreement that the evidence for predictive utility of any of these variables is still inconsistent or equivocal" (p.272). Finally, Westover and Lanyon (1990) wrote a review in which they stated that across 22 studies, only 6 of 31 variables were shown to predict outcome in two or more studies. These six variables were 1) restricting caloric intake after treatment, 2) consistent exercise after treatment, 3) enrollment in further weight loss programs, 4) problem solving training, 5) regular weighing, and 6) client-therapist contact. Although not a particularly impressive showing, what is interesting are the types of variables found to replicate. These findings might be restated as "those people who do what their dieticians tell them to do, lose weight." Unfortunately, this is not a very informative statement. Although most people would agree with it, it does not predict which people will follow their dietician's advice.

POSSIBLE REASONS FOR OUR POOR PREDICTION

Given the consensus that we cannot really predict treatment outcome, it may be fruitful to explore some possible reasons for this. First it is possible that we can predict outcome, but we just do not realize it. Second, we may have relied too much on univariant methods and eschewed multivariant prediction. A third possibility is that we have failed to systematically replicate and validate our prediction models. A fourth is that we have problems with knowing when to use dimensional versus categorical predictors. The final two suggestions we have as to why we cannot predict treatment outcome are that we have failed to consider theory, and that we have failed to consider the possibility of attribute-treatment interactions. We will attempt to explain and discuss each of these in turn.

Possibility I. We Can Predict Outcome But Do Not Realize It

The following is a statement by Robert Rosenthal, a leader in the area of meta-analysis.

> *Poor cumulation does not seem to be due primarily to lack of replication or failure to recognize the need for replication. Indeed, the calls for further research with which we so frequently end our articles are carried wherever scholarly journals are read. It seems rather that we have been better at issuing such calls than at knowing what to do with the answers. (1991, p. 4)*

In science, many are quick to end their research reports with a statement that "more research is needed." Rosenthal argues that for many questions, more research is not needed. In many instances, if one simply compiled all of the studies done, one would have confidence intervals so tight that one would never need to study that question again. Unfortunately, this is not realized because data is often accumulated poorly.

Let us see what happens when this is done in the field of prediction. For illustration purposes, we will focus on locus of control. We choose locus of control for two reasons, the first being that it has been cited as something that may be a valid predictor (Weiss, 1977). Secondly, there have been many studies on locus of control and consequently, there is much data to work with. Locus of control is a construct that characterizes a person's way of viewing sources of reinforcement. An individual with an internal locus of control believes that outcomes tend to be under their own control. A person with an external locus of control tends to believe that outcomes are the result of powerful others or chance.

In Table 2, one can see eleven studies regarding locus of control as a predictor of weight loss. The association between locus of control has been converted to a correlation. Taking a weighted mean, a positive value of 0.19 is obtained. Given a total of 858 subjects, this is clearly a significant finding. This means that, on average, the correlation between locus of control and weight loss is 0.19, indicating that people with a more internal locus of control are more successful at losing weight.

However, as indicated by the significant value of the chi-square, this is also a heterogeneous finding and suggests that across studies, researchers are not all obtaining the

Table 2. A "Mini-Meta-Analysis" of Locus-of-Control as a Predictor of Weight Loss

Study	N	Result (r)
Nir & Neuman (1991)	113	+NS (.12)
Kincey (1981)	131	.28
Rodin et al. (1977)	204	-.03
Kincey (1983)	58	.31
Epstein et al. (1986)	41	NS*
Hartigan et al. (1982)	27	.62
Chavez & Michaels (1980)	43	.40
Cohen & Alpert (1978)	15	.60
Bolocofsky et al. (1984)	156	.31
Balch & Ross (1975)	34	+S (>.34)
Harris et al. (1980)	36	ND
	858 total	.19 weighted mean

Note. Hartigan et al. & Cohen et al. cluster together.
Chi-Square = 29.7, df=10, p<.001
Correlation between N and r=-.458
*NS = not significant

Table 3. Studies Predicting Weight Loss in "Behavioral" Programs with Multiple Regression

Study	N	k[1]	R
Bolocofsky et al. (1984)	78	25	0.68
Carroll et al. (1980)	24	11	0.64
Gormally et al. (1980)	40	6	0.51
Flanery & Kirschenbaum (1986)	23	25	0.61

[1]k is calculated as the total number of predictors tried, not necessarily the total number that were retained in the model.

same results. When one explores further, one finds that all of the heterogeneity is accounted for by the studies done by Cohen and Alpert (1978) and Hartigan, Baker-Strauch and Morris (1982), which yield higher correlations than the other studies, using more focused measures. These researchers were not just using measures of general locus of control but more specifically, weight locus of control and health locus of control.

These results suggest two things. First, "focused" predictors tend to work better than "shotgun" predictors. Second, when research is appropriately accumulated with meta-analytic techniques, one obtains clear evidence of the ability to predict treatment outcome. Unfortunately, treatment outcome is still predicted weakly, so that one only accounts for a small amount of the variance in weight loss.

Possibility II. Univariate versus Multivariate Prediction

Harold Yuker, one of our graduate professors, warned, "People aren't simple, don't do simple research." One needs to recognize that obesity and weight loss, like most human traits and behaviors, are multifactorial conditions. This suggests the use of multivariant prediction rather then univariant prediction. Table 3 displays multivarient prediction equations.

As can be seen, when using multivariant prediction one tends to get modest R's. These values average about 0.60 but are larger than the univariate r values typically seen. However, one should note that the N's are very small (Table 3) and the number of variables in the prediction equation, the k values, are very large. It is quite interesting to see that, in one case, k exceeds N. This is a statistician's worst nightmare. Moreover, no study cross validated their prediction equation. Using certain analytical formulae, one can compute the expected cross validity coefficient, known as a shrunken R^2, for these equations. Assuming that one used this equation in an independent sample and has used k predictors and N subjects, what is the expected R? The expected R is approximately zero for all of the equations in table 3. This is because they used too many predictors in relation to the number of subjects.

Possibility III. Dimensional versus Categorical Prediction

We will now look at dimensional versus categorical prediction, but in the interest of space, focus primarily on the advantages of dimensional prediction. The main advantage of the dimensional system, that is treating continua as continua and not dichotomizing them, is that statistical power is preserved. People often prefer to dichotomize continuous variables. For example, it is easier to say, "restrained eaters did this more than unrestrained eaters" than "people who tend to be higher in restraint tend to score higher on such and such." Unfortunately, dichotomizing results in a considerable loss of power.

To illustrate this, consider a hypothetical correlation coefficient between a predictor and an outcome, with the predictor being restrained eating and the outcome being weight loss. Assume that the r is 0.50, with an r^2 of 0.25. If one were to dichotomize the predictor at the median, (assuming the distribution is normal, this is also at the mean) half of the subjects are "high," and the other half are "low," and the resulting r value will be reduced to about 0.40 and the r^2 to about 0.16. As this "effect size" drops, the power drops correspondingly. The situation worsens when one classifies "high" as two standard deviations above the mean, a common criterion for "abnormal." If one takes anywhere from two standard deviations above the mean and calls that "high," while all other values are considered "low," the r value is less than 0.20 and one is explaining less than 4% of the variance even though the actual r explains 25%. In other words, any chance of having a reasonably powered study is destroyed. Consequently, one may conduct the study and fail to find an effect even though there is one. Alternatively, if one increases the power with a large enough N, one will find an effect and conclude that it accounts for only 2% of the variance when, in fact, it really accounts for 25% of the variance. In sum, if we can keep continuous variables continuous in our studies, we are likely to increase power, increase effect size, and predict more successfully.

Possibility IV. Failure to Consider Theory

In our opinion, the most important reason for the lack of ability to predict outcome may be a general failure to consider theory. The literature is pervaded with papers about prediction (e.g. Barnstuble, Kesges, & Terbizan, 1986; Bonato & Boland, 1987; Abrams, 1991;) yet, it seems rare to read one by a researcher who set out initially to do a study of prediction and thought to randomize people to a weight loss trial and measure putative predictors to see if they predict weight loss. Rather, many people seem to go back into their file cabinets after the fact and publish something that has been sitting around, rather then utilizing more theoretical prediction. In the absence of theory, most past attempts at prediction can be seem as simply data dredging. One should not expect them to replicate and in fact, it would be surprising if they did on a regular basis. In the absence of theory, there is little reason to expect things fortuitously found in one situation to be effective in another.

Now, in order to use theory to make predictions, one must have a theory. So, let us look at what we know about theory. We may not have many strong theories of obesity, but we do know in a very broad sense that there is a genetic component and that there is an environmental component. From our reading of the data, the genetic component explains about 60-70% of the within population phenotype variance (Stunkard, Harris, Pederson & McClearn, 1990; Allison, Heshka, Neale, Lykken, & Heymsfield, in press). It is also known that the most important of the environmental components seem to be fleeting and tend to be unique environmental components, rather than shared familial environmental components (Fabitz, Carmelli & Hewitt, 1992). The environment that influences an individual at Time 1 does not seem to be active at Time 2, when new environmental influences are at play. Therefore, if one wants to look at environmental influences one must look at aspects of the current environment and look at them continuously.

The above suggests if the past environment is not crucial, then the current environment is and therefore, environmental malleability may be important. Rena Wing (this volume) has told us that as good behavior modifiers, we need to modify the environment, not the individual. Instead of asking questions with the 16PF and the MMPI about the individual, perhaps we need to ask questions about the environment. In other words, one must "give the environment a questionnaire." However, it is not immediately clear how to give an environment a questionnaire. In this light, it is interesting that locus of control, as mentioned earlier, is one of the few constructs that is a reliable predictor of treatment outcome. Perhaps, when people say they have some expectancy for success, they could be saying something about their environment. That is, we may be indirectly tapping a notion they have that their environment is somehow malleable. If one can find people who are in situations where they do have some control of their environment or in which their environment could be intervened upon, one would have greater success in producing weight loss. This is a promising direction for the future.

The degree of genetic liability for obesity may also be an important factor. We know that a large genetic component is involved (Stunkard, Harris, Pedersen, & McClearn, 1990). We are frequently reminded that genetics does not mean predetermination, but rather predisposition. However, we are probably misleading ourselves if we think that someone with an enormous genetic push toward obesity can just as easily make a choice not to be obese as someone without such a push. When it is possible to quantify genetic liability, we might be able to use genetic liability as a predictor.

Until then, one might draw on the work of Price and his colleagues, suggesting that early onset obesity is a marker for familial obesity (Price, Stunkard, Ness, Wadden, Heshka, Kanders & Cormillot, 1990). This information and the possibility that age of onset is a predictor of outcome, implies that genetics are involved. Returning to the treatment setting, a genetic liability by environmental malleability interaction might be important, in that those people who have a low genetic liability are likely to have a high environmental influence on their obesity. If one can identify people who have a high environmental influence and have a malleable environment, then perhaps one could accurately predict that they will be successful in losing weight. This hypothesis remains to be tested.

Possibility V. Failure to Consider Attribute-Treatment Interactions

The last reason we would like to consider is the failure to consider attribute treatment interactions. The idea of the attribute treatment interaction is that no one treatment works equally well for everyone. Many people have discussed the heterogeneity of obesity (Allison & Heshka, 1991, 1992) however, it is difficult to know how to place some people into one treatment and some people into another. Unfortunately, there is little research regarding any attempt to target specific treatments to specific kinds of individuals to see if differential effects are attainable.

From what little research there is in this area, we will discuss two particular studies (Renjilian, Perri, Nezu, McKelvey & Schein, 1990; Murray, 1976). Although not quite a traditional attribute treatment interaction, this study illustrates our point. Seventy-five obese people were assigned to 1 of 4 groups. All were asked whether they preferred group therapy or individual therapy. Half of those who expressed a preference for individual therapy were placed in individual therapy and the other half were placed in group therapy. Of those who preferred group therapy, half were placed in group therapy while the remaining half were placed in individual therapy.

One would expect that people who preferred group therapy and received it should have better results than those people who preferred group therapy and did not, and visa versa. However, there was no such "attribute-treatment interaction" at all in this study, an all too common occurrence (Dance & Neufeld, 1988). Interestingly, there was a significant and fairly large main effect favoring group therapy over individual therapy. Regardless of what people preferred, group therapy was more successful in promoting weight loss.

In the last study we will discuss, 12 overweight females were asked if they prefer self-control training or treatment involving increasing determination to lose weight and motivation coaching (Murray, 1976). Both groups lost a significant amount of weight regardless of which group they were in or their preference.

Unfortunately, because the power was low (with an N of only 12) one may make only the most tentative conclusions. There was no significant interaction, but the probability of Type-II error is high. So stands the stage of the research on attribute interactions. Obviously, this area is in need of further study.

CONCLUSION

We would like to conclude with the idea that if outcome is to be predictable, what we need in this field is a better accumulation of findings. We need well-designed multivarient studies in which we recognize the complexity of people and allow for multiple factors to be important. Of course, we need to systematically validate our prediction equations to determine whether or not they hold true in more than one instance. We need to make intelligent and explicit decisions as to whether predictors would be treated as dimensional or categorical. It is markedly inappropriate to continue to simply cut-off dimensional variables in research without an extremely strong rationale based on both data and theory.

Most importantly, we need to have theoretically based predictors. We need to think about what we know about psychology, physiology, and genetics, and use that information in trying to predict outcome. Finally, we need well-designed, sophisticated research on evaluating potential attribute-treatment interactions.

REFERENCES

Abrams, M. (1991). The eating disorder inventory as a predictor of compliance in a behavioral weight-loss program. International Journal of Eating Disorders, 10(3), 355-360.

Allison, D. B. (in press). Methodological Issues in Obesity Research with Examples from Biometrical Genetics. Proceedings of the symposium Obesity and Weight Control Advances in the Medical and Psychosocial Management of the Nation's Most Prevalent Life-Threatening Illness. Charles Press.

Allison, D. B., & Heshka, S. (1991). Toward an empirically derived typology of obese persons. International Journal of Obesity, 15, 741-754.

Allison, D. B., & Heshka, S. (1992). Toward an empirically derived typology of obese persons: Derivation in a nonclinical sample. International Journal of Eating Disorders, 13, 9: 108.

Allison, D. B., Heshka, S., Neale, M. C., Lykken, D. T., & Heymsfield, S. B. (in press). A genetic analysis of weight residualized for height among 4020 twin pairs with an emphasis on sex specific effects. Health Psychology.

Allison, D. B., Neale, M. C., Heshka, S., & Heymsfield, S. B. (in press). Race effects in the genetics of adolescents' body mass index. International Journal of Obesity.

Balch, P., & Ross, A. W. (1975). Predicting success in weight reduction as a function of locus of control: A unidimensional and multidimensional approach. Journal of Consulting and Clinical Psychology, 43, 119.

Barnstuble, J. A., Klesges, R. C., & Terbizan, D. (1986). Brief reports: Predictors of weight loss in a behavioral treatment program. Behavior Therapy, 17, 288-294.

Bolocofsky, D. N., Coulthard-Morris, L., & Spinler, D. (1984). Prediction of successful weight management from personality and demographic data. Psychological Reports, 55, 795-802.

Bonata, D. P., & Boland, F. J. (1987). Predictors of weight loss at the end of treatment and 1-year follow-up for a behavioral weight loss program. International Journal of Eating Disorders, 6(4), 573-577.

Borden, B. L. (1974). Variables related to success in the behavioral treatment of obesity. Paper presented at the annual meeting of the Western Psychological Association, San Francisco, CA.

Brownell, K. D., & Wadden, T. A. (1986). Behavior therapy for obesity: Modern approaches and better results. In K. D. Brownell & J. P. Foreyt (Eds.), Handbook of eating disorders: Physiology, psychology, and treatment of obesity, anorexia, and bulimia (pp. 180-197). New York: Basic Books.

Brownell, K. D., & Wadden, T. A. (1991). The heterogeneity of obesity: Fitting treatments to individuals. Behavior Therapy, 22, 153-177.

Carroll, L. J., Yates, B. T., & Gray, J. J. (1980). Predicting obesity reduction in behavioral and nonbehavioral therapy from client characteristics: The self-evaluation measure. Behavior Therapy, 11, 189-197.

Chavez, E. L., & Michaels, A. C. (1980). Evaluation of the health locus of control for obesity treatment. Psychological Reports, 47, 709-710.

Cohen, N. L., & Alpert, M. (1978). Locus of control as a predictor of outcome in treatment of obesity. Psychological Reports, 42, 805-806.

Dance, K. A., & Neufeld, R. W. (1988). Aptitude-treatment interaction research in the clinical setting: A review of attempts to dispel the "patient uniformity" myth. Psychological Bulletin, 104(2), 192-213.

Dubbert, P. M., & Wilson, T. (1983). Failures in behavior therapy for obesity: Causes, correlates, and consequences. In E. B. Foa, & P. M. G. Emmelkamp (Eds.), Failures in Behavioral Therapy (pp. 263-288). New York: John, & Wiley, & Sons.

Epstein, L. H., Wing, R. R., Koeske, R., & Waloski, A. (1986). Effect of parent weight on weight loss in obese children. Journal of Consulting and Clinical Psychology, 54(3), 400-401.

Fabsitz, R. R., Carmelli, D., & Hewitt, J. K. (1992). Evidence for independent genetic influences on obesity in middle age. International Journal of Obesity, 16, 657-666.

Flanery, R. C., & Kirschenbaum, D. S. (1986). Dispositional and situational correlates of long- term weight reduction in obese children. Addictive Behaviors, 11, 249-261.

Gormally, J., Rardin, D., & Black, S. (1980). Correlates of successful response to a behavioral weight control clinic. Journal of Counseling Psychology, 27(2), 179-191.

Harris, M. B., Sutton, M., Kaufman, E. M., & Carmichael, C. W. (1980). Correlates of success and retention in a multifaceted, long-term behavior modification program for obese adolescent girls. Addictive Behaviors, 5, 25-34.

Hartigan, K. J., Baker-Strauch, D., & Morris, G. W. (1982). Perceptions of the causes of obesity and responsiveness to treatment. Journal of Counseling Psychology, 29(5), 478-485.

Johnson, S. F., Swenson, W. M., & Gastineau, C. F. (1976). Personality characteristics in obesity: Relation of MMPI profile and age of onset of obesity to success in weight reduction. The American Journal of Clinical Nutrition, 29, 626-632.

Kelly, A. H. (1975). A comparison of learning-theory based approaches in the treatment of obesity. Dissertation Abstracts International, 36, 912 B. (University Microfilms No. 75-17, 225).

Kincey, J. (1981). Internal-external control and weight loss in the obese: Predictive and discriminant validity and some possible clinical implications. Journal of Clinical Psychology, 37(1), 100-103.

Kincey, J. (1983). Compliance with a behavioural weight-loss programme: Target setting and locus of control. Behavioral Research and Therapy, 21(2), 109-114.

McRenolds, W. T., & Lutz, R. N. (1974). Weight loss resulting from two behavioral modification procedures with nutritionists as therapists. Paper presented at the annual convention of the Association for the Advancement of Behavior Therapy, Chicago, IL.

Murray, D. C. (1976). Preferred versus nonpreferred treatment, and self-control training versus determination raising as treatments of obesity: A pilot study. Psychological Reports, 38(1), 191-198.

Nir, Z. & Neumann, L. (1991). Self-esteem, internal-external locus of control, and their relationship to weight reduction. Journal of Clinical Psychology, 47(4), 568-575.

Perri, M. G., Nezu, A. M., Patte, E. T., & McCann, K. L. (1989). Effect of length of treatment on weight loss. Journal of Consulting and Clinical Psychology, 57, 450-454.

Price, R. A., Stunkard, A. J., Ness, R. Wadden, T., Heshka, S., Kanders, B., & Cormillot, A. (1990). Childhood onset (age < 10) obesity has a high familial risk. International Journal of Obesity, 14, 185-195.

Renjilian, D. A., Perri, M. G., Mezu, A. M., McKelvey, W. F., & Schein, R. L. (1990). Individual versus group therapy for obesity: Matching clients with treatments. Paper presented at the American Psychological Association Convention, Boston, MA.

Rodin, J., Bray, G. A., Atkinson, R. L., Dahms, W. T., Greenway, F. L., Hamilton, K., & Molitch, M. (1977). Predictors of successful weight loss in an outpatient obesity clinic. International Journal of Obesity, 1, 79-87.

Rosenthal, R. (1991). Meta-Analysis Procedures for Social Research. Newbury Park, CA: Sage.

Stein, P. M., Hassanein, R. S., & Lukert, B. P. (1981). Predicting weight loss success among obese clients in a hospital nutrition clinic. The American Journal of Clinical Nutrition, 34, 2039-2044.

Stunkard, A. J., Harris, J. R., Pedersen, N. L., & McClearn, G. E. (1991). The body-mass index of twins who have been reared apart. New England Journal of Medicine, 322, 1483-1487.

Wadden, T. A., & Bell, S. J. (1990). Obesity. In A. S. Bellack, M. Hersen, & A. E. Kazdin (eds.), International handbook of behavior modification and therapy (2nd ed.) (pp. 449-473). New York: Plenum.

Weiss, A. (1977). Characteristics of successful weight reducers: A brief review of predictor variables. Addictive Behaviors, 2, 193-201.

Westover, S., & Lanyon, R. (1990). The maintenance of weight loss after behavioral treatment. Behavior Modification, 14, 123-127.

Yang, M. U. (1988). Body composition and resting metabolic rate in obesity. In R. T Frankle & M. U. Yang (Eds.), Obesity and weight control (pp. 71-96). Rockville, MD: Aspen Systems Corporation.

PREDICTION IN WEIGHT MANAGEMENT OUTCOME: IMPLICATIONS FOR PRACTICE

John P. Foreyt and G. Ken Goodrick

Nutrition Research Clinic
Department of Medicine
Baylor College of Medicine
Houston, TX 77030

Despite hundreds of published, controlled studies reporting the treatment of obesity, results with all of those reporting long-term data are identical: virtually all patients treated regain the lost weight within five years (NIH Technology Assessment Conference Panel, 1993). This finding has contributed to the concept of obesity as a chronic disorder, requiring treatment in a continuing care model (Perri, Nezu, & Viegener, 1992; Goodrick & Foreyt, 1991). But even using this model, which requires the utilization of considerable resources and time, results are modest at best.

In order to improve treatment outcome, it has been suggested that patients be matched to treatments based on client and program factors. The idea is that only certain programs are effective with certain patients, and that matching would result in better outcome (Brownell & Wadden, 1991). Unfortunately, there is no research to date to support any improvement in outcome through assignment of patient profiles to matched treatments. Matching at its most basic level involves sending those patients with the most weight to lose to programs which produce the greatest losses. However, recent analysis of the literature has found no long-term difference between very-low-calorie-diet interventions and less intensive programs (National Task Force on the Prevention and Treatment of Obesity, 1993).

IMPLICATIONS OF PREDICTABILITY OF SUCCESS

It can be assumed hypothetically that there is a treatment for obesity which is effective in producing significant and lasting weight loss in some patients, and that the profile of these successful patients could be identified before treatment began. This assumption leads to a discussion of the implications for practice, and then to a discussion of what such speculative thinking might reveal for the current scenario of ineffectiveness.

Table 1. Predictors of Weight Loss

PREDICTOR	RELATIONSHIP
Patient Factors	
Initial body weight	+
Resting metabolic rate	+
Adipocyte hyperplasia	+
Self-efficacy	+
Body fat distribution	?
Personality/psychopathology test results	?
Dietary restraint	?
Weight cycling	?
Binge eating	?
Process Variables	
Early weight loss	+
Attendance	+
Behavioral Changes	
Self-monitoring	+
Goal-setting	+
Slowing rate of eating	+
Treatment Factors	
Length	+
Social support	+
Physical activity	+

Data from Blair, 1993; Foreyt & Goodrick, 1993; Perri, Nezu, & Viegener, 1992; Wadden & Letizia, 1992.

+ Positive correlation
? Mixed findings

SUCCESS FACTORS

Many factors have been associated with success in weight loss and maintenance (cf. reviews by Blair, 1993; Foreyt & Goodrick, 1993; Perri, Nezu, & Viegener, 1992; Wadden & Letizia, 1992). These are summarized in Tables I and II.

Other predictive factors include self-efficacy (Edell, Edington, Herd, O'Brien, & Witkin, 1987; Rodin, Elias, Silberstein, & Wagner, 1988), history of success in weight loss (Black 1989), greater weight loss early in program (Black, 1989; Rodin et al, 1988), and agreement with treatment philosophy (Rodin et al, 1988).

Continuing attendance at weight loss programs has been predicted by Organization,

Table 2. Predictors of Maintenance of Weight Loss

FACTOR	RELATIONSHIP
Physical activity	+
Self-monitoring	+
Positive coping style	+
Continued contact	+
Negative life events	−
Family dysfunction	−
Data from Blair, 1993; Foreyt & Goodrick, 1993; Perri, Nezu, & Viegener, 1992; Wadden & Letizia, 1992. + Positive correlation − Negative correlation	

Responsibility, Anxiety, and Energy Level scores on the Jackson Personality Inventory, and higher depression as assessed by the D30 Scale (Pekarik, Blodgett, Evans, & Wierzbicki, 1984). Attendance has also been associated negatively with higher Hunger and Restraint Scores of the Eating Inventory (LaPorte & Stunkard, 1990), and by binge eating, stress, and smaller initial weight loss (Wadden et al, 1992).

Each of these factors accounts for only a small part of the outcome variance, and the number of factors is large relative to study sample size. The notoriously large outcome variance in weight-loss studies also makes it virtually impossible to develop a predictive profile that has clinical utility.

CONCEPTUALIZING SUCCESS

Success can be conceptualized as the simultaneous satisfaction of two criteria in any patient: 1) Long-term adherence to prudent and tolerable eating and exercise regimens; and 2) Physiological/cellular responsivity to these regimens which will result in significant reduction of excess adipose tissue. Prediction, then, can be conceptualized as having two dimensions: 1) A psychosocial dimension for prediction of adherence, and 2) A physiological dimension for the prediction of the body's response. The psychological aspects of adherence may be ultimately caused by some underlying physiological condition, i.e., some aspect of physiological functioning might make exercise less enjoyable for some patients. However, this would become manifest by subjective reports on a psychological level if there was no biological marker for exercise dyshedonia. Likewise there is the possibility that psychological processes mediate physiological processes through the stress/ exogenous depression responses. The physiological profile could include prediction of success with the use of drugs.

To simplify matters, we assume that a prediction profile would have psychosocial as well as physiological factors. If the physiological profile indicated very little likelihood of successful weight management, no amount of adherence would be likely to produce weight loss or maintenance. On the other hand, if the patient showed a physiologically optimal profile for weight management but had a psychosocial profile indicating very little likelihood of behavioral compliance, what is the clinician to do? The four possible cases of the profile matrix are shown in Figure 1.

		Physiological Prediction	
		Success	Failure
Psychosocial Prediction	Success	I. Prudent exercise and eating.	II. Prudent exercise and eating. Therapy to accept limitations. Social support
	Failure	III. Therapy to alter adherence factors *or* Therapy to accept limitations. Social support	IV. Therapy to alter adherence factors *and* Therapy to accept limitations. Social support

Figure 1. Prediction Matrix and Interventions

The intervention for quadrant I is obvious. These patients will adhere to and respond to exercise and reduced-fat eating. These are the individuals who are used as testimonials in weight clinic advertising. These are the persons least likely to present at a weight clinic since they experience little difficulty in weight management.

In quadrant II are those who can adhere to a reduced- fat diet and who can exercise regularly, but who do not experience appreciable fat loss. If this outcome were predictable, patients would be assigned to therapy to help them accept the fact that they will never be thin (Ciliska, 1990; Polivy & Herman, 1992). One aspect of this therapy is the structuring of social support from others who are in the same predicament. Without such support they may be in a continuing struggle with their limitations resulting in psychological and physiological damage. Care should be taken to prevent patients in this category from attempts at weight loss through excessive exercise or restrictive dieting, since this may lead to eating disorders, amenorrhea, and osteoporosis. They would be encouraged to maintain prudent exercise and eating in order to reap the health benefits obtainable apart from weight loss.

Individuals found to be in Quadrant III might be candidates for psychotherapy and structured social support designed to change their psychosocial profile in the direction of successful adherers. However, some of the factors used in making the prediction, such as the triad of low educational level/low socioeconomic status/high life stress often found in urban areas, may be very difficult to change. If efforts to move these patients into Quadrant I fail, then the intervention would revert to helping the patient accept their weight management limitations.

In Quadrant IV one finds the case of the patient whose profile indicates little chance of reducing adipose tissue size, or of adopting healthful habits. As in Quadrant III, an attempt might be made to move the patient up into Quadrant II so that the benefits of prudent eating and exercise could be gained. Whether it proves feasible to improve adherence or not, this patient might still benefit from therapy to accept weight management limitations because of psychophysiological intransigence.

As depicted in Figure 1, the physiological and psychosocial predictions for success are binary variables; however, the predictive methodology would most likely result in patients being placed on a bi-dimensional continuum, placing them at various points in the grid. This begs the question of where to draw the triage lines to determine who gets what treatment. These decisions would be based on two considerations: 1) The cost/benefit ratio derived from an analysis of the predicted effort and time involved to engender and maintain success (both for the clinician as well as the patient) and the predicted psychophysiological benefit/risk reduction associated with success; and 2) Given limited treatment resources, how this cost/benefit ratio compares with the ratios of other patient groups seeking the same treatment resources.

The cost/benefit ratio for patients in Quadrant I is quite favorable. According to the hypothetical prediction model, the cost of motivating patients in Quadrant II would be the same as those in Quadrant I, but patients would not experience weight loss. Their risk reduction would be that associated with exercise and reduced-fat eating, which might be less than risk reduction with weight loss and prudent lifestyle.

Patients in Quadrant III need psychological support to modify the factors which keep them from adhering to lifestyle changes. This form of therapy is relatively expensive; these patients might have to wait in line behind those whose predictive profiles show more promise for behavioral change. If the psychological intervention was successful, they would alter lifestyle and experience the benefits of prudent living as well as weight loss.

Those in Quadrant IV would need the expensive psychological intervention. However, they could only hope to experience the benefits of exercise and reduced-fat eating, but not weight loss per se, should the psychological intervention prove effective. Thus those in this quadrant would have the lowest priority for treatment.

IMPLICATIONS OF THE MODEL

What can be learned from this hypothetical model? It is clear that most patients presenting to a clinic with the complaint of obesity fall into Quadrant IV; they have excess fat which will not appreciably disappear, and they are unlikely to maintain prudent behavior indefinitely (Perri, 1992); most patients regain lost weight. Because of this likely outcome, some have advocated that weight loss treatment should not be given since it only provides an occasion for another failure experience (Wooley & Garner, 1991).

Many clinics appear to operate (at least if one is to judge from advertising) on the assumption that patients fall into Quadrant I. The fact that most of those treated regain in a way that is discordant with the direct or implied promises made by therapists poses an ethical question (Lustig, 1991) which is currently an issue for governmental regulatory agencies (Begley, 1991).

While the treatment outcome research shows that patients tend to fall into Quadrant IV, and clinics would have them in Quadrant I, it is likely that most patients see themselves as falling into Quadrant II or III. Those seeing themselves in Quadrant II are looking for the "magic pill" treatment that will move them physiologically into Quadrant I. Those who see themselves in Quadrant III believe they can have success if only they could be motivated to change their behaviors. They go to clinics to receive psychological interventions and group support.

This confusion among clinicians and patients about what is possible and what is expected from treatment needs to be clarified. Furthermore, the health benefits associated with prudent lifestyle without appreciable weight loss (Goldstein, 1992) need to be better understood and communicated to patients, since altered lifestyle with very modest weight loss may be the most likely outcome even for those who maintain behavioral changes.

IMPLICATIONS FOR PRACTICE

Since prediction of treatment outcome is not yet possible, clinicians need to help their patients with a flexible approach which is designed to optimize psychological as well as physical health. The approach we recommend (Foreyt & Goodrick, 1994) is most applicable to the typical quadrant II and IV patient. It starts with the assumption that a health professional should use treatments which have the best potential for healing the emotional damage caused by dieting failure, and for ending the social isolation often associated with obesity.

This non-dieting approach to weight management involves five components which are applied in the following order:

1) Development of therapist and peer support;
2) Cessation of dieting and normalization of eating patterns;
3) Gradual increase in exercise;
4) Gradual reduction of fat in eating; and
5) Acceptance of whatever weight is achieved with prudent eating and exercise habits.

The task of the therapist and therapy group members is to provide an environment in which self-acceptance can be developed independent of perceptions about appearance, and in which social skills can be improved. Because our culture idealizes thinness and ostracizes on the basis of fatness, many overweight individuals grow up socially isolated with deficiencies in social skills. They struggle alone to become thin so that they will become acceptable and loved. However, failure at dieting only adds to feelings of self-hatred and increased feelings of isolation. The way out of this cycle is to learn to develop loving relationships, first with oneself and then with others. The group forms an artificial world of acceptance and understanding, two commodities which are in scant supply for the overweight in the real world.

The eating regimen in this approach involves two phases to normalize eating patterns. In the first phase, which may need to last from 6 to 12 months, participants are directed to eat 3 meals a day of whatever they want in order to get out of the habit of restrictive dieting. After they become more comfortable with food, the second phase involves motivating them to reduce the amount of fat in their food gradually and without feelings of deprivation. The reduction in fat is associated with a spontaneous reduction in calorie intake and weight loss (Lissner et al., 1987). With training by a dietitian in small groups, women have been able to achieve a reduction from 39 to 21 percent calories from fat without feelings of deprivation, and to maintain this level at a two-year follow-up (Insull et al., 1990). Another important component of the plan is reteaching the subjects what true hunger is, as distinguished from cravings.

Soon after entering treatment, patients are helped to develop an aerobic exercise program. Exercise is emphasized as mandatory, since it is one of the most reliable predictors of success in weight loss maintenance. Exercise burns calories and allows more flexibility in eating choices. The development of an exercise habit may also be associated with a reduction in preference for fat, and an increased preference for carbohydrates. In rat studies, dieting with weight fluctuation has been shown to increase preference for fat, and exercise has been shown to reduce this preference (Reed et al., 1988; Gerardo-Gettens et al., 1991). Exercise may also be beneficial for the overweight since it is associated with elevated mood, enhanced self-esteem, and an improved body image. Considering that weight loss treatments result at best in modest sustained weight loss, then a "healthy weight" is defined as that weight which can be achieved and maintained with the eating and exercise regimens associated with these approaches. We tell our patients that they can have good control over their eating and their exercise, but that they cannot have direct control over their weight. The weight they achieve with prudent lifestyle depends in part on genetic factors, their metabolism, their number of fat cells, and possibly on the effects of many years of dieting. Counseling is directed at helping them accept the weight that is associated with a prudent and tolerable lifestyle.

ACKNOWLEDGEMENTS

Preparation of this paper was supported in part by grant DK43109 from the National Institute of Diabetes and Digestive and Kidney Diseases.

REFERENCES

Begley, C.E. (1991). Government should strengthen regulation in the weight loss industry. Journal of the American Dietetic Association, 91, 1255-1257.

Black, D.R. (1989). Identifying predictor variables of weight loss outcome: Implications for a stepped program and weight management. Psychology and Health, 3, 207-216.

Blair, S.N. (1993). Evidence for success of exercise in weight loss and control. Annals of Internal Medicine, 119, 702-706.

Brownell, K.D., & Wadden, T.A. (1991). The heterogeneity of obesity: Fitting treatments to individuals. Behavior Therapy, 22, 153-177.

Ciliska, D. (1990). Beyond dieting. New York: Brunner/Mazel.

Edell, B.H., Edington, S., Herd, B., O'Brien, R.M., & Witkin, G. (1987). Self-efficacy and self-motivation as predictors of weight loss. Addictive Behaviors, 12, 63-66.

Foreyt, J.P., & Goodrick, G.K. (1993). Evidence for success of behavior modification in weight loss and control. Annals of Internal Medicine, 119, 698-701.

Foreyt, J.P., & Goodrick, G.K. (1994). Living without dieting. New York: Warner Books.

Gerardo-Gettens, T., Miller, G.D., Horwitz, B.A., McDonald, R.B., Brownell, K.D., Greenwood, M.R., Rodin, J., & Stern, J.S. (1991). Exercise decreases fat selection in female rats during weight cycling. American Journal of Physiology, 260, R518-524.

Goldstein, D.J. (1992). Beneficial effects of modest weight loss. International Journal of Obesity, 16, 397-415.

Goodrick, G.K., & Foreyt, J.P. (1991). Why treatments for obesity don't last. Journal of the American Dietetic Association, 91, 1243-1247.

Insull, W., Henderson, M.H., Prentice, R.L., Thompson, D.J., Clifford, C., Goldman, S., Gorbach, S., Moskowitz, M., Thompson, R., & Woods, M. (1990). Results of a randomized feasibility study of a low-fat diet. Archives of Internal Medicine, 150, 421-427.

LaPorte, D.J., & Stunkard, A.J. (1990). Predicting attrition and adherence to a very-low-calorie diet: A prospective investigation of the Eating Inventory. International Journal of Obesity, 14, 197-206.

Lissner, L., Levitsky, D.A., Strupp, B.J., Kalkwarf, H.J., & Roe, D.A. (1987). Dietary fat and the regulation of energy intake in human subjects. American Journal of Clinical Nutrition, 46, 886-892.

Lustig, A. (1991). Weight loss programs: Failing to meet ethical standards? Journal of the American Dietetic Association, 91, 1252-1254.

National Task Force on the Prevention and Treatment of Obesity. (1993). Very low-calorie diets. Journal of the American Medical Association, 270, 967-974.

NIH Technology Assessment Conference Panel. (1993). Methods for voluntary weight loss and control. Annals of Internal Medicine, 119, 764-770.

Pekarik, G., Blodgett, C., Evans, R.G., Wierzbicki, M. (1984). Variables related to continuance in a behavioral weight loss program. Addictive Behaviors, 9, 413-416.

Perri, M.G. (1992). Improving maintenance of weight loss following treatment by diet and lifestyle modification. In T.A. Wadden, & T.B. VanItallie, (Eds.), Treatment of the seriously obese patient (pp. 456-477). New York: Guilford.

Perri, M.G., Nezu, A.M., & Viegener, B.J. (1992). Improving the long-term management of obesity: Theory, research, and clinical guidelines. New York: Wiley.

Polivy, J. & Herman, C.P. (1992). Undieting: A program to help people stop dieting. International Journal of Eating Disorders, 11, 261-268.

Reed, D.R., Contreras, R.J., Maggio, C., Greenwood, M.R., & Rodin, J. (1988). Weight cycling in female rats increases dietary fat selection and adiposity. Psychology and Behavior, 42, 389-395.

Rodin, J., Elias, M., Silberstein, L.R., & Wagner, A. (1988). Combined behavioral and pharmacologic treatment for obesity: Predictors of successful weight maintenance. Journal of Consulting and Clinical Psychology, 56, 399-404.

Wadden, T.A., Foster, G.D., Wang, J., Pierson, R.N., Yang, M.U., Moreland, K., Stunkard, A.J., & VanItallie, T.B. (1992). Clinical correlates of short- and long-term weight loss. American Journal of Clinical Nutrition, 56(1 Suppl.), 271S-274S.

Wadden, T.A., & Letizia, K. (1992). Predictors of attrition and weight loss in patients treated by moderate and severe calorie restriction. In T.A. Wadden, & T.B., VanItallie (Eds.), Treatment of the seriously obese patient (pp. 383-410). New York: Guilford.

Wooley, S.C., & Garner, D.M. (1991). Obesity treatment: The high cost of false hope. Journal of the American Dietetic Association, 91, 1248-1251.

NEUROENDOCRINE ASPECTS OF HUMAN OBESITY AND FAT DISTRIBUTION: POTENTIAL FOR INTERVENTION

Per Bjorntorp

Department of Heart and Lung Disease
University of Goteborg
Sahlgren's Hospital
Goteborg, Sweden

Obesity treatment is often too much focused on the number of kg of body fat lost only. It is at least equally important to follow the effects of treatment on the obesity-associated metabolic complications. If they were not coupled to the obese state, the increased mass of adipose tissue might only be regarded as an extra rucksack which has to be carried around. This summary is focusing on the possibilities to treat the Metabolic Syndrome associated with visceral obesity.

Visceral obesity is followed by a multiple endocrine abnormality which is found along the hypothalamo-adrenal, -gonadal and growth hormone axes, as well as the central sympathetic nervous system. There is considerable evidence to suggest that these abnormalities provide a background to understand how several of the abnormalities of the Metabolic Syndrome, particularly insulin resistance, are caused. Furthermore, these aberrations may provide an understanding of the shift of excess body fat accumulation to visceral depots (Bjorntorp, 1993).

In order to test whether this presumed chain of cause-effect events is correct, several intervention studies against these abnormalities have been performed. First, in preliminary studies, the hyperandrogenicity following abdominal obesity in women has been treated with oral 17~ estradiol in women with non-insulin dependent diabetes mellitus. This seems to be followed by marked improvements of their diabetes (Andersson, Hahn, Mattsson, & Bjorntorp, 1993). Furthermore, the hypogonadism following abdominal obesity in men has been treated with testosterone (T) to substitute the hypogonadism. This was followed by a marked improvement of the components of the Metabolic Syndrome, decreasing insulin resistance, lowering plasma lipids and blood **pressure,** as well as diminishing visceral fat depots significantly (Marin, & Bjorntorp, 1993). **Growth hormone** has been administered to hypophysectomized patients, fully substituted with other hormones, resulting in marked diminution of **visceral fat depots** (Bengtsson, Eden, Lonn, Kvist, Stokland, Lindstedt, Bossaeus, Tolli, Sjostrom, & Isaksson, 1993). These results support the notion that the Metabolic Syndrome following visceral obesity is indeed caused by the hormonal deficiencies in question.

The background to this multiple endocrine abnormality is most likely of neuroendocrine origin, and has the character of a hypothalamic arousal, seen after certain forms of reaction to stress (Henry, & Stephens, 1977). When placed in a situation where subjects can not cope with the stressful environment an endocrine reaction follows, similar to the abnormalities seen in visceral obesity with the Metabolic Syndrome, including hyperactivity along the hypothalamoadrenal axis, and inhibitory effects on sex hormone secretions (Bjorntorp, 1993). A decrease of growth hormone secretion, and elevated activity in the central sympathetic nervous system might be other abnormalities. This neuroendocrine reaction also follows smoking and alcohol consumption.

There are several signs suggesting that the background to the multiple endocrine abnormalities in visceral obesity with the Metabolic Syndrome is indeed a stress reaction with poor coping, perhaps based on socio-economic handicaps due to a low degree of education and poorly paid employment (Lapidus, Bengtsson, Hallstrom, & Bjorntorp, 1989; Larsson, Seidel, Svardsudd, Welin, Tibblin & Wilhelmsen, 1989). This might be followed by frequent periods of sick-leave, often in psychosomatic type of diseases, alcohol consumption, smoking and use of anxiolytic and antidepressive drugs (Ibid). Based on the finding of these characteristics in subjects in the general population with abdominally localized body fat mass (Ibid), this possibility has been suggested (Bjorntorp, 1987). It is, for obvious reasons difficult to test this hypothesis by intervention experiments in humans, both by attempts to improve the situation, and, particularly to induce such stress situations chronically. This has, however, recently been performed in monkeys (Shivley, Clarkson, Miller, & Weingard, 1987; and Shively and Jayo, this symposium). Exposing monkeys to a stressful environment, followed by a poor coping with the situation, is followed by a neuroendocrine reaction similar to that seen in humans with visceral obesity and the Metabolic Syndrome. Recent experiments of the same type have shown that such monkeys accumulate visceral fat, and previous reports have shown that these monkeys also obtained the full-blown Metabolic Syndrome, including insulin resistance, impaired glucose tolerance, elevated **plasma lipids and** blood pressure as well as coronary atherosclerosis. The results of these experiments lend strong support to the presumed chain of events in humans with visceral obesity and the Metabolic Syndrome. In fact the condition in monkeys and humans is identical, although the abnormalities in androgen and growth hormone secretions in humans have not yet been studied in the monkeys.

With this background, suggesting a neuroendocrine dysfunction in visceral obesity, we have recently determined the concentrations of neuropeptides and catecholamine metabolites in the cerebrospinal fluid of obese women. A number of abnormalities were found including decreased concentrations of corticotropin releasing hormone and metabolites of serotonin (unpublished). Although not possible yet to fully interpret, these results demonstrate that a neuroendocrine aberration is present in human obesity. These findings may also provide new ideas for intervention at the level of the central nervous system .

REFERENCES

Andersson, B., Hahn, L., Mattsson, L-A, & Bjorntorp, P. (1993). Female sex steroids and the metabolic syndrome. In Proc. of the Novo Nordisk International Symposium. Copenhage, Denmark, Wells Medical Ltd., Novo Copenhagen, 85-92.

Bengtsson, B-A, Eden, S., Lonn, L., Kvist, H., Stokland, A., Lindstedt, G., Bossaeus, I, Tolli, J., Sjostrom, L., Isaksson, O. G. P. (1993). Treatment of adults with growth hormone deficiency with recombinant human growth hormone. Journal of Clinical Endocrinology and Metabolism, 76, 309-317.

Bjorntorp, P. (1987). The associations between obesity, adipose tissue distribution and disease. Acta Medica Scandinavia, 723, 121-134.

Bjorntorp, P. (1993). Visceral obesity: A "Civilization Syndrome". Obesity Research, 1.

Henry, J. P. & Stephens, P. M. (1977). Stress, Health , and the Social Environment: A Sociobiological Approach to Medicine. Springfield, NY.

Lapidus, L., Bengtsson, C., Hallstrom, T., & Bjorntorp, P. (1989). Obesity, adipose tissue distribution and health in women: Results from a population study in Gothenbury, Sweden, Appetite, 12, 25-35.

Larsson, B., Seidell, J., Svardsudd, K., Welin, L., Tibblin, G., & Wilhelmsen, L. (1989). Obesity, adipose tissue distribution and health in men: The study of men born in 1913. Appetite, 13, 37-44.

Marin, P., & Bjorntorp, P. (1993). Androgen treatment of middle-aged obese men: Effects on glucose tolerance, insulin sensitivity, and fat distribution. Obesity Research, in press.

Shively, C. A., Clarkson, R. B., Miller, C., & Weingard, K. W. (1987). Body fat distribution as a risk factor for coronary artery atherosclerosis in female, Cynomolgus monkeys. Atherosclerosis, 7, 226-231.

SOCIAL STRESS EFFECTS ON REGIONAL FAT DISTRIBUTION IN MALE AND FEMALE MONKEYS

J.M. Jayo, C. Shively, T. Clarkson, and J. Kaplan

Wake Forest University
The Bowman Gray School of Medicine
Department of Comparative Medicine
Medical Center Boulevard
Winston-Salem, NC 27157

We have studied the factors which influence the development of coronary heart disease (CHD) several decades. One of our major interests has been gender differences in CHD morbidity and mortality. Even though CHD is the number one killer of women, men are twice as likely to die of CHD than women. As most of you are aware, a major pathogenic process underlying the development of clinically relevant coronary heart disease is atherosclerosis of the coronary arteries (CAA). If you feed monkeys diets that contain fat and cholesterol in amounts similar to that consumed by people, they get atherosclerosis. Men have twice as extensive CAA as women, and male monkeys have twice as extensive CAA as female monkeys.

As you know, traditional risk factors only account for a portion of the variance observed in CHD and CAA, so we are always on the lookout for new risk factors. Well, with that in mind you can understand that we were very excited when adipose tissue distribution was found to predict CHD. We immediately began considering this variable in our own studies.

Cynomolgus monkeys come in all shapes and sizes. Knowing that there is natural variability in amounts of body fat, and because visual inspection suggested to us that there may also be natural variation in fat distribution we set out to examine the relationships between body fat distribution and CAA in cynomolgus monkeys. First we looked at females because it was clear at that time that fat distribution was making an independent contribution to CHD risk in women, and because we have a lot more females than males available for study.

We measured body mass index, subscapular, suprailiac, and triceps skinfolds on 36 female monkeys. We investigated all of these, and all possible combinations of these, as potential predictors of CAA extent. We found that the ratio of truncal fat - measured as the subscapular skinfold, to peripheral fat - measured as the triceps skinfold, was a significant predictor of CAA. In fact, females with a greater than average truncal to peripheral fat ratio had more than three times the CAA than those that were below average in the truncal:peripheral fat ratio. Furthermore, none of the other measures were significant predictors - including body mass index. The implication that we can draw from these data is that it is likely that the reason women with truncal fat are at greater risk for CHD is because they have worsened CAA rather than any of a number of other circulatory system disturbances that may be contributing to risk of MI (Shively et al 1987).

These monkeys live in complex societies which are organized. One of the basic organizing mechanisms of monkey society is the social status or dominance hierarchy. Dominant animals have priority of access to resources such as food, water, favorite resting places and mates. Whereas, subordinates maintain a highly vigilant state to keep track of dominants in order to avoid aggressive interactions. In spite of that, subordinates receive more aggression, and spend more time alone than dominants.

These monkeys have menstrual cycles like women. The cycles are about the same length and include hormonal fluctuations that are similar to those of women. One of the most interesting phenomenon in many mammalian species is the social suppression of reproductive function. Socially subordinate female monkeys have poor reproductive function, that is more abnormal menstrual cycles, compared to dominant females. By abnormal I mean that the luteal phase is characterized by low progesterone concentrations and the follicular phase is characterized by low estrogen concentrations. In many cases ovulation does not occur.

Subordinate females with poor ovarian function have significantly more CAA than dominant females with good ovarian function. In fact, subordinate females are indistinguishable from ovariectomized females in CAA extent. Subordinate and ovariectomized females also have relatively low HDL cholesterol concentrations- a risk factor for CAA and CHD (Adams et al., 1985).

We know that there is a relationship between patterns of fat distribution in females and sex steroids. Truncal fat deposition is often associated with a more androgenic hormone profile in women. Since subordinate females have aberrant ovarian function, we compared their fat distribution patterns to those of dominant females. Subordinate females were significantly more likely than dominants to fall in the top half of the distribution of truncal to peripheral fat, whereas the reverse was true for dominant females. We conclude that stress can deleteriously effect fat distribution patterns in females, probably, at least in part, through the suppression of ovarian function (Shively et al., 1988).

In summary, female primates the stress of social subordination causes deleterious changes in a number of systems. Note that these systems include the reproductive system, which we talked about; the autonomic nervous system as reflected in heart rate which we did not have time to talk about; the hypothalamic-pituitary-adrenal system which we also did not have time to talk about; and adipose tissue distribution. All of these may contribute to exacerbated CAA. Potential mechanisms by which stress may alter adipose distribution include but are not limited to the autonomic nervous system, the hypothalamic-pituitary-adrenal axis, and the reproductive system. The mechanism of stress effects on adipose tissue has yet to be determined.

Males have the most extensive CAA, and healthy, nonstressed, dominant females with good ovarian function have the least CAA. In terms of CAA extent, subordinate females that are stressed, and have poor ovarian function are indistinguishable from females with no ovaries, and males.

It is intriguing that there are also gender differences in responses to stressors. In one experiment half of the males lived in stable social groups for 2 years and half of the males lived in social groups that were disrupted and reorganized monthly by the introduction of social strangers-unstable social groups. Likewise, half of the females lived in stable social groups and half of the females lived in unstable social groups. CAA extent was measured at the end of the two year period. Males who are socially dominant and live in unstable social groups have exacerbated CAA. So social instability and social status interact to effect CAA risk in males (Kaplan et al., 1982). Among females we see a different pattern. Females are unaffected by social instability, however, as we saw in previous data, subordinates have exacerbated CAA.

Our next experiment addressed the effects of stress on CAA in 80 male monkeys, half of which were sedentary and half of which exercised (Jayo et al., in press). Within each of these treatment groups, half of the males were stressed by repeated social reorganization-social instability; and half were not stressed, living in stable social groupings for the duration of the experiment.

We provided half of the animals with exercise by training them to run in a motorized wheel for 40 min 3x/week at 17 rpm. We chose this level of exercise to approximate moderate long-term exercise in people. This exercise regimen did not attempt to model the effects of intensive exercise training, however, for the monkeys it represented a significant increase in activity level.

The study was conducted in 3 phases. Phase 1 was about 5 months in length. During this phase the monkeys were habituated to their new environment and to their new social groups, and baseline measures were made. Phase 2 was about 10 months in length. During this phase all animals learned to run in the motorized running wheel. They were conditioned to run for 30 min at 17 rpm. In phase 3 the monkeys were assigned to either the sedentary or the exercising group based on their running ability, and plasma lipid concentrations. They began consuming an atherogenic diet containing 0.25 mg cholesterol/Cal with 40% of calories from fat, and continued to do so, ad libitum, for the remainder of the experiment. Phase 3 lasted for 9 months. The final phase, phase 4, was about 3 years in length. During this phase the stress of social instability was introduced. Also, the exercising monkeys increased to 40 min at 17 rpm 3x/week.

The exercise caused significant decreases in heart rates, recorded by telemetry, while the animals were free to move about in their social groups. Exercise also caused increased cardiac output measured by echocardiography, larger hearts, and significantly thicker walls of the ventricles measured by echocardiography and at necropsy. Our goal with this exercise was to achieve significantly improved cardiac fitness, and these data suggest that goal was achieved.

Anthropometric measures were made once during the baseline period, 4x/year during phase 2, and 2x/year during phases 3 and 4. We measured the subscapular, triceps, suprailiac and posterior thigh skinfolds, as well as BW and body length. We also measured the waist, arm, hip and upper thigh circumferences at all time periods except baseline. At the end of the experiment intra-abdominal and subcutaneous abdominal adipose tissue was measured by computed tomography in 10 animals from each treatment group for a total of 40 animals.

We have previously validated this measure of abdominal adipose tissue in monkeys and demonstrated that a 1 cm section at the level of the umbilicus is as representative of abdominal fat measured at several levels above and below the umbilicus as it is in people. Also monkey adipose has about the same density as the adipose tissue of people and so we use density ranges similar to those used to measure adipose tissue in people (-140 - -40 hounsfield units) (Labor-Laird et al., 1991). The area for intra-abdominal fat was defined by outlining the transversus abdominous muscle with a cursor. Total fat was defined by outlining the body margin. Subcutaneous fat was calculated by subtracting the intra-abdominal fat from the total abdominal fat.

We corrected for any baseline differences between the monkeys in total or regional obesity by putting significant baseline predictors into the analysis as covariates. Exercise and stress did not have any effect on BW or BMI. These animals were eating as much as they wished.

There were only two measures that were affected by exercise only: the posterior thigh skinfold thickness, and the ratio of the waist:thigh circumference. Exercise decreased the thigh skinfold and the ratio of waist to thigh circumference.

In the rest of the measures stress interacted with exercise to affect regional adiposity in male monkeys. Waist circumference was reduced by exercise but only in monkeys that were not stressed. Similarly, the ratio of waist to hip circumference was reduced by exercise, but only in the nonstressed group. Exercise reduced the ratio of suprailiac to triceps skinfold thicknesses in unstressed males only and this was due to a reduction in subcutaneous abdominal fat. There was no effect on peripheral fat measured at the triceps either as a circumference or a skinfold thickness. Similarly, the ratio of subscapular:triceps skinfolds appears to be reduced by exercise, but in the nonstressed group only. Note that this is the skinfold ratio that predicts CAA in female monkeys. The effect on the ss:tri ratio was due to a reduction in truncal subcutaneous fat measured below the scapula. Again, there was no effect of exercise or stress on peripheral fat deposition measured by the triceps skinfold thickness or the arm circumference.

Thus, the effects of exercise and stress on anthropometric measures of whole and regional adiposity are highly consistent: stress abolishes the beneficial reduction in truncal fat caused by exercise. There were no effects of stress on peripheral measures of fat. There were also no effects of exercise on peripheral fat deposit - except the thigh skinfold. Stress and exercise had different effects on Ct measurements of abdominal fat.

Stress appeared to cause increased intra-abdominal or visceral fat measured by CT in both the exercise and the nonexercise group. There were no significant effects of stress or exercise on subcutaneous abdominal fat measured by CT. However, when the proportion of total abdominal fat that was located subcutaneously was considered we found that monkeys that were stressed deposited less of their abdominal fat in the subcutaneous depot. Monkeys that were stressed preferentially deposited fat in the visceral or intra-abdominal fat depot (Jayo et al., in press).

The mechanisms through which social stress causes deleterious patterns of fat distribution are not well understood. Three possible physiologic characteristics of stressed females are also known to effect adipocyte metabolism. These were increased secretion from the HPA axis, increased SNS tone as evidenced by increased heart rate, and decreased ovarian function. We have not characterized the physiological effects of stress as completely in males. However, we will be examining the relationships between physiologic stress responses and fat deposition in future.

REFERENCES

Adams, M. R. et al. (1985). Ovariectomy, social status, and atherosclerosis in cynomolgus monkeys. Arteriosclerosis, 5, 192-200.

Jayo, J. et al (in press). Effects of exercise and stress on body fat distribution in male cynomolgus monkeys. International Journal of Obesity.

Kaplan, J. R. et al (1982). Social status, environment, and atherosclerosis in cynomolgus monkey. Arteriosclerosis, 2, 359-368.

Labor-Laird, K. et al. (1991). Assessment of abdominal fat deposition in female cynomolus monkeys. International Journal of Obesity, 15, 213-220.

Shively, C. A. et al. (1987). Body fat distribution as a risk factor for coronary artery atherosclerosis in female cynomolus monkeys. Arteriosclerosis, 7, 226-231.

Shively, C. A., et al. (1988). Regional obesity and coronary artery atherosclerosis in females: A non-human primate model. Acta Medica Scandinavia Suppl, 723, 71-78.

THE SEARCH FOR OBESITY GENES

R. Arlen Price

Department of Psychiatry
University of Pennsylvania
422 Curie Boulevard
Philadelphia, PA 19104-6141

Evidence from a variety of sources indicate that genes play a major role in determining proneness to obesity (Price, in press). Family, twin and adoption studies indicate that genes also play a role in determining levels of fatness or thinness in the normal range (Price, in press; Price & Gottesman, 1991; Sorensen, Price Stunkard, & Schulsinger, 1989). At least in adults, environmental influences appear to originate outside the family (Price & Gottesman, 1991; Sorensen, Price, Stunkard, & Schulsinger, 1989) and genes mediate response to the environment (Bouchard, Tremblay, Despres, Nadeau, Lupien, Theriault, Dussault, Moorgani, Pinault, & Fornier, 1990). Obesity associated with single gene mutations in animals and chromosome abnormalities in humans indicate that disruption or deletion of single genes or several contiguous genes can result in obesity, even in the absence of special obesity promoting diets (Friedman, Leibel, & Bahary, 1991; Johnson, Greenwood, Horwitz, & Stern, 1991; Price, in press). Possibly of more relevance to extreme obesity in humans are multi-genic models of obesity that appear to depend on both genotype and exposure to high fat diets (West, Waguespack, & Price, 1994). Thus, genes appear to influence proneness to obesity across a broad range of fat and thin phenotypes and to possess a range of susceptibility to the environmental influences of diet and exercise.

There appears to be no simple Mendelian mechanism for the inheritance of obesity genes (Price, in press). Single gene effects are apparent for certain animal obesity mutants and are suggested even for some human syndromes. Moreover, several segregation studies appear to suggest a recessive mode of inheritance for normal variation in obesity (Price, Ness & Laskarzewski, 1990). However, these apparent recessive effects could also be due to temporal increases in prevalence and levels of obesity between generations (Price, Charles, Pettitt, & Knowler, 1993). In any case, no single model can explain the inheritance of obesity in all families, and it is likely that several different genes are needed to account for most human variation (Price, in press).

Gene locus and allele effect sizes are likely to vary considerably. In rare cases of extreme obesity that is independent of diet, there may well be genes with large effects that account for most of the risk for obesity in the families in which they are segregating. This is a heterogeneity

Obesity Treatment, Edited by D.B. Allison
and F.X. Pi-Sunyer, Plenum Press, New York, 1995

model. These genes would be analogous to obesity mutants such as <u>ob</u> and <u>fa</u> or chromosome abnormalities such as the Prader-Willi syndrome. More common genes may have relatively smaller effects, are likely to be diet dependent and may act in combination with other genes in either an additive (oligogenic model) or interactive (epistatic model) manner. These genes may be causes of diet sensitive obesity in animals and may account for cases of extreme obesity in human families. Genes accounting for variation of body fatness within the normal range are likely to be more numerous and to have even smaller individual effects (polygenic model). On the other hand, mapping studies of quantitative traits in plants and animals suggest that even for polygenic obesity only a few genes, say, 6-10, could account for most normal variation (Lander, & Botstein, 1989).

Based on studies in a number of species, one would expect a negative curvilinear relationship between gene effect sizes and gene frequencies. For example, if the human equivalents of the ob or fa genes are expressed in much the same way as their rodent counterparts, then the gene effect sizes would be extremely large in the families in which the genes are segregating, and the gene effects would appear regardless of diet. However, the gene frequencies in human populations might be extremely low. In other words, human homologs of mouse obesity mutants could be rare except in the most extreme forms of obesity. Obesity genes causing more common forms of obesity should have less extreme effects and may depend on diet for expression. The rationale for this assertion comes in part from the high prevalence of obesity and in part from the parallel temporal changes in obesity, diet and exercise (Price, & Gottesman, 1991) over the last half century. Together, these observations suggest very common obesity genes that have become increasingly penetrant with modern living conditions (Price, in press; Price, & Gottesman, 1991). Some polygenes are likely to have even smaller effects on the obesity phenotype. Currently, it is impossible to know just how many genes with each magnitude of effect are present, but, as noted, several single gene obesities have already been identified in animals and additional genes probably contribute significantly to common human obesities and to normal variation in levels and distribution of body fat.

Different measures of obesity may reflect different mixtures of genes and environmental influences. Most epidemiologic studies of obesity have used indices of obesity that are derived from weight corrected for height, e.g., the body mass index. Other estimates of total obesity can be made from skinfold measures, both individually and in combination, bioelectrical impedance, underwater weighing, and whole body imaging with CT and MRI. All such indices of obesity are highly correlated. However, there appear to be unique variances associated with individual measures which may be genetically based. All these phenotypes are appropriate ones for identifying obesity genes, and there is no way of predicting in advance which are likely to have the strongest relationship with specific obesity genes. When possible it will be important to examine several alternative phenotypes in attempting to map obesity genes. However, care should be taken to adjust statistical criteria for the multiple phenotypes examined. Such an approach will increase the probability of finding true genetic effects and minimize spurious reports of linkage.

Previous research has not been able to resolve the number and type of genes involved in common forms of obesity. However, the studies do suggest hypotheses that are necessary to guide linkage, biochemical and molecular genetic studies. Genetic linkage studies of obesity are well justified but should exercise care the sampling and analytic methods selected are compatible and the approaches chosen maximize the efficiency of the search for human obesity genes. Moreover, large numbers of families will be needed.

As much as feasible, approaches should take into account what we know about the causes of human obesity. For example, one possible sampling design is as follows. Selecting families with extreme obesity (for example, at least 80% overweight in one individual and 50% overweight in another) and some normal weight individuals (for example, at least one parent and one adult sibling who never have been more than 20% overweight) will optimize the probability of genetic differences between selected families and the general population as well as maximize gene segregation within families under a range of modes of inheritance. Focusing only on the obese siblings within such families will avoid problems associated with reduced gene penetrance and expression due to genetic background and environmental conditions. However, our simulation studies have shown that inclusion of a normal weight adult sibling also increases gene segregation and thus information for linkage analyses. Utilizing a sibling design also makes it feasible to use analytic methods that do not require genetic homogeneity among families. This family sampling design should be useful for identifying genes with a wide range of effect sizes from major genes to quantitative trait loci, since power will depend on sample size and not on idiosyncrasies of specific family structures.

In some highly stable populations with large family sizes, extended pedigree structures may also be of value in mapping obesity genes. These structures will be most useful when they are drawn from population isolates with limited genetic variability and, possibly, inbreeding. Furthermore, the most informative families will be those with obesity descending from a single branch, i.e., from only one of the four grandparents in the case of three generation families. Some large families should be selected in any case, since they will be useful in clarifying questions about gene expression, gene penetrance and gene-environment interactions in particular families.

Genome searches aimed at finding linkage between obesity and random genetic markers offer the best strategy for mapping obesity genes. More biologically based "candidate gene" approaches have intuitive appeal but in most cases will be inefficient because of the complexity of the "candidate" biological systems. The best candidates for mapping obesity genes in humans will be homologous genes or chromosome regions linked to obesity in animals.

Overall, previous research suggests that there are several, relatively rare genes that have large effects in particular families. Common genes are likely to have smaller effects, and the inherited polygenic background against which single obesity genes segregate will be made up of many genes with smaller quantitative effects. Studies aimed at identifying obesity predisposing genes should adopt strategies that take into account genetic heterogeneity, varying gene effect sizes and environmentally mediated gene penetrance and expression. One design which appears to be robust in the face of such complexities requires the sampling of families with at least two extremely obese siblings with one normal weight parent and a normal weight adult sibling. Finally, random gene mapping approaches to identifying obesity predisposing genes appear to have greater efficiency than more biologically intuitive candidate gene approaches. Candidate gene approaches can work if a homologous gene or region has been identified in an animal model.

ACKNOWLEDGEMENTS

Supported in part by National Institute of Health Grant R01-DK44073 to Dr. Price. Dr. Danielle Reed made useful comments on an earlier draft.

REFERENCES

Bouchard, C., Tremblay, A., Despres, J.-P., Nadeau, A., Lupien, P. J., Theriault, G., Dussault, J., Moorjani, S., Pinault, S., and Fournier, G. (1990). The response to long-term overfeeding in identical twins, New England Journal of Medicine, 322, 1477.

Friedman, J. M., Leibel, R. L., and Bahary, N. (1991). Molecular mapping of the mouse ob mutation, Mammalian Genome, 1, 130.

Johnson, P. R., Greenwood, M. R. C., Horwitz, B. A., and Stern, J. S. (1991). Animal models of obesity: genetic aspects, Annual Review of Nutrition, 11, 325.

Lander, E.S., and Botstein, D.(1989). Mapping Mendelian factors underlying quantitative traits using RFLP linkage maps. Genetics, 121, 185-99.

Price, R.A.(1994, in press). The case for single gene effects on human obesity. In C Bouchard (Ed.), The Genetics of Obesity. Boca Raton, Florida: CRC Press.

Price, R. A., Charles, M. A., Pettitt, D. J., and Knowler, W. C. (1993, in press). Obesity in Pima Indians: Large increases among post-World War ll birth cohorts, American Journal of Physical Anthropology.

Price, R. A., and Gottesman, I.l. (1991). Body fat in Shields' cohort of identical twins reared apart, Behavioral Genetics.

Price, R. A., Ness, R., and Laskarzewski, P. (1990). Common major gene inheritance of extreme overweight, Human Biology, 62, 747.

S0rensen, T. I. A., Price, R. A., Stunkard, A. J., and Schulsinger, F. (1989). Genetics of obesity in adult adoptees and their biological siblings, British Medical Journal, 298, 87.

West, D.B., Waguespack, J, Price, R.A. (1994, under revision following peer review) A genetic model for the control of dietary obesity in AKR/J and SWR/J mice. Mammalian Genome, 4.

DEFINING THE GENETIC BASIS OF OBESITY: CHALLENGES AND OPPORTUNITIES

Claude Bouchard

Physical Activity Sciences Laboratory
PEPS, Laval University
Quebec, Canada G1K 7P4

CURRENT STATUS

Attempts to define the genetic basis of obesity in the present century probably began with the study of Davenport reported in 1923. A number of papers were published on the topic based on weight for height data prior to the 1970s. Bray (1981) has summarized a good number of these studies which quite consistently demonstrated that obese children had frequently obese parents. Thus, in about 30% of the cases both parents of obese children were obese, with a range in frequency of 6% to 43%. Of course, one can readily observe that the fit between the obese state of the children and that of the parents is variable and not very tight. Following this period, the field of genetic epidemiology began to contribute new methods and research strategies in the efforts to define the genetic basis of quantitative multifactorial phenotypes. For the past 15 years or so, a good number of reports have been published regarding the heritability level and the segregation pattern of body mass for stature, and other indicators of obesity. Unfortunately, much less has been reported on the determinants and intermediate phenotypes of obesity or fat topography phenotypes.

Seventy years after the paper by Davenport, some progress has been made in the understanding of the genetic basis of human obesities. What have we learned from genetic epidemiology ? First, the estimates of heritability are quite heterogeneous. However, a trend in the size of the heritability levels is apparent: the estimates based on twins are the highest (as high as 80 percent and more of the phenotype variance) while those derived from adoption data are the lowest, with a range from about 10 to 30 percent. Heritability values (total transmission effect) computed from nuclear family data fall in between these extremes.

Second, several studies based on familial data have considered the hypothesis that a single major gene for high body mass was segregating based on familial data. If one considers only the studies that have used body mass adjusted for height in one way or another, several have found evidence for a major effect compatible with a major gene (Mendelian transmission). However, three studies did not find support for Mendelian transmission unless age and/or gender variations in the major gene were taken into account. From this small body of data, the trend seems to be for a major recessive gene accounting for about 20 to 25 percent of the variance, but with age-associated effects, with a gene frequency of about 0.2. From these studies, one can also estimate that the homozygotes for the recessive gene may represent about 4 to 6 percent of the samples.

Third, from some epidemiological studies, it can be estimated that about 25% of the obese cases occur in families with normal weight parents despite the fact that the risk of becoming obese is much higher if the person had obese parents. Moreover, the obese persons tend to be much heavier than those of the previous generation and the prevalence of obesity is clearly increasing from generation to generation.

Fourth, manipulating energy balance conditions in short term and long term intervention studies conducted with pairs of identical twins has indicated that there were considerable individual differences in body weight, body fat and fat topography changes. However, the between pairs variance in response was consistently at least 3 times greater than the within pairs variance. But the within identical twin pairs variation in weight gain or weight loss (or fat mass or fat free mass) remains quite large.

While the above suggests that the current body of knowledge on the genetic basis of human obesities is quite limited, the situation can also be seen as one which offers a multitude of opportunities. Let us briefly define some of them.

AN IMPORTANT DISTINCTION

Most cases of human obesities are complex multifactorial traits evolving under the interactive influences of dozens of affecters from the social, behavioral, physiological, metabolic, cellular and molecular domains. Segregation of the genes is not easily detected in familial or pedigree studies and whatever the influence of the genotype on the etiology, it is generally attenuated or exacerbated by nongenetic factors.

Efforts to understand the genetic causes of human obesities will stand a better chance to be successful if they are based on an appropriate conceptual framework, and adequate phenotype and intermediate phenotype measurements. In this context, the distinction between "necessary" genes and "susceptibility" genes proposed recently by Greenberg (1993) seems particularly relevant. Although there are several examples of necessary loci resulting in excess body mass or body fat for height, that is carriers of one or two copies of the deficient alleles have the disease, they represent only a small fraction of the obese population (Bouchard and Pérusse, 1988). An example of a necessary locus for human obesity is the paternally imprinted locus on chromosome 15q11-13 causing the Prader-Willi syndrome (McKusick, 1993).

Of particular importance for the human obesity phenotypes is the susceptibility gene concept. A susceptibility gene is defined as one that increases susceptibility or risk for the disease but that is not necessary for disease expression (Greenberg, 1993). An allele at a susceptibility gene may make it more likely that the carrier will become obese, but the presence of that allele is not sufficient by itself to explain the occurrence of the disease. It merely lowers the threshold for a person to develop the disease (Greenberg, 1993). As suggested by Greenberg, if the deficient allele at a susceptibility locus carries a relative risk for the disease which is less than about 10 times the risk observed with the normal allele, linkage analysis is not likely to be successful. Association studies may be more productive.

METHODOLOGICAL ADVANCES

Recent progress in animal genetics, transfection systems, transgenic animal models, recombinant DNA technologies applied to positional cloning, and methods to identify loci contributing to quantitative traits have given a new impetus to this field. The stage is now set

Table 1. Families of Research Strategies to Define the Genetic Basis of a Multifactorial Phenotype

---

1. Genetic epidemiology (top down) :
heritability, segregation pattern, etc.

2. Association studies with candidate genes.

3. Linkage studies with candidate genes and other markers.

4. Quantitative trait loci (QTL) approach.

5. Positional cloning.

6. Transgenic models.

7. DNA sequencing.

---

for major advances to occur in the understanding of the genetic and molecular basis of complex diseases such as human obesities. Table 1 provides an overview of some of the methods that can now be harnessed to bear upon the task of uncovering the genes and molecular mechanisms pertaining to the causes of human obesities and of the genetic susceptibility to the metabolic complications of obesity.

Most of the data accumulated so far have been generated by genetic epidemiologists. However, a small body of knowledge derived from association and linkage research is emerging. It is fair to conclude that no major advances have been made thus far from these areas of research, but association and linkage studies are now more frequently reported. Based on the current understanding of the pathophysiology of human obesity, including upper body fat obesity and abdominal visceral obesity, we expect that the candidate gene approach will yield useful association and linkage results. Moreover, with the advent of a comprehensive human genetic linkage map (NIH/CEPH Collaborative Mapping Group, 1992), linkage studies with a large number of markers covering most of the chromosomal length of the human genome are likely to be helpful in the identification of putative obesity genes or chromosomal regions. However, these approaches have also their limitations particularly when confronted with a complex multifactorial phenotype.

An important methodological advance in this area has been the development of the quantitative trait loci (QTL) approach (Lander and Botstein, 1989). The method allows the identification of the loci linked with a phenotype, such as obesity, and to isolate the loci by genetic crosses so that the genes can be eventually defined by positional cloning (Warden and Fisler, 1993; Warden et al, 1992). We anticipate that major progress will be made by a combination of the QTL and positional cloning technologies, particularly as more is learned about the mouse and rat genetic linkage maps.

Another area that will undoubtedly contribute in a major way to our understanding of the genetic and molecular basis of human obesity is that of the transgenic models (Jaenisch, R., 1988; Merlino, G.T., 1991; Metsäranta and Vuorio, 1992). Several studies are currently in progress with a variety of transgenes and the preliminary data reported at meetings in the past year or so suggest that much will be learned about gene expression and perhaps about dysfunction as a common feature of obesity by this approach. Indeed, it is progressively becoming apparent that dysregulation in the expression of an otherwise normal gene product, even in pathways that appear to be totally unrelated to the disease, has the potential to cause obesity. A recent intriguing example is the report about the dysregulation in the expression of the gene potentially responsible for the obesity in the Yellow mouse (Bultman et al, 1992). One of the lessons from the latter paper, and from the findings of transgenic animals, is in our view that the genes that play a role in the etiology of human obesities may turn out to be markedly different from those that are listed in the panel of the most promising candidate genes, as envisaged by the geneticists interested in this common disease

CHALLENGING PROBLEM AREAS

Are there genotype-environment effects and/or gene-gene effects that influence the events leading to the various obesity phenotypes or to some of their undesirable outcomes. These questions remain very difficult to investigate even with the present-day technology. Using the unmeasured genotype approach, we recently proposed (Bouchard et al, 1990) that one way to test for the presence of a genotype-environment (diet, exercise and others) effect in humans was to challenge several genotypes in a similar manner by submitting both members of monozygotic (MZ) twin pairs to a standardized treatment and compare the within- and the between-pair variances of the response to the treatment.

The finding of a significantly higher variance in the response between pairs than within pairs suggests that the changes induced by the treatment are more heterogeneous in genetically dissimilar individuals. In a series of experiments conducted on MZ twins over the last 10 years in our laboratory, we used either exercise training with or without negative energy balance or chronic overfeeding as treatments to investigate these effects. In general, these studies have revealed that genotype-environment interaction effects seem to be ubiquitous (Bouchard et al, 1990; Bouchard et al, 1992).

The study of the genotype-environment effect in humans can be extended to a measured genotype approach. An important advantage of the measured genotype approach over the unmeasured genotype approach is that it makes eventually possible the identification of the responsible genes, thereby providing a mean of detecting individuals at a higher risk because of differences in susceptibility. Molecular markers can thus be used in the MZ twin intervention design defined above to delineate both the quantitative importance of the genotype-treatment interaction effect and its molecular basis. This approach can be extended to several genes or molecular markers in order to look for evidence of gene-gene interaction effects on quantitative phenotypes or common multifactorial diseases such as obesity.

In the search for genes associated with genotype-environment effects, one could also use the method proposed by Berg (1981, 1990). The method is clearly less demanding from an experimental point of view as it can be carried out on cross-sectional observations made in pairs of MZ twins of the same sex. However, a relatively large number of MZ pairs is required for the findings to be robust and conclusive.

Briefly, since MZ brothers or sisters have the same genes, any difference between two members of a given pair in a multifactorial phenotype is caused by nongenetic factors. One can then compare the mean within-pair difference in the phenotype between MZ pairs who have a given allele at a locus with those who have other alleles of the same gene. Berg has argued that if an allele has a permissive effect, the within pair variance would be greater in those pairs with the allele than in those lacking the particular allele. The opposite would be true for an allele with a restrictive effect.

This amounts to a method allowing to test for genotype-environment interaction effect considering one gene at a time. Berg (1988) has applied this approach to plasma lipids

Table 2. Human Obesities are Not Simple Entities

- PROBLEMS WITH ASSESSMENT OF THE PHENOTYPES
- INCREASED PREVALENCE WITH AGE, GENERATION
- MULTIFACTORIAL PHENOTYPES
- MAJOR ROLE OF NONGENETIC FACTORS
- MULTIGENIC SYSTEMS
- STRONG POSSIBILITY OF LARGE NUMBER OF SUSCEPTIBILITY GENES
- POSSIBLY WEAK SIGNALS FROM EACH GENE
- GENE-GENE INTERACTIONS
- GENE-ENVIRONMENT / LIFESTYLE INTERACTIONS
- AGE AND GENDER RELATED EFFECTS
- GENOMIC AND / OR PRENATAL IMPRINTING
- CHAOS!

and lipoproteins in a series of studies and has reported several cases of apolipoprotein genes having significant effects on within MZ pairs phenotype variability. The method has not been used yet to any extent in the investigation of the genetic determinants of obesity.

Among the issues that have not been considered at all so far, one needs to mention the problem of gene-gene interaction effects. It seems to us that the whole field of the genetic basis of human obesities and of the genetic susceptibility to metabolic derangements in the presence of an obese state is one in which gene-gene interactions are ubiquitous. There is no doubt that the topic will attract a lot of attention over the next decade. It will likely be a complicated area of research, however, in the sense that large sample sizes will be needed if several genes are to be considered in the same analysis, new and innovative experimental designs will have to be developed, and the panel of the most important genes to investigate will probably emerge only when strong data become available from association, linkage, QTL, positional cloning or transgenic studies.

WORST CASE SCENARIO

In the opening address to the European Association for the Study of Obesity meeting held in Nice, France, in 1991, we argued that the task of uncovering the genetic basis of human obesities was a daunting one because some of the most pessimistic scenarios (from the standpoint of genetic determinism) remained quite plausible (Bouchard, 1992). Indeed, human obesity phenotypes are not simple entities and scientists of all schools interested by the topic of the genetic basis of human obesities must come to terms with the characteristics identified in Table 2.

The full complement of the characteristics listed in the table represents the equivalent of a worst case scenario for those attempting to define the genetic basis of a complex multifactorial phenotype. Indeed, the noise to signal ratio in the relation between a given gene and a relevant obesity phenotype is likely to be quite high, even more so if the phenotype is assessed only by means of a surrogate measurement. We will need all the power of the new technologies and imaginative experimental designs if we want to be successful in meeting the challenge of uncovering the genetic and molecular basis of an excessive body content, of the android body fat distribution phenotype, and of abdominal visceral obesity as well as of the metabolic complications associated with a persistent obese state. Our optimism is, however, somewhat dampened by the thought that the worst case scenario may apply here.

REFERENCES

Berg, K. (1988). Variability gene effect on cholesterol at the Kidd blood group locus, Clinical Genetics, 33, 102.

Berg, K. (1981). Twin research in coronary heart disease, in Twin Research 3: Part C, Epidemiological and Clinical Studies, Gedda, L., Parisi, P. and Nance, W. E., Eds., Liss, New York, 117.

Berg, K. (1990). Molecular genetics and nutrition, in Genetic Variation and Nutrition, Simopoulos, A. P. and Childs, B., Eds., Basel, Karger, 63, 49.

Bouchard, C., Dionne, F. T., Simoneau, J. A. and Boulay, M. R. (1992). Genetics of aerobic and anaerobic performances, in Holloszy, J. O. (ed.), Ener. Sport Scientific Review, William & Wilkins, 20, 27.

Bouchard, C., Tremblay, A., Després, J. P., Nadeau, A., Lupien, P. J., Thériault, G., Dussault, J., Moorjani, S., Pineault, S. and Fournier, G. (1990). The response to long-term overfeeding in identical twins. New England Journal of Medicine, 322, 1477.

Bouchard, C. and Pérusse, L. (1988). Heredity and body fat. Annual Review of Nutrition, 8, 259.

Bouchard, C. (1992). Human obesities: Chaos or Determinism? In: G. Ailhaud, B. Guy-Grand, M. Lafontan and D. Ricquier. (eds). Obesity in Europe 91. Proceedings of the 3rd European Congress on Obesity. John Libbey & Company Ltd, pp. 7-14.

Bray, G. A. (1981). The inheritance of corpulence. In The body weight regulatory system: Normal and disturbed mechanisms. L. A. Cioffi, W. P. T. James & T. B. Van Itallie, Eds, Raven Press, New York, 185.

Bultman, S. J., Michaud, E. J. and Woychik, R. P. (1992). Molecular characterization of the mouse Agouti Locus. Cell, 71, 1195.

Davenport, C. B. (1923). Body build and its inheritance. Carnegie Institution of Washington, 329.

Greenberg, D. A. (1993). Linkage analysis of "necessary" disease loci versus "susceptibility" loci, American Journal of Human Genetics, 52, 135.

Jaenisch, R. (1988). Transgenic animals, Science, 240, 1468.

Lander, E. S. and Botstein, D. (1989). Mapping Mendelian factors underlying quantitative traits using RFLP linkage maps, Genetics, 121, 185, 1989.

McKusick, V. A. (1993). Catalogs of Autosomal Dominant, autosomal Recessive, X-Linked, Y-Linked, and Mitochondrial Phenotypes. OMIM (Online Mendelian Inheritance in Man), The Johns Hopkins University, Baltimore, Maryland.

Merlino, G. T. (1991). Transgenic animals in biomedical research. FASEB Journal., 5, 2996.

Metsäranta, M. and Vuorio, E. (1992). Transgenic mice as models for heritable diseases, Annals of Medicine, 24, 117.

NIH/CEPH Collaborative Mapping Group. (1992). A comprehensive genetic linkage map of the human genome. Science, 258, 67.

Warden, C. H. and Fisles, J. S. (in press). Identification of genes underlying polygenic obesity in animal models, in Genetics of Obesity, Bouchard, C., Ed., Boca Raton: CRC Press Inc.

Warden, C. H., Daluiski, A. and Lusis, A. J. (1992). Identification of new genes contributing to atherosclerosis: the mapping of genes contributing to complex disorders in animal models. In Molecular genetics of coronary artery disease. Candidate genes and processes in atherosclerosis. Monogram of Human Genetics. Lusis, A. J., Rotter, J. I. and Sparkes, R. S., Eds., Basel, Karger, 419.

RESEARCH DESIGN AND METHODS TO STUDY THE GENETIC
EPIDEMIOLOGY OF OBESITY

Michael C. Neale and Lindon Eaves

Medical College of Virginia
Richmond, VA 23200

INTRODUCTION

As discussed elsewhere in this volume, obesity is associated with increased risk of cardiovascular disease. Besides its apparent health consequences, obesity can be a source of psychosocial stress. The overweight may worry about their future health, and may be subject to direct or indirect social pressures to be thin. To understand the causes of individual differences in body composition is therefore an important scientific objective.

Although the classification of certain individuals as obese is useful for clinical purposes, most measures of body composition, such as body mass index (BMI), skin folds and percent body fat are continuously distributed. Study of these continuous measures has two important advantages: (i) statistical power is much greater with continuous than ordinal or binary variables; and (ii) statistical methods for continuous variables are often simpler and require less computer time than those for ordinal data.

While we do not rule out the possibility that the population may contain a mixture of distinct groups --- such as may arise from the effects of a major genetic or environmental factor --- most of the methods we shall describe are primarily based on the assumption that variation is *multifactorial*. Thus individual differences are assumed to arise from the effects of many factors each of small effect, which, under the central limit theorem, would generate a normal distribution. Most indices of obesity either closely approximate a normal distribution or may be transformed to do so. Even if there are some genetic or environmental factors of large effect, these seem sufficiently rare that they do not account for large proportions of the population variance. If such factors were identified --- through studies of genetic linkage for example --- the methods we describe may be extended to incorporate them.

In this chapter we shall outline research designs and methods for the analysis of data collected from relatives, including nuclear families, twins, and adoptees. We shall examine some results that we and others have found and consider reasons for discrepancies where they occur.

Finally, we shall outline some new methods, including models for genotype $\times$ environment interaction, and for the study of multivariate and longitudinal data, which are likely to prove valuable in future research.

Obesity Treatment, Edited by D.B. Allison
and F.X. Pi-Sunyer, Plenum Press, New York, 1995

DESIGN AND METHODS

The statistical analysis of resemblance between relatives has a long history, going back to studies by Pearson (1904), Fisher (1918), and Wright (1921). Here we focus on structural equation modeling and path analysis, which have become very popular in many areas of human research during the past twenty years. Our treatment will be brief since many excellent general texts exist (Bollen, 1989; Loehlin, 1987; Everitt, 1984). A more thorough account of the application of structural equation models to data collected from twins may be found in Neale & Cardon (1992).

Path Analysis

Sewall Wright is credited with the invention of path analysis, a graphical system for representing mathematical models of causal and correlational relationships between variables (Wright, 1921). A good modern description of the mathematical axioms of the system may be found in McArdle & Boker (1990). Essentially, the method distinguishes between latent and observed variables. *Latent variables,* drawn in circles, are not observed and typically cannot be measured; examples include the residual variance of the dependent variable in multiple regression, measurement error, and the genotype in a multifactorial model. *Observed variables* are those that have been measured in the study. When they are continuous and normally distributed, the sample data will usually be summarized as a covariance matrix. Because genetic models predict covariances between relatives, the analysis of covariance structure through structural equation modeling is a natural choice of method.

The investigator may specify that two variables in a system are directly related in one of two ways: either through a *causal* path (drawn as a single-headed arrow from cause to effect) or through a *correlational* one (drawn as a double-headed arrow). Two variables that are not directly related in this way may still be predicted to correlate due to indirect pathways through other variables, or because they share a common cause. Note that the distinction between causal and correlational paths is usually made *ex hypothesi*. Specifying a causal path instead of a correlational one may or may not lead to different predicted covariances among the observed variables. For a mathematically complete description, the residual variances of every variable in the system should be specified by a double-headed arrow leading from the variable to itself. However, many popular accounts omit these arrows, assuming that they have a value of unity for exogenous variables (those that do not have causal arrows pointing at them), or zero for endogenous variables (which do have causal arrows pointing at them). Here we shall include them explicitly because it greatly simplifies definition of the rules of path analysis.

Derivation of the covariances between the observed variables in a path model may be done by a variety of means. Perhaps simplest is to trace *bridges* between variables, by:

1. tracing causal arrow heads backwards (from arrow head to tail)
2. passing through a double-headed correlational arrow
3. tracing causal arrows forwards to the secondary variable

The covariance due to the bridge in question - which we term a bridge effect - is calculated by multiplying the constituent paths together. The total covariance between two variables is computed as the sum of all possible bridges between the pair. Note that steps 1 and 3 may involve any number of causal arrows, from zero to many. We recognize that the method may be used to calculate the variance of a variable; the only difference when calculating a variance is that bridges are considered distinct if either their constituent paths are different *or the order of the paths is different*. We shall illustrate this method with the genetic models described below.

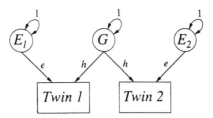

Figure 1. Genetic (G) and Environmental (E) effects on a pair of separated MZ twins. G represents all genetic effects, additive and non-additive.

Twins

Twins form a very natural approach to the resolution of genetic and environmental effects, though their use involves several assumptions. To highlight these methodological issues, consider the following unusual experiment. Imagine that *in vitro* fertilization had been used to fertilize ova from a random sample of potential mothers in the population of interest. Also, assume that this was done with sperm from fathers in the same population. Then, the few zygotes that spontaneously divided to form monozygotic (MZ) twins were selected after division and implanted into different mothers, again selected at random from the population. Except for environmental factors shared during the first few cell divisions before the MZ twinning process, the only source of similarity between the twins would be their genotype. Being monozygotic, their genotypes are identical, which we can represent as a single latent variable. Their environments are essentially uncorrelated. A simple diagram to represent this model is shown in Figure 1. Statistically speaking, this is an additive model, because variation in the phenotype is assumed to arise from the sum of the environmental and genetic sources. Using the rules of path analysis, we can obtain the predicted covariance matrix of the pairs of twins. The bridges from P1 to P1 are $h \times 1.0 \times h$, and $e \times 1.0 \times e$, which gives $var(P1) = h^2 + e^2$, which is also the variance of P2. The covariance of P1 and P2 is simply $h \times 1.0 \times h = h^2$. Thus we have

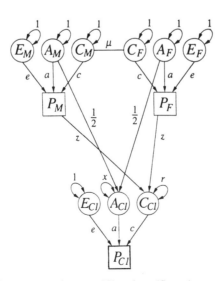

Figure 2a. Additive genetic(A), common environment (C), and specific environment (E) effects on phenotypes (P) of mother, father and child. Phenotypic assortative mating is represented by the headless arrow u.

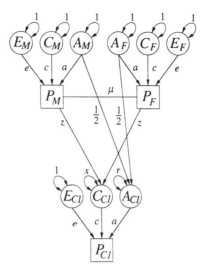

Figure 2b. Consequences of phyenotypic assortative mating (shown in Figure 2a). The latent variables of the parents become correlated. A-C covariance, which may arise from cultural transmisison, is not shown.

two predicted quantities in terms of two parameters. If we were to measure a sample of pairs of twins created in this way, we could readily calculate covariance matrices from the data. These observed statistics could then be used to estimate parameters of the model.

In reality, this odd experiment is not likely to occur often enough to yield a sample of sufficient size to estimate h^2 accurately. Some moderate-sized samples of MZ twins separated at birth do exist (Bouchard, 1992), but these confound the intrauterine factors shared by twins with genetic variance. Fortunately, it is not necessary to manipulate either biology or the rearing environment of humans to achieve roughly the same ends. An appropriate `control' for MZ twins exists --- dizygotic (DZ) twins. Biologically derived from two sperm and two ova, DZ twins are related as ordinary brothers and sisters and, under random mating their genotypes correlate one-half. Environmentally, their shared experiences are likely to be about as similar as those of MZ twins. Some small variance may be attributed to chorionicity (whether the twins share the same fluid-filled sac in the womb), because MZ twins may be either mono- or dichorionic but DZ twins are dichoronic only. Beyond these early experiences, the home-environments and treatment of the twins as children are likely to be roughly equally similar whatever their zygosity. This is the `equal environments' assumption of twin research, which has generally been found to hold when tested empirically (Loehlin & Nichols, 1976; Kendler et al, 1993). Doubtless the twins within a pair receive different treatment from time to time, and, quite possibly, DZ twins are more often treated differently than are MZ. However, it is most likely that such differential experiences are *the result of the twins eliciting different treatment*. The alternative that MZ twins are treated more alike by their parents and others simply due to their perceived zygosity would be most surprising, and has not received empirical support (Scarr & McArtney, 1983). Thus the challenge that greater MZ twin similarity is due to greater treatment rather than greater genetic similarity is generally overthrown.

To the extent that shared environmental factors have an effect on the outcome or phenotype of interest, they will increase both MZ and DZ covariances by the same amount. This amount may be estimated from the three observed statistics: the variance of twins, the MZ covariance and the DZ covariance. Therefore, the estimation of heritability from studies of MZ and DZ twins reared together is an attractive place to begin the analysis of the cause of individual differences. It should not be thought of as a complete study for it carries several assumptions - particularly regarding assortative mating and genetic dominance - that should be tested with data from other sources.

Nuclear Families

Another popular research design is to study nuclear families consisting of parents and their children. This design provides data on three varieties of familial resemblance: sibling, parent-offspring, and husband-wife. While covariances between these types of relative may be compared under simple models, they are all very different in nature and therefore do not provide a natural control for each other. Husband-wife or `marital' correlations may arise from assortment (which can be from either direct mate selection or `social homogamy' as might be caused by sociodemographic stratification), marital interaction, or sharing of relevant environmental factors during marriage. Of these various causes, only direct marital assortment has marked consequences for genetic variation. As originally shown by Fisher (1918), positive marital assortment for a trait will increase its genetic variance in the population. If there is transmission of environmental variance from parent to child, direct marital assortment will also increase trait variance --- and so will social homogamy. These conclusions are not easy to grasp without the aid of some formal modeling, so we present path diagrams for two types of homogamy in Figures 2a, 2b and 3. Each of these figures features two parents and one child for simplicity - larger sibship sizes may be drawn by adding further offspring. In Figure 2a, we show marital resemblance through direct assortment and cultural transmission from parent phenotype to the environment of the child. The headless arrow reflects a sort-merge process that generates covariance between the P_M and P_F. Because these variables are entirely caused by their latent variables (A, C, and E), the consequences of inducing covariance between the phenotypes is to induce covariances between the latent variables, as shown in Figure 2b. Note that the parents' genotypes are now correlated and this therefore increases the variance of the offspring genotype. Thus genetic variance will increase from generation to generation, once phenotypic assortative mating has begun. It can be shown that this process will lead to

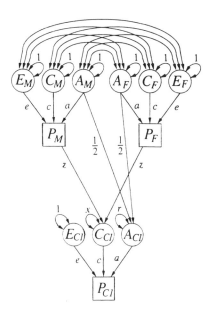

Figure 3. Model of social homogamy, genetic and cultural transmission. A-C covariance will arise if there is both genetic and P to C cultural transmission. This in turn will lead to covariance betwen genotypes.

a stable equilibrium with increased genetic variance proportional to the degree of assortative mating (i.e., the size of μ). This result contrasts with the consequences of social homogamy (Figure 3), which only affects genetic variance if there is G-E covariance. Relative to the path from genotype to phenotype, G-E covariance is usually small, so the genetic consequences of social homogamy are practically negligible.

Because parents and children share 50% of their genes, these relatives may well resemble each other because of genetic factors, and it is here that we encounter a problem with studies of nuclear families. The effects of genes and environment are confounded. Siblings may resemble each other because of genetic and environmental factors, as may parents and children. However, unlike the classical twin study, the environmental similarities between parents and children are wildly different from those shared by siblings, so there is no appropriate control. The marital resemblance data do not help resolve genetic from environmental effects. They are useful, however, because assortative mating (like marrying like) can inflate the effects of genetic or environmental transmission. There is evidence for modest (r=1. to .3) assortative mating for weight and relative weight in a number of studies (Price & Vandenberg, 1980; Plomin et al, 1977; Annest et al, 1983; Price, 1987). Quite unlike genetic theory, there is rarely good *a priori* reason to suppose that one form of sharing of environmental factors is equivalent to another. Very different types of relative are expected to share the same proportion of genes, e.g., grandparents and grandchildren, half-siblings, cousins related through MZ twins. We have no environmental theory that predicts the environmental similarity of these diverse relationships.

Twins and Parents

Because twins reared together are readily available from the population, their parents make a natural extension to the classical twin study. All the power of the twin study to resolve genetic and environmental effects is retained, and we gain two types of information: husband-wife and parent-offspring covariances. The former allows the assessment of possible effects of assortative mating or marital interaction, both of which lead to husband-wife similarity. Although it may be possible to distinguish between assortment and interaction if we have data on length of marriage, the power to do so is usually low unless sample sizes are very large. For blood pressure, we found no evidence for increasing marital similarity with length of marriage in a large sample (Tambs et al, 1992). Similarly, albeit in a smaller sample, we find no relationship between length of marriage and marital resemblance for BMI (Allison et al, submitted). Therefore, the assumption that husband-wife similarity is due to *phenotypic assortative mating*, seems justified. This process generates correlations between parents' genotypes and environments (see, e.g., Fisher, 1918; Eaves et al, 1978, Carey, 1986 or Fulker, 1988 for the mathematical details of this effect). The parent-offspring data provide something of a test of elements of the model. From genetic theory we know that the additive genetic correlation between parents and children is .5 --- the same as for DZ twins or siblings. Therefore we could predict the parent-child correlation from the MZ and DZ covariances. Departures from the predicted value might be interpreted in different ways. If there is genetical non-additivity such as dominance, then the parent-child correlation will be less than the predicted value. Likewise, if there are age-dependent genetic effects (`genotype × age interaction'), the parent-child correlation will usually be decreased relative to those of twins, because parents and children are assessed at different ages. On the other hand, if the parents' phenotypes form a significant part of the twins' environment (`cultural transmission') the parent-child correlation may exceed the DZ twin one.

Adoption Studies

From the methodological standpoint, the ideal adoption study is where the adoptees come from a representative sample of parents in the population, are separated from their parents and other relatives at birth, and are placed into families selected at random from the population. In reality, these conditions are rarely, if ever, met (and for good reason!). First, parents who give up their children for adoption are typically younger and less wealthy than those who do not. Second, separation from parents does not always take place at birth, and subsequent placement into the adoptive home may occur only after a period of rearing in temporary foster homes or institutions. Third, sound ethical principles guide the placement of adoptees into homes where good parenting practices and a healthy rearing environment is apparent. Fourth, there may also be some tendency to match the adoptees to fit their future families. Nevertheless, despite these departures from random sampling and placement, adoption studies can be useful since these shortcomings are either (i) not relevant to the phenotype under study, or (ii) statistically controlled. Quite often, it is necessary to use methods developed for (ii) to test whether (i) is the case.

To some extent, the full adoption study yields more information than the study of twins and their parents. We may compare unrelated children reared in the same family (UT) with full siblings (FS) raised the same way --- this corresponds to the MZ-DZ comparison of the twin study. The methods both yield husband-wife and parent-natural child correlations. However, the adoption study may also provide covariances of biological parent with adopted-away child (BPAC) and adoptive parent with adopted child (APAC). In principle, these statistics resolve the effects of genetical non-additivity from those of cultural transmission. However, careful control of the effects of age, age at placement, selective placement, and non-random sampling should be made before these parameters may be estimated accurately. To date, most studies have attempted to test for the effects of selective placement by examining the correlation between BP and AP. When these are significant, their effects may be statistically modelled using equivalent methods to those described above for assortative mating. The effects of non-random sampling may be assessed by comparison of the means and variances of the BP, AP and BC and AC groups. Some discussion of the possible effects of sampling bias may be found in Neale et al, 1989. Attempts to dealing with non-random sampling are comparatively rare in this area, at least in part because of the methodological complexity involved. Nevertheless, advances in software development and computer hardware performance make statistical correction of sampling bias more feasible than has been the case in the past.

CHANGE IN GENE EXPRESSION AS A FUNCTION OF AGE AND GENDER

A priori, parsimony would lead us to prefer a model in which there are no changes in gene expression with age or gender, but there are some theoretical reasons to suggest that a more complex model may be required. Natural selection is strongest during the reproductive years. Furthermore, genes relevant to fitness tend to show directional dominance (Fisher, 1928). Haldane (1941) combined these ideas to develop theories for change in genetic architecture with age. If body composition were related to reproductive fitness, these theories would predict that:

1. The expression of genetic effects on normal and abnormal body mass will change with age.
2. Additive genetic effects (`genetic noise') and environmental effects will increase with age
3. Dominant genetic effects will become less marked with increasing age
4. These changes will be more sudden in women than men.

Unfortunately, testing these hypotheses requires very large sample sizes in addition to sophisticated statistical methodology. However, we can review some recent findings that suggest some support for the theory.

EMPIRICAL SUPPORT FOR HALDANE'S THEORY FROM BMI DATA

This article does not intend to offer a thorough review of studies of the inheritance of body mass; such accounts may be found elsewhere (Grilo & Pogue-Guile, 1991; Meyer & Stunkard, 1993). Rather, we shall discuss two contradictory reports in the light of our description of methods, and then examine some recently published data for their support of Haldane's theory.

Perspective on the Conflicting Reports of Bouchard & Stunkard

Most researchers in the field are aware of the reports of Bouchard (1989) and Stunkard (1991); most are puzzled by the contrary conclusions. Stunkard estimates the total (additive

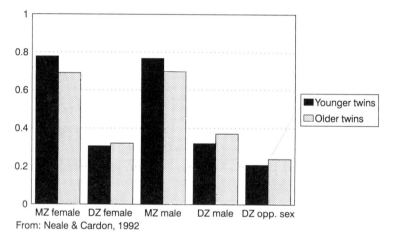

From: Neale & Cardon, 1992

Figure 4. Twin Correlations for BMI. Young and older cohorts. 1981 Australian survey.

and non-additive) heritability of BMI to be around 70% whereas Bouchard's figure is only 5%. The key difference may be in the methods rather than the data, which, for the most part, agree. Bouchard uses a modified Beta model of Rice et al (1978), which is essentially a structural equation model for data from parents and their offspring. In addition to parameters for assortative mating and cultural and genetic transmission, the model uses two 'special twin environment' factors, one for MZ and one for DZ twins. These factors effectively ignore the twin data, because any values of the MZ and DZ correlations (e.g. if both were .999) would not affect the estimates of other parameters of the model. For many of the body-mass related variables studied by Bouchard, these parameters are large and highly significant, particularly for MZ twins. Such estimates would also seem unrealistic. It is difficult to imagine what factors could possibly be so much more similar for MZ and DZ twins. If there are non-linear age interactions, the estimates from twins, who are usually assessed at the same age, will generally be more accurate than those computed from relatives measured at different times in their lives. It is also difficult to imagine what non-genetic factors could possibly lead to vastly greater similarity of MZ than DZ twins. Could it be function of much more similar treatment of MZ

Table 1. Results of Fitting Models to Twin Pair Covariance Matrices and Twin Means for Body Mass Index (from Neale & Cardon, 1992).

| | | FEMALE | | | |
| | | Young | | Older | |
Model	df	x^2	p	x^2	p
1. No heterogen. + of means or variances	11	8.16	.70	20.62	.08
2. Heterogeneity + of means	9	6.03	.74	17.84	.09
3. Heterogeneity + of variances	9	5.70	.77	7.76	.74
4. Heterogeneity of means and variances	7	3.93	.79	5.74	.77
Genetic Model		ADE		AE#	
Means Model		MZ ≠ DZ		MZ = DZ	

| | | MALE | | | |
| | | Young | | Older | |
Model	df	x^2	p	x^2	p
1. No heterogen. + of means or variances	11	54.97	.001*	48.55	.001*
2. Heterogeneity + of means	9	29.22	.001*	44.58	.001*
3. Heterogeneity + of variances	9	22.76	.01	7.68	.74
4. Heterogeneity of means and variances	7	7.72	.36	5.69	.77
Genetic Model	ADE		AE#		
Means Model	MZ ≠ DZ		MZ = DZ		

+ Between concordant-participant versus discordant-participant twins
* p < .001
# AE models have two more degrees of freedom thal shown in the df column

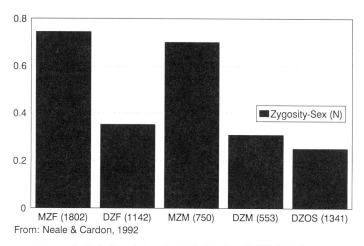

From: Neale & Cardon, 1992

Figure 5. Twin Correlations for BMI. Virginia 30,000 1987 Survey.

Table 2. Parameter Estimates Obtained by Fitting Genotype x Sex Interaction Models to Virginia and AARP Body-Mass Index (BMI) Twin Data.

Parameter	MODEL				
	I	II	III	IV	V
h_f	0.449	0.454	0.454	0.454	0.346
d_f	0.172	0.000	--	--	0.288
e_f	0.264	0.265	0.265	0.267	0.267
h_m	0.210	0.240	0.240	0.342	--
d_m	0.184	0.245	0.245	--	--
e_m	0.213	0.213	0.213	0.220	--
h'_m	0.198	--	--	--	--
k	--	--	--	--	0.778
\hline					
x^2	9.26	11.80	11.80	38.53	19.62
d.f.	8	9	10	11	11
p	0.32	0.23	0.30	0.00	0.05
AIC	-6.74	-6.20	-8.20	16.53	-2.38

than DZ twins? This seems highly unlikely given the arguments made above about the effects of similarity of treatment based on perceived zygosity per se. What we seem to require is an alternative model that does not rely on the exclusion of the twin data. One such model simply involves the addition of genetical dominance which can give rise to considerably increased MZ twin and slightly increased full sibling & DZ twin correlations without changing other predicted correlations.

Bouchard may be right when he challenges the proportion of additive genetic variance, estimates of which may be biased in analyses that ignore the effects of genetical dominance. However, it seems more plausible that there is genetic dominance rather than an enormous effect of MZ twin special environment.

Age Effects in the Australian NH\\&MRC Twin Data

For part of our book on methodology for genetic studies (Neale & Cardon, 1992) we analyzed BMI data collected from a mailed questionnaire survey of volunteer twins from the Australian National Health and Medical Research Council (NH\\&MRC) registry. The sample of 3808 pairs in which both twins responded was divided into those above and below thirty years, and covariance matrices were computed for each of the sex, zygosity and age groups (ten in all). Except for the relatively small sample of DZ male pairs, in each case the total variance is greater in older than younger twins, *in accordance with the above predictions 1 and 2 of Haldane's theory*. Figure 4 shows twin correlations for BMI in this dataset. Evidently, the MZ twin correlation declines somewhat from old to young cohort, while the DZ twin correlations do the opposite. Model-fitting results are tied to this pattern, such that for the younger cohort, models including dominant genetic effects fit better than those without. In contrast, there was no evidence for significant dominant genetic effects in the older cohort. These effects were consistent across gender, and *support the prediction 3* .

Sex-Limitation in Body-Mass Index in Older Twins.

Although the change in genetic architecture from both additive and dominant genetic effects in those under thirty to additivity alone in the older cohort was found in both males and females in the Australian data, the possibility that different genetic factors were operating in males and females was not tested. In a volunteer sample of twins aged over fifty-five obtained through the American Association of Retired Persons (AARP; Truett, 1993, Truett et al. 1994) there is evidence of sex-limitation.

This may be seen by examining the correlations as shown in Figure 5. Note that these data are in broad agreement with those of the Australian survey. It appears that the most parsimonious explanation of the data, using Akaike's Information Criterion (Akaike, 1987) as a guide, is given by a model that consists of additive genetic and random environment effects in females, but *both additive and dominant genetic effects in males*. These results are detailed in Chapter 11 of Neale & Cardon (1992).

Although the finding of some dominant genetic variation in the older males does not agree with the results from the Australian sample, we note that the power to discriminate these effects is low in data from twins (Martin et al, 1978). However, the result *agrees with prediction 4 above*. We are aware that these results are based on samples whose ascertainment was not ideal for epidemiological purposes because they consist of volunteers. However, unless the samples are extremely unrepresentative of BMI scores in the general population (which they do not appear to be) these results may well be robust. Their replication with a population sample and the testing of further hypotheses would be well justified.

First, both the total and the additive genetic variance of BMI in women was larger than in men. For this age group, 28 to 52 years, we would expect more additive variance in women, whose genetic architecture should be changing more rapidly according to Haldane's theory. Again the study found a model of additive and dominant genetic effects to be the most parsimonious explanation of the data. However, the estimated dominance component was smaller in this study, and there was no tendency for genetic dominance to be greater in males than in females.

FUTURE DIRECTIONS

Methods for Modeling Genotype × Age Interaction

As we have seen, many current approaches to the analysis of data from relatives are based on structural equation modeling (Neale & Cardon, 1992). Models may be fitted to data with a variety of commercial packages such as LISREL (Jöreskog & Sörbom, 1989) EQS (Bentler, 1989) or LISCOMP (Muthèn, 1987), or with 'shareware' packages such as Mx (Neale, 1991), or with purpose-built FORTRAN programs. However, except for Mx, the packages require some form of data summary, such as covariance matrices, for analysis. The structure of the data from most studies defies such summary if we wish to account for possible age effects. Only studies where all subjects are assessed at the same age --- and where there is no variation in age at placement or length of time spent living together --- can be handled this way. A partial strategy would be to subset the data into different groups according to age strata, which will allow a broad examination of the possibility of age interaction.

This can be done in Mx for many age strata using the variable-length record structure and maximum likelihood estimation based on the raw data. In its current version, fitting such a model would require definition of the covariance structure for all possible combinations of ages (or times of placement). Each pedigree would then have its covariance matrix extracted from the global one, and the likelihood function calculated accordingly.

Clearly, for truly continuous measures of age, this method is impractical. Models for such data have been called 'data specific' (Neale & Cardon, 1992). Further developments of the Mx code are planned to facilitate this type of modeling.

Multivariate Methods

Univariate genetic analysis of body mass provides only the first step in understanding the genetic epidemiology of obesity. Many methods for multivariate analysis of data collected from unrelated individuals gain power when they are adapted for use in genetically informative design. The most obvious example is confirmatory factor analysis in which general and specific factors are defined to account for variance and covariance in many measures. In a genetic context, such hypotheses about the nature of covariation between measures can be tested at the level of the latent genetic and environmental variables, so that, e.g., we can test whether the same genetic component underlies both BMI and skinfold measures (Maes, 1992). Another example is Latent Class analysis, which postulates probabilities of observing particular outcomes that vary between a few separate classes in the population. In obesity, we might look for specific classes of body mass related variables that appear to cluster among relatives according to mendelian ratios, in a way similar to segregation analysis.

The analysis of cause is central to scientific endeavors, and the genetic study provides a unique opportunity to test certain simple hypotheses about direction of causation (Neale & Cardon, 1992; Heath et al, 1993; Neale et al, 1994). For traits with equivalent reliability yet different genetic architecture, it is possible to reject certain models of direct cause between variables, e.g., that amount of 'junk food' eaten causes body mass. {BMI & BP in review} Similarly, we could analyze the other side of the equation by the simultaneous measurement of health variables such as cardiovascular function or physical fitness. We should also be alert to the possibility that certain variables are best modeled as mediators which modify the impact of one variable on another. Measures of metabolic rate are fine candidates for mediating the relationship between calorific intake and fat storage. We require similar methods to those described above for genotype × environment interaction to fit models of this type.

Finally, no discussion of the study of human individual differences would be complete without consideration of longitudinal data. The workshop showed that there are many fine datasets consisting of repeated measures of body mass related variables assessed on different occasions. These multiple measures may be made at intervals of days, weeks, months or years and each may require separate types of model to describe their pattern of change over time. Again, this will demand careful statistical methods that can deal with missing data and variable intervals between assessments (and, in genetic studies, variable intervals between assessment of relatives. We have begun the development of software to simplify the application of growth curve and other mathematical modeling of change to complex, incomplete data structures, but there is much yet to be done.

In conclusion, therefore, genetic studies can tell us far more than whether or indices of obesity are heritable. Rather, they provide a powerful tool for unraveling the causes of individual differences, be they genetic, environmental or some additive or non-additive function thereof. We see the potential to resolve genuine external environmental factors from those that are selected or elicited by the subject themselves. Another example is the analysis of an association between some parental characteristic such as rearing style or diet, and body mass in their children. This association might come from a direct environmental impact of the parent on the child, but could be indirect if some of the genes for obesity also effect differences in rearing style. Such basic epidemiological research is essential for the development of effective procedures for interventionand recommendations for nutrition and diet. It is fair to say that genetic studies are the best way to study the environment. Yet it should be recognized that strongly heritable characteristics are not immutable; the effects of genes may change over time, or we may be able to find ways to interrupt the pathway from genotype to obesity. We must bear in mind the classic example is phenylketonuria or "PKU". Without treatment, those people with two copies of the phenylketonuria gene suffer severe mental retardation. However, by studying the pathway from gene to disease, scientists were able to discover that one particular amino acid - phenylalanine - which is broken down by normal metabolism, was not being broken down in phenylketonurics. Restriction of the diet to exclude this amino acid - if done early enough in development - stops the mental retardation altogether. Imagine if such a simple cure were to be found for obesity! This may be unlikely, but we will never know unless we study our genetic blueprint.

REFERENCES

Akaike, H. (1987). Factor analysis and ARC. Psychometrika, 52, 317-332.

Allison, D.B., Heshka, S., Neale, M.C., Lykken, D.T. \& Heymsfield, S.B. (In press) A genetic analysis of relative weight among 4020 twin pairs with an emphasis on sex effects. Health Psychology.

Annest, J. L., Sing, C. F., Biron, P., & Mongeau, J. G. (1983). Familial aggregation of blood pressure and weight in adoptive families. III. Analysis of the role of shared genes and shared household environment in explaining family resemblance for height, weight and selected weight/height indices. American Journal of Epidemiology, 117, 492-506.

Bentler, P. M. (1989). EQS: Structural equations program manual. Los Angeles: BMDP Statistical Software.

Bollen, K. A. (1989). Structural Equations with Latent Variables. New York: John Wiley.

Bouchard, C. (1989). Genetic factors in Obesity. Medical Clinics of North America, 73, 67-81.

Carey, G. (1986). A general multi variate approach to linear modeling in human genetics. American Journal of Human Genetics, 39, 775-786.

Eaves, L. J., Last, K. A., Young, P. A., & Martin, N. G. (1978). Model-fitting approaches to the analysis of human behavior. Heredity, 11~ 249-320.

Everett, B. S. (1984). An introduction to latent variable models. Chapman and Hall.

Fisher, R. A. (1918). The correlation between relatives on the supposition of Mendelian inheritance. Translations of the Royal Society, Edinburgh, 52, 399-433.

Fulker, D. W. (1988). Genetic and cultural transmission in human behavior. In B. S. Whir, E. J. Risen,M. M. Goodman, & G. Namkoong weds.), Proceedings of the second international conference on quantitative genetics (pup. 318-340). Sunder land, MA: Sinauer.

Grilo, C. M. and Pogue-Guile, M. F. (1991) The nature of environmental influences on weight and obesity: A behavior genetic analysis. Psychological Bulletin, 110, 20-537

Haldane, J. B. S. (1941). The relative importance of principal and modifying genes in determining some human diseases. Journal of Genetics, 41, 149-157.

Heath, A. C., Kessler, R. C., Neale, M. C., Hewitt, J. K., Eaves, L. J., & Kendler, K. S. (1993). Testing hypotheses about direction-of-causation using cross-sectional family data. Behavior Genetics. (pup. 29-50) .

Jöreskog, K. G. & Sörbom, D. (1989). LISREL 7: A Guide to the Program and Applications (end ed.). Chicago: SPAS, Inc.

Kendler, K.S., Neale, M.C., Kessler, R.C., Heath, A.C. & Eaves, L.J. (1993) A test of the equal-environment assumption in twin studies of psychiatric illness. Behavior Genetics 23:21-28.

Loehlin, J. C. (1987). Latent Variable Models. Hillsdale: Lawrence Erlbaum Associates.

Loehlin, J. C. & Nichols, R. C. (1976). Heredity, Environments and Personality. Austin: University of Texas Press.

Maes, H. H. M. (1992). Univariate and multi variate genetic analysis of physical characteristics of loinsand parents. Unpublished doctoral dissertation, Katholieke Universiteit Leuven, Leuven, Belgium.

Martin, N. G., Eaves, L. J., Kearsey, M. J., & Davies, P. (1978). The power of the classical twin study. Heredity, 40, 97-116.

McArdle, J J and Boker, S M (1990) RAMpath path diagram software. Denver, CO: Data Transforms Inc.

Meyer, J.M. & Stunkard, A.J. (1993) Genetics and human obesity. In A.J. Stunkard and T. A. Wadden (Eds.) Obesity: Theory and Therapy (pp. 137-149). New York: Raven Press

Muthèn (1987) LISCOMP: Analysis of Linear Structural Equations with a Comprehensive Measurement Model. Mooresville, IN: Scientific Software, Inc

Neale, M. C. (1991). Mx: Statistical Modeling. Box 710 MCV, Richmond, VA 23298: Department of Human Genetics.

Neale, M. C. & Cardon, L. R. (1992). Methodology for Genetic Studies of Tw ins and Families. Kluwer Academic Publishers.

Neale, M.C., Eaves, L.J., Kendler, K.S. \& Hewitt, J.K. (1989) Bias in correlations from truncated samples of relatives. Behavior Genetics, 19, 163-169.

Neale, M.C., Eaves, L.J., Hewitt, J.K., MacLean, C.J., Meyer, J.M. \& Kendler,K.S. (1989). Analyzing the relationship between age of onset and risk torelatives {\it American Journal of Human Genetics;}{\bf 45:}226-239

Neale, M. C., Walters, E. W., Heath, A. C., Kessler, R. C., Perusse, D., Eaves, L. J., & Kendler, K. S. (1994). Depression and parental bonding: cause, consequence, or genetic covariance? Genetic Epidemiology, In press.

Pearson, K. (1904). On a generalized theory of alternative inheritance, with special references to Mendel's laws. Phil. Trans. Royal Society A, 203, 53-86.

Price, R. A., Cadoret, R. J., Stunkard, A. J., & Troughton, E. (1987). Genetic contributions to human fatness: An adoption study. American Journal of Psychiatry, 144, 1003-1008.

Price, R. A., & Vandenberg, S. G. (1980). Spouse similarity in American and Swedish couples. Behavior Genetics, 10, 59-71.

Rice, J., Cloninger, C. R., & Reich, T. (1978). Multifactorial inheritance with cultural transmission and assortative mating. I. Description and basic properties of the unitary models. American Journal of Human Genetics, 30, 618-643.

Scarr, S. & McCartney, K. (1983) How people make their own environments: A theory of genotype-environment effects. Child Development, 54, 424-435

Stunkard, A. J. (1991). Genetic contributions to human obesity. In Genes, Brain and Behavior (pp. 205-218). Raven Press Ltd.

Tambs, K., Moum, T., Holmen, J., Eaves, L.J., Neale, M.C., Lund-Larsen, P.G. & Næss, S., (1992) Genetic and environmental effects on blood pressure in a Norwegian sample. Genetic Epidemiology, 9, 11-26

Truett, K. R. (1992) Age differences in conservatism. Personality & Individual Differences 14(3):405-411

Truett, K. L., Walters, E. E., Eaves, L. J., Heath, A. C., Hewitt, J. K., Meyer, J. M., Silberg, J. L., Neale, M. C., Martin, N. G., & Kendler, K. S. (1994). A model system for analysis of family resemblance in extended kinships of twins. Behavior Genetics. In press.

Wright, S. (1921). Correlation and causation. Journal of Agricultural Research, 20, 557-585.

MODELLING AND DATA ANALYSIS FOR LONGITUDINAL DIETARY INTERVENTION

Robert M. Elashoff and Kwan-Moon Leung

Department of Biostatistics
University of California
Los Angeles, CA 90007

Two trials essentially designed to reduce weight will be used as illustrations of modelling issues and data analyses. The first study is a randomized trial intervening on percent fat calories and exercise to bring weight, percent fat calories and specific lipid measures to appropriate levels. The study was designed principally by David Heber and Robert M. Elashoff. Certain aspects of this study were reported in *Preventive Medicine*, 1992. Up to five measurement times are to be observed. The second study is a weight reduction single arm trial, which, except for the specific intervention, has a rather standard design. The first 100 days of the study will be considered; observations were to be carried out weekly as is customary in such trials. Both of these trials were designed and implemented is a state-of-the-art way.

Figure 1 shows 6 different individual time trend curves for weight from the first study where subjects were assigned to the intervention strategy of the Women's Health Trial. Clearly, subjects do not follow the same time trend curve. In addition, one notes that not all subjects are observed the same number of times. Thirdly, while not clear from these curves, the time points at which subjects were observed fails to agree with the specified times at which each subject is to be observed according to the design. These three comments vitiate the standard pre-1986 statistical approaches to the modelling and data analyses for longitudinal data (also called repeated measurements data).

This talk will focus on statistical models and data analyses that deal specifically with the three comments or three departures from standard approaches as given for example in *An Introduction to Applied Multivariate Statistics*, Srivastava and Carter; *Applied Computational Statistics in Longitudinal Research*, Rovine and von Eye; *Multivariate Analysis-III*, Krishnaiah.

MODELLING LONGITUDINAL DATA

Fixed Effects Models

To fix ideas, consider the weight data for Study 1. In standard time trend models, we

Obesity Treatment, Edited by D.B. Allison
and F.X. Pi-Sunyer, Plenum Press, New York, 1995

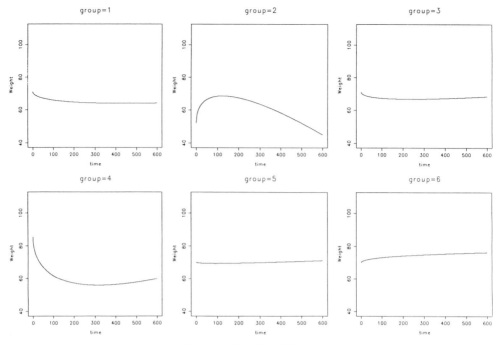

Figure 1. Time Trend Cluster

have for subject i at time t, suppose a quadratic fits the weight by time graph. Then,
weight = treatment effect + time trend + error

$$y = \alpha x + \beta_0 + \beta_1 t + \beta_2 t^2 + \epsilon \qquad (1)$$

$$x = \begin{array}{ll} 1 \text{ if} & \text{treatment 1} \\ 0 & \text{treatment 2} \end{array}$$

This relationship assumes each individual follows this time trend, where $\beta_0, \beta_1, \beta_2$ are fixed, unknown constants to be estimated from all the subject data. The data would look like this:

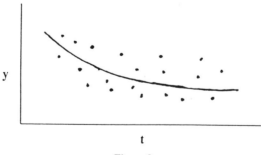

Figure 2.

We would <u>not</u> plot the curves for each of the 280 subjects.

To provide estimates of $\alpha, \beta_0, \beta_1, \beta_2$ and to test hypotheses concerning α or the β's, the statistician requires additional assumptions (A. Sen and M. Srivastava, 1990). These assumptions must include that each subject follows (1) above; also, certain requirements concerning the times observed, normality of y, variance and independence assumptions about the y.

Random Coefficient Regression Models (RCR)

Let us consider the weight data from Study 1. Let us assume that each individual i has a time trend curve that is a quadratic. We now have

$$y - \alpha x + b_{0i} + b_{1i}t + b_{2i}t^2 + \epsilon , \qquad (2)$$

where y, x, ϵ have the same meaning as in (1). The fixed, unknown constants are α and the variance of ϵ. The quantities b_{0i}, b_{1i}, b_{2i} are terms specific to subject i. The number of time points and their specific times are constrained only weakly. Figure 3 shows this new setup.

Recall Figure 1. Clearly, the RCR model should represent the weight by time trend curves more realistically than the single curve of Figure 2.

One problem: there exist 280 subjects in Study 1 and 241 subjects in Study 2. Do we produce a curve for each subject? How can we determine the significance of a trend? How do we estimate and test hypotheses about the treatment effect α? And many more questions?

We must answer these questions. Before we do so, we should complete the formulation of the statistical model. Most writers on RCR models assume that we cannot estimate so many time trend curves so that the regression coefficients (b_{0i}, b_{1i}, b_{2i}) follow a normal distribution. Also, many writers assume that the weights y_i at time t given the regression coefficients are statistically independent--though this is not necessary.

With these additional assumptions, model 2 now has a nickname--the linear RCR model. The most commonly asked inference questions such as hypothesis testing for the treatment effect α and assessment of the population mean weight time trend have explicit answers.

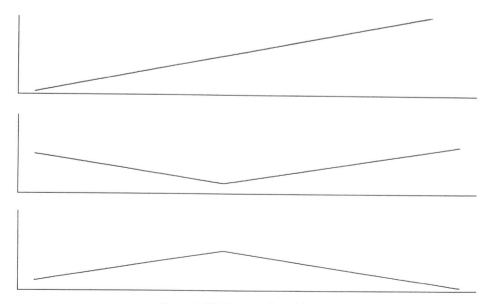

Figure 3. Weight curves that might occur

Study 1: Comparison of the Fixed Effects Model and the Linear RCR Model

The following model gave good fit to the data:

$$y_{it} - \alpha_1 X_{1i} + \alpha_2 X_{2i} + b_{0i} + b_{1i}t + b_{2i}t^{1/2} + \epsilon \quad , \tag{3}$$

variance $\epsilon = \sigma^2$, and $x_{1i} = 1$ or 0 depending on the treatment group and $x_{2i} =$ baseline weight. Parameter estimates and standard errors are:

Parameter	Fixed Effect	Linear RCR
α_1	-0.335 (0.215)	-0.134 (0.272)
α_2	0.989 (0.009)	0.987 (0.012)
b_0	1.57 (1.15)	1.473 (0.948)
b_1	0.013 (0.004)	0.012 (0.002)
b_2	-0.373 (0.133)	-0.351 (0.069)
σ^2	11.36	2.0

For this study, there is quite a difference on σ^2 between these two models.

What are We Doing?

Essentially, the results up to the present for the linear RCR model are these:

a) Development of a time trend model to fit the subject, time data
b) Estimation of a population time trend curve
c) Estimation of a treatment effect
d) Estimation of standard errors and error variance
e) In addition, highly variable estimated time trend curves for each subject.

With the moderate sample sizes available to us, we should be able to obtain the following results:

a) Determine the number and type of different time trend curves for weight
b) Classify subjects into one of these clusters of time trend curves
c) Explore how these clusters might be associated to additional variables, behavioral or lipid.

Thus, only one of the goals of the study should be estimating the mean treatment effect.

Towards a More General RCR Model

Let us assume that the equation linking weight to time is correct. Now, we will assume that only m distinct time trend curves exist. The quantity m must be estimated. We also assume a more general distribution for weight (non-normal). We do not need to know the correct correlation structure of weight in a given individual over time. We need to correctly specify the variance. From this broadening of the assumptions in the previous RCR Model, let us now return to Study 1 and, then, Study 2.

Data Analyses for Study 1

Applying our generalized RCR model we obtain these results. Table 1 indicates that

Table 1.

Outcome : Weight (DATASET=CINDY)

Sample size : # of Subjects=280, # of Observation=1030

Model 1 : $Y_{it} = \alpha_1 X_{1i} + \alpha_2 X_{2i} + b_{0i} + b_{1i}t_{it} + b_{2i}t_{it}^{1/2} + \epsilon_{it}$

where Y_{it} = weight for subject i at time t
X_{1i} = group indicator, 1 for WHEP and 0 for WHT
X_{2i} = Baseline weight

$P(m=3|data) = 1.28 \times 10^{-52}$
$P(m=4|data) = 3.42 \times 10^{-15}$
$P(m=5|data) = 2.40 \times 10^{-14}$
$P(m=6|data) = 0.99999$
$P(m=7|data) = 1.27 \times 10^{-5}$

Estimates :
$\alpha_1 = 0.10\ (0.198)$
$\alpha_2 = 0.98\ (0.008)$
$\phi = 0.32$

		(2.31, 0.0165, -0.69)	w.p. 0.153
		(-16.82, -0.1328, 2.97)	w.p. 0.008
		(2.29, 0.0186, -0.57)	w.p. 0.260
(b_{0i}, b_{1i}, b_{2i})	=	(16.17, 0.092, -3.28)	w.p. 0.018
		(1.01, 0.008, -0.153)	w.p. 0.507
		(0.91, -0.0037, 0.345)	w.p. 0.055

Table 2.

Comparison of Methods; Outcome=Weight
Outcome : Weight (DATASET=CINDY)

Model : $Y_{it} = \alpha_1 X_{1i} + \alpha_2 X_{2i} + b_{0i} + b_{1i}t_{it} + b_{2i}t_{it}^{1/2}$

Parameters	Fixed Effect	Normal Random Effect	Robust Random Effect
α_1	-0.335(0.215)	-0.134(0.272)	0.10 (0.198)
α_2	0.989(0.009)	0.987(0.012)	0.982(0.008)
b_{0i}	1.57(1.15)	1.473(0.948)	1.670(Mean)
b_{1i}	0.013(0.004)	0.012(0.002)	0.012(Mean)
b_{2i}	-0.373(0.133)	-0.351(0.069)	-0.348(Mean)
σ^2	11.36	1.995	3.14

m=6 time trend curves (from a possible 280) are all that is required to specify the number of types of time trend curves. Also, a hypothesis test of $H_o = \alpha_1 = 0$ vs. $H_1 = \alpha^1 \neq$ would be accepted (no treatment difference). Baseline weight is an important predictor of weight at time t. Table 2 compares estimators. Figure 4 gives the 6 types of curves. Figure 5 shows the results of classifying each subject into the cluster with the highest probability. We have not related our lipid measurements to these clusters at the present time. Figure 6 gives a sample of 30 subject curves.

Data Analyses for Study 2

Study 2 is a one-arm trial, effectively an efficacy trial in weight reduction. Table 3 presents the general RCR model. Table 3 gives the parameters (fixed effects). The estimated value of m=12, and shows the strong effect of baseline departure from ideal weight to predict weight departure from ideal at later time t. Table 4 presents comparisons between the three approaches with the change in σ^2 being the most pronounced and the inconsistency of the gender effect. Figure 7 shows the 12 time trends; while Figure 8 shows all subject fitted curves. I will be making adjustments through penalty constraints in our estimation algorithms to show

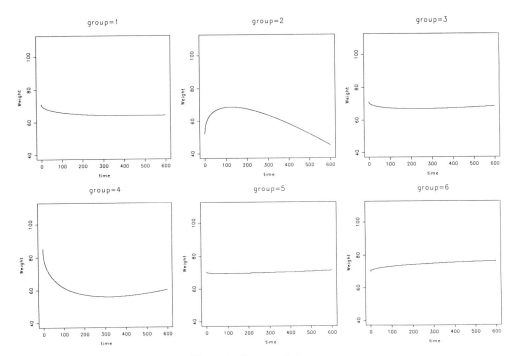

Figure 4. Time Trend Cluster

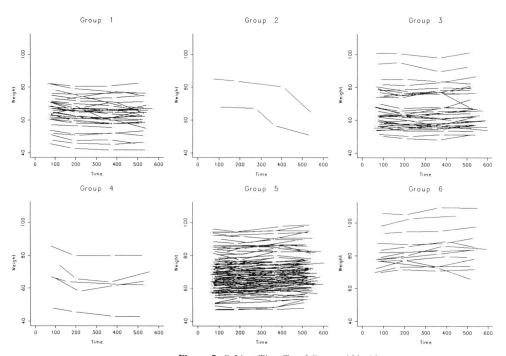

Figure 5. Subject Time Trend Curve within Cluster

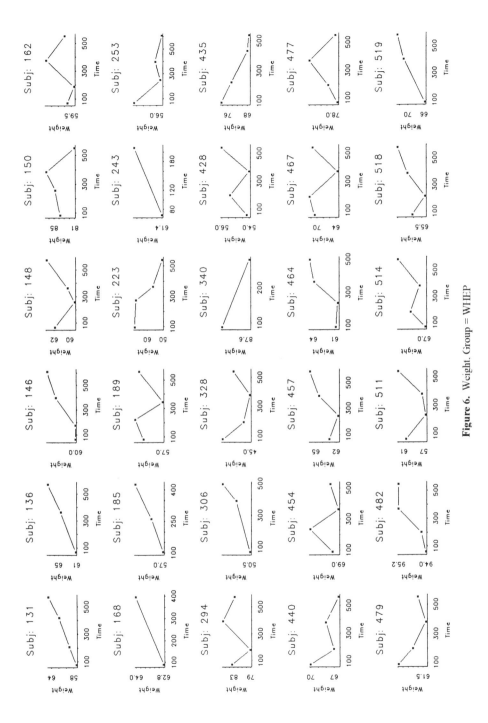

Figure 6. Weight. Group = WHEP

245

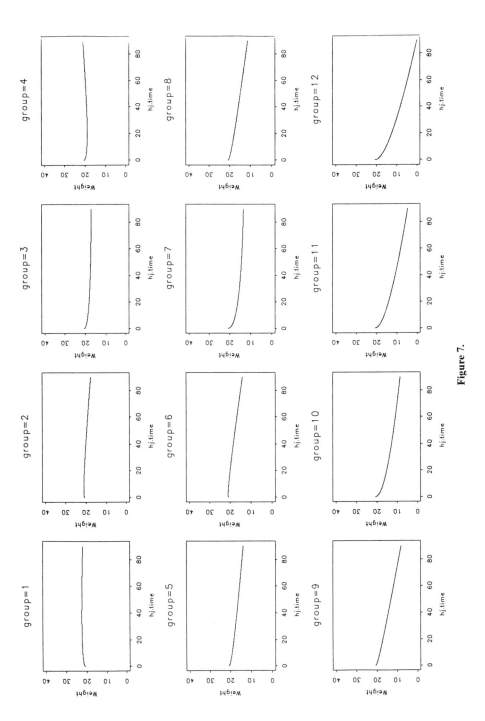

Figure 7.

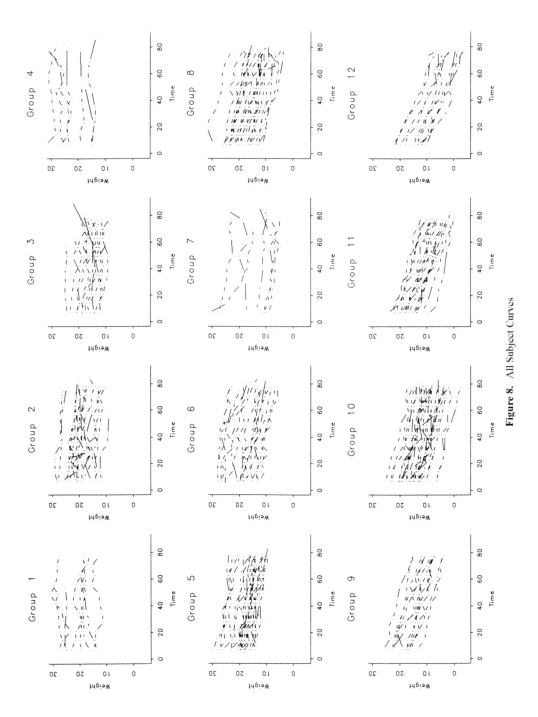

Figure 8. All Subject Curves

247

Table 3.

Outcome : Weight (DATASET=HE-JING)

Sample size : # of Subject=241, # of Observations=2447

Model : $Y_{it} = \alpha_0 + \alpha_1 X_{1i} + \alpha_2 X_{2i} + b_{1i}t_{it} + b_{2i}t_{it}^{1/2} + \epsilon_{it}$

where Y_{it} = (Weight-IBW)/IBW*100%
        X_{1i} = Gender
        X_{2i} = (WT0-IBW)/IBW*100%

$P(m= 9|data) = 9.72 \times 10^{-27}$
$P(m=10|data) = 8.94 \times 10^{-14}$
$P(m=11|data) = 1.05 \times 10^{-7}$
$P(m=12|data) = 0.99939$
$P(m=13|data) = 6.08 \times 10^{-4}$

Estimates :

$\alpha_0 = -1.665\ (0.284)$
$\alpha_1 = -0.753\ (0.083)$
$\alpha_2 = 1.018\ (0.008)$
$\phi = 0.736$

	$(b_{1i}, b_{2i}) =$		
	(-0.046, 0.558)	w.p.	0.034
	(-0.071, 0.355)	w.p.	0.087
	(0.035, -0.706)	w.p.	0.062
	(0.085, -0.763)	w.p.	0.042
	(-0.038, -0.374)	w.p.	0.151
	(-0.109, 0.319)	w.p.	0.114
	(0.052, -1.274)	w.p.	0.051
	(-0.066, -0.374)	w.p.	0.133
	(-0.103, -0.353)	w.p.	0.081
	(-0.008, -1.216)	w.p.	0.126
	(-0.039, -1.324)	w.p.	0.073
	(-0.067, -1.553)	w.p.	0.045

Table 4.

Comparison of Methods
Outcome : Weight (DATASET=HE-JING)

Model : $Y_{it} = \alpha_0 + \alpha_1 * X_{1i} + \alpha_2 * X_{2i} + b_{1i} * t_{it} + b_{2i} * t_{it}^{1/2} + \epsilon_{it}$

Parameters	Fixed Effect	Normal Random Effect	Robust Random Effect
α_0	-1.159(0.75)	-2.42 (0.61)	-1.665(0.28)
α_1	-1.223(0.169)	0.071(0.269)	-0.753(0.083)
α_2	0.983(0.016)	1.048(0.025)	1.018(0.008)
b_{1i}	-0.060(0.02)	-0.037(0.076)	-0.042(Mean)
b_{2i}	-0.344(0.24)	-0.549(0.084)	-0.509(Mean)
σ^2	11.93	0.99	1.36

what we are all seeing. Essentially, there are too many clusters--needlessly. All subjects are classified into one of the clusters.

Comments on the Theory

A review of several RCR models is to be published in *Statistics in Medicine* by C. Rutter and R.M. Elashoff under the title of "Analysis of Longitudinal Data: Random Coefficient Regression Modelling." The theory for the more general RCR model described in this paper is under development by Kwan-Moon Leung and R.M. Elashoff, where clustering of time trend curves receives emphasis.

In general, many RCR models are easily checked for validity by the developing methodology on model verification. The work of R.E. Weiss and R.D. Cook and was helpful to us. When an RCR model is appropriate, the estimators of the fixed effects is increased generally. Of course, the RCR models that permit clusters of subjects to be identified breaks new ground in the analysis of longitudinal data.

REFERENCES

Heber, D, Ashley ,J.M., McCarthy, W.J., Solares, M.E., Leaf, D.A., Chang, L.F., & Elashoff, R.M. (1992). Assessment of Adherence to a Low-Fat Diet for Breast Cancer Prevention. Preventive Medicine, 21, 218-227.

Krishnaiah, P.R. (1972). Multivariate Analysis-III. New York: Academic Press, Inc.

Rovine, M..J. & von Eye, A. (1991). Applied Computational Statistics in Longitudinal Research. San Diego: Academic Press, Inc.

Rutter, C.M. and Elashoff, R.M. Analysis of Longitudinal Data: Random Coefficient Regression Modelling. To appear in Statistical Science.

Srivastava, M.S. & Carter, E.M. (1983). An Introduction to Applied Multivariate Statistics. New York: Elsevier Science Publishing Co., Inc.

Sen, A. & Srivastava, M. (1990). Regression Analysis: Theory, Methods, and Applications. New York: Springer-Verlag.

Weiss, R.E. & Cook, R.D .(1992). A Graphical Case Statistic for Assessing Posterior Influence. Biometrika, 79, 51-55.

MULTILEVEL ANALYSIS IN OBESITY RESEARCH

David Rindskopf

City University of New York Graduate Center
33 West 42nd Street
New York, NY 10036

ABSTRACT

In obesity research it is common to have repeated measures on subjects. Traditional statistical analyses of repeated measures data are analysis of variance (ANOVA) for random effects, and multivariate analysis of variance (MANOVA). Each assume that every subject was measured (i) the same number of times, and (ii) at the same time points. Another typical complication of many research designs is the presence of time-varying covariates. The usual ANOVA approach to repeated measures does not allow such covariates, and the MANOVA approach usually treats them as dependent variables. Hierarchical linear models deal with all of the above issues in a natural manner, making them an important tool for obesity research. This paper discusses some simple hierarchical models, and shows their application using two real data sets.

INTRODUCTION

In a wide variety of research areas, including obesity research, study designs typically call for the collection of repeated measures data. In obesity research this would include not only outcome variables such as weight indices and body fat, but also concommitant physiological measures such as serum electrolytes. These may be treated as outcomes, or they may be treated as control or predictor variables for weight.

Traditional statistical analyses of repeated measures data are analysis of variance (ANOVA) for random effects, and multivariate analysis of variance (MANOVA). Each assume that every subject was measured (i) the same number of times, and (ii) at the same time points. Often, however, researchers are unable to implement such a design because of practical considerations concerning the inability to collect data on a large number of subjects at one time, or because subjects cannot adhere to the desired schedule.

Another typical complication of many research designs is the presence of time-varying covariates. The usual ANOVA approach to repeated measures does not allow such covariates,

Obesity Treatment, Edited by D.B. Allison
and F.X. Pi-Sunyer, Plenum Press, New York, 1995

and the MANOVA approach usually treats them as dependent variables.

The problems listed above would be enough to cause unhappiness with the traditional approaches, but they are mere technical problems. A more important issue is that the traditional methods focus on group behavior, because they analyze the mean (average) measurement of a group. A more interesting approach is to model the behavior of individuals, to characterize the course of their changes, and to then model the changes as a function of stable individual characteristics such as age, sex, personality traits, or treatment group. This approach involves (at least) two levels of analysis; first is the analysis of individual behavior over time, and second is the modeling of the time-course of behavior as a function of stable characteristics. Such methods are called multilevel (or hierarchical) statistical models.

Multilevel (or hierarchical) linear models provide a statistical approach to deal with all of the problems discussed above in a natural manner, making such models an important tool for obesity research. This paper discusses some simple hierarchical models, and shows their application using two real data sets.

OVERVIEW OF MULTILEVEL MODELS

We begin with the simplest possible design that will show the general principles involved. Suppose that body fat measures are available on a number of individuals, but the measurements are made a different number of times and at different time points for different individuals. Each person is measured over a period of several months during which they are following a treatment regimen, with the initial measurement coinciding with the start of treatment. For each person, the time since the beginning of treatment is available for each measurement (initial measures will thus be at time 0). (We will see that other choices are available for scaling the time variable, and may be preferable in some situations.)

Within-person (Observation-level) Model

Figure 1 shows the measurements for three subjects in the study. The horizontal axis

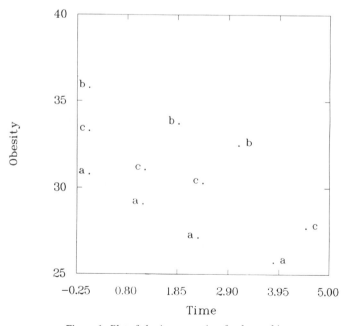

Figure 1. Plot of obesity versus time for three subjects.

is time from the initiation of treatment, and the vertical axis is the a measure of obesity, such as body mass index (BMI). Individuals are denoted by letters of the alphabet, so that all the points labelled "a", for example, refer to measurements made on the same person. For each person, his or her data can be fit rather well by a straight line. (Nonlinear data are common, and will be discussed later.) A straight line is commonly characterized by two numbers, an intercept and a slope, which we will denote as b_0 and b_1 respectively. Obviously people may have different intercepts and different slopes. To allow this in the statistical model, we will use the subscript j for individuals, so that the intercept and slope for individual j will be written as b_{0j} and b_{1j}.

As usual, in writing the statistical model for each person we will include a residual term, r_{ij}, to indicate that the outcome variable (here, body mass index) is not perfectly predictable by time of measurement. The within-person model developed thus far for individuals can be written:

$$y_{ij} = b_{0j} + b_{1j} t_{ij} + r_{ij} \qquad (1)$$

where y_{ij} is the body mass index of subject j on measurement occasion i, and t is the amount of time since the beginning of treatment. In this example, the intercept represents the body mass index of an individual at the beginning of the study, and the slope represents the rate of change in BMI per unit of time. The slope is a primary outcome measure in the next level of the analysis.

An important but subtle issue is that we do not <u>know</u> the intercepts and slopes for each individual, but can only <u>estimate</u> them from the (usually limited) data available. Therefore, there will be variation from person to person in our <u>sample</u> estimate of the slopes (and intercepts) even if the <u>population</u> values of the slopes (or intercepts) are the same for each individual. The statistical method used must be able to test whether there is true variation in the slopes and intercepts, over and above what is due to sampling variability.

If a straight line does not provide an accurate description of the change of an individual over time, typical methods can be used to improve the model. The best choice, when it works, is to transform the outcome variable (and/or the time measurement). Such a transformation is preferable because a straight line can still be fit, and the parameters of a straight line are easily interpretable. Another choice is to fit a polynomial model, such as a quadratic curve; the interpretation of the parameters of the model is more difficult in this case, but such a curve may be necessary to describe subjects who lose and then regain weight.

A third possibility is to fit a nonlinear model, such as a logistic or exponential curve, with non-zero asymptotes. In some cases this will be the most appropriate course of action. No new general principles are involved, but computer software for these models is not yet generally available.

Between-Person (Individual-level) Model.

As mentioned above, one of the first statistical tests we will do is to determine whether the observed variation in intercepts and slopes is greater than would be expected due to sampling variability. If this is the case, the next step is to develop models to explain the variation over individuals in their intercepts and slopes (although the slopes are probably most important from a substantive point of view). Differences among individuals may be accounted for by personal characteristics such as age, sex, race, blood type, treatment condition in an experiment, or personality traits. Notice that these are all time-invariant characteristics of individuals.

In our hypothetical example, consider what would be expected if rate of weight loss (the slope in the statistical model) were related to a personality trait such as locus of control. Figure 2 shows a possible outcome of plotting each person's slope on the vertical axis, and their score on a locus-of-control instrument on the horizontal axis. In this figure, locus of control is

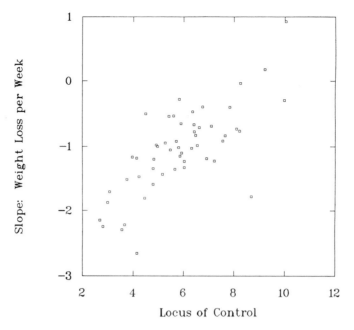

Figure 2. Plot of regression slopes versus locus of control.

assumed to be scaled so that (in spite of the location of the axes) the average score is zero.

In this figure, those with an internal locus of control (on the left) tend to lose weight at a higher rate than those with an external locus of control (on the right). The relationship between slopes and locus of control measurements is well-approximated by a straight line, which can be characterized by a slope and an intercept.

To put this into the context of a statistical model, a second type of equation is needed, in which the intercepts and slopes are modeled as functions of individual characteristics (in this case, locus of control). The between-person equations for this example are:

$$b_{0j} = g_{00} + g_{01} L_j + u_{0j} \tag{2}$$
$$b_{1j} = g_{10} + g_{11} L_j + u_{1j} \tag{3}$$

In these equations, the b_{0j} and b_{1j} are the same intercepts and slopes for individuals as in Equation (1). L_j is the locus of control score for individual j; the g_{ij} are regression coefficients; and the u_{ij} are residuals.

If the right-hand sides of Equations (2) and (3) are substituted for b_{0j} and b_{1j} in Equation (1), the result is a single equation for the complete model:

$$y_{ij} = g_{00} + g_{01}L_j + g_{10}t_{ij} + g_{11}L_jt_{ij} + u_{1j}t_{ij} + u_{0j} + r_{ij} \tag{4}$$

in which the g_{ij} are parameters in what are called the fixed effects part of the model, and the variance of r_{ij} and the variances and covariances among the u_{ij} are parameters for the random effects in the model. This representation is similar to what has been called a mixed model in the traditional analysis of variance literature, although early versions of the mixed model did not allow continuous variables as predictors.

The slope of the straight line describing the data in Figure 2 would be an estimate of g_{11}, and the intercept would be an estimate of g_{10}. What is the interpretation of these numbers? The intercept g_{10} is the predicted rate of BMI loss for a person who has a zero on the locus-of-control scale, and is (by virtue of the scaling of the scores) average on locus of control. The slope g_{11} is the predicted change in rate of BMI loss for each unit change on the locus of control scale.

Table 1. Simple Hierarchical Model for Body Mass Index as a Function of Time

---

FIXED EFFECT ESTIMATES:

	ESTIMATE	STANDARD ERR	T STATISTIC	p-VALUE
FOR INTERCEPT COEFFICIENT				
g_{00}	33.074055	.562405	58.808	.000
FOR TIME SLOPE				
g_{10}	-.898962	.091344	-9.841	.000

RANDOM EFFECT ESTIMATES:

PARAMETER	ESTIMATED PARAMETER VARIANCE	DEGREES OF FREEDOM	CHI SQUARE	P-VALUE
INTERCEPT	15.73548	52	873.03	.000
TIME SLOPE	.24328	52	561.27	.000

RELIABILITY ESTIMATES:

INTERCEPT	.924
TIME SLOPE	.448

Now it is obvious why locus of control was scaled so that its average was zero; if it had not been scaled, the intercepts g_{00} and g_{10} in Equations (2) and (3) would represent the intercept and slope of individuals with a score of zero on the locus of control scale. If a score of zero is not meaningful, then the estimates of g_{00} and g_{10} have no substantive interest. In the same vein, the measurement of time may be scaled so that a value of 0 indicates a certain amount of time after the beginning of treatment, rather than the beginning of treatment as we have done in this example.

Example 1: Obesity and QT Waves

A real example illustrating the use of these techniques was developed using data kindly provided by David Allison. A group of people undergoing treatment using a partial liquid diet were measured up to six times on a number of variables. Subjects varied on the number of measurements available and the timing of the measurements. Variables included measures of obesity; for these analyses body mass index (BMI) was used. Other variables were serum electrolytes (sodium, potassium, and calcium), and EKG measurements. For some analyses, an index involving the length of the QT segment on the EKG was used. For each person in the study time-invariant variables such as sex, race, and age were also recorded.

Analysis of Growth Patterns. The initial analyses investigate the status of BMI over time for each subject. While there is good reason to believe that using a straight line to summarize the growth or decline in BMI is not strictly correct for these data, we will do so to keep the discussion at a relatively simple level. For this simple model, Equation (1) has the form discussed in the previous section, while Equations (2) and (3) have no predictor variables on the right-hand side:

$$b_{0j} = g_{00} + u_{0j} \tag{5}$$
$$b_{1j} = g_{10} + u_{1j} \tag{6}$$

These equations indicate that the intercepts (b_{0j}) and slopes (b_{1j}) vary across individuals, but no individual-level predictors (such as race, sex, or age) are used to account for this variation.

The results of fitting this model are displayed in Table 1, which shows some of the (edited) output from the computer program HLM. The first section of the table displays the

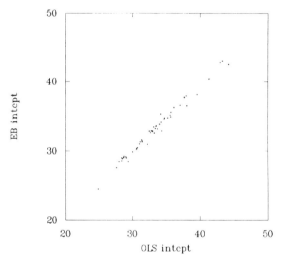

Figure 3. Model: BMI = b0 + b1 Time. Estimated true (EB) intercepts versus observed (OLS) intercepts for model of body mass index (BMI) as a function of time.

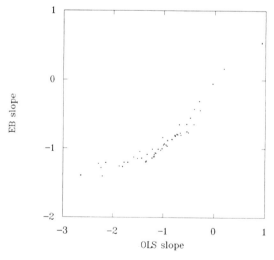

Figure 4. Model: BMI = b0 + b1 Time. Estimated true (EB) slopes versus observed (OLS) slopes for models of body mass index (BMI) as a function of time.

fixed effect results. The most important finding is that g_{10} is significantly different from zero. This means that, on average, there is a change in BMI over time. Since time is measured in months, the change is a loss of about .90 in BMI per month, so on average the subjects are losing weight. The estimated value of g_{00}, 33.07, is the average value of BMI at time 0, which is the beginning of treatment.

Of course, there is variability from person to person in the initial value of BMI, as well as in the rate of weight loss (slope). The reliability estimates in the table are the proportion of the observed variation in the intercept and slope that are true variation, rather than due to sampling fluctuations. For the intercept the reliability is rather high, while for the slopes it is rather modest. To illustrate this point, Figure 3 shows the plot of estimated true intercepts (labelled EB, which stands for Empirical Bayes, on the plot) versus observed intercepts (labelled OLS, for Ordinary Least Squares, on the plot), while Figure 4 shows a similar plot for slopes. The observed values come from doing a simple regression for each person of their BMI measurements versus time. Figure 3 shows that the true intercepts are not very different from the observed intercepts.

However, in Figure 4 the observed slopes range from near -3 to about 1, while the estimated true slopes range only from about -1.5 to .5. This "shrinkage" is due to the relatively low reliability of the estimated slopes.

The Random Effects section of Table 1 provides estimates of the true (rather than observed) variability in the intercepts, and tests of whether these are significantly different from zero. The estimated true variance of the intercepts is 15.73; the square root of this value, 3.97, is the estimated standard deviation of the intercepts. The estimated true varince of the slopes is .24328; the estimated standard deviation is therefore .49. Rounding off slightly, we estimate that an approximate 95 percent confidence interval for the slopes (rate of weight loss) is -.90 plus or minus 2(.5), or from -1.9 to .1.

The hypothesis test shows that the variability of both slopes and intercepts are significantly greater than zero, so the possibility exists to explain some of this variation in terms of individual characteristics. The results of an exploratory analysis displayed in Table 2 help in the search for variables that might explain why people have different slopes and intercepts.

Three possible predictors were used in the exploratory analysis: WHITE is coded 1 for whites, 0 for nonwhites; MALE is coded 1 for males, 0 for females; and AGE is age in years. For this analysis the estimates of the residuals u_{0j} and u_{1j} in Equations (2) and (3) are regressed on the potential predictors WHITE, MALE, and AGE. The results show that the only value close to being significant is the effect of race (WHITE) on the slope b_{1j}. In other words, it may be that whites and nonwhites differ in their rate of weight loss, with whites losing at a faster rate (i.e., their slope is more negative than for nonwhites)

To test more precisely the effect of race on weight loss, a model was fit in which the variable WHITE was included on the right-hand side of an equation like (3):

$$b_{1j} = g_{10} + g_{11} W_j + u_{1j} \tag{7}$$

Table 2. Exploratory Analysis for Simple Hierarchical Model of Body Mass Index

	WHITE	MALE	AGE
INTERCEPT	.359	-.203	.052
S. E.	1.191	1.192	.044
T VALUE	.301	-.170	1.169
	WHITE	MALE	AGE
TIME SLOPE	-.208	.051	.002
S. E.	.110	.113	.004
T VALUE	-1.893	.451	.510

Table 3. Modified Hierarchical Model for BMI as a Function of Time

FIXED EFFECT ESTIMATES:

	ESTIMATE	STANDARD ERROR	T STATISTIC	p-VALUE
FOR INTERCEPT				
g_{00}	33.081470	.562307	58.832	.000
FOR TIME SLOPE				
g_{10}	-.652645	.157525	-4.143	.000
g_{11}	-.352591	.190519	-1.851	.073

RANDOM EFFECT ESTIMATES:

PARAMETER	ESTIMATED PARAMETER VARIANCE	DEGREES OF FREEDOM	CHI SQUARE	P-VALUE
INTERCEPT	15.73538	52	876.05	.000
TIME SLOPE	.22526	51	416.31	.000

RELIABILITY ESTIMATES:

INTERCEPT	.924
TIME SLOPE	.430

The results, shown in Table 3, are that the effect is not quite significant at the .05 level. As the analysis was based on 53 people, the power may not have been enough to detect a difference. The estimate of g_{10} shows that nonwhites had a rate of loss of BMI of about .65 per month, while g_{11} indicates that the rate for whites was greater than that for nonwhites by .35, for a total rate of about 1.00 per month for whites.

Analysis of Within-Individual Relationships

Another important aspect of this study was the relationship between EKG measurements (in particular, the length of the QT segment) and weight (as measured here by body mass index). A traditional approach might be to compute the correlation between length of QT segment and BMI. Because there are several measurements for each person, we might only want to use one (say the first) from each person to avoid the problem of dependence among observations. In this data set, the correlation between QT (adjusted for RR interval) and BMI, both measured at baseline, is .34. Therefore we can say that heavier people have longer QT intervals, but this tells us nothing about what might happen to the length of the QT segment for an individual whose weight changes. To address this issue we must have several measurements on each person as the person's weight changes. Hierarchical linear models provide a natural framework to model this relationship within individuals, and to see how the relationship varies across people.

Figure 5 shows a plot of adjusted QT interval versus BMI for a single individual. The relationship appears to be slightly positive; the correlation for this subject is .22. A regression line through the points for this (and every other) individual would have an intercept and a slope.

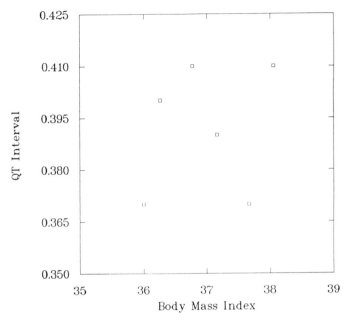

Figure 5. Adjusted QT interval versus body mass index (BMI) for a single individual measured six times.

The statistical model for individuals is written in a form similar to Equation (1), but now BMI rather than TIME is the predictor variable:

$$QT_{ij} = b_{0j} + b_{1j} BMI_{ij} + r_{ij} \qquad (8)$$

In this equation, $\underline{i}$ represents the occasion of measurement, and $\underline{j}$ represents the subject. Each individual is characterized by an intercept (b_{0j}) and slope (b_{1j}).

The simplest between-individual equations would be Equations (5) and (6) described above. The coefficient g_{10} is the most important parameter of this part of the model, because if it differs from zero then changes in BMI are related to changes in QT interval <u>within an individual</u>. Another important parameter is the variance of u_{1j}. If it is significantly greater than zero, then the relationship between BMI and QT interval varies across individuals.

The results of fitting this model are presented in Table 4. The estimates of the fixed components have only one interesting part, the test of g_{10}. This is nearly significant at the .05 level, and we will treat it as significant for purposes of discussion. The value of 1.19 for the estimate of this parameter indicates that when an individual's BMI changes by 1 unit, the length of the (adjusted) QT segment increases by 1.19. Because of the scaling used for QT (it was multiplied by 1000), this is a very small amount. In contrast with the usual between-person correlation and regression coefficients, this tells us what happens <u>within an individual</u> as he or she changes in weight.

The reliability estimates for both the intercept and slope indicate that most variability across individuals is sampling error. Even so, the random effects part of the table shows that the true variability in the intercepts (but not the slopes) differs from zero. The variance of the slope estimates is 3.614; the standard deviation is the square root of this, or about 1.90. If the slopes were normally distributed, we would expect about 95 percent of the true slopes to be between 1.19 - 2(1.9) = -2.61 and 1.19 + 2(1.9) = 5.01.

Figure 6 plots the estimated true slopes versus the observed slopes for individuals. The range of the observed slopes is much greater than the range of the estimated true slopes, confirming the low reliability of the slope estimates. The probable reason for this is that EKG

Table 4. Simple Hierarchical Model for QT Interval as a Function of BMI.

FIXED EFFECT ESTIMATES:

	ESTIMATE	STANDARD ERROR	T STATISTIC	p-VALUE
FOR INTERCEPT				
g_{00}	2.387543	3.224324	.740	.301
FOR BMI SLOPE				
g_{10}	1.194676	.582405	2.051	.051

RANDOM EFFECT ESTIMATES:

PARAMETER	ESTIMATED PARAMETER VARIANCE	DEGREES OF FREEDOM	CHI SQUARE	P-VALUE
INTERCEPT	252.80432	49	86.934	.001
BMI SLOPE	3.61387	49	52.864	.327

RELIABILITY ESTIMATES:

INTERCEPT	.088
BMI SLOPE	.047

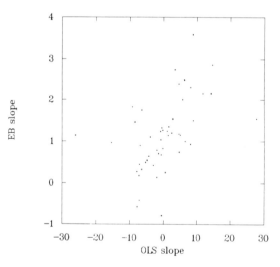

Figure 6. Model: QT = b0 + b1 BMI

measurements were not taken as often as weight, so there are fewer values for each subject in this analysis than there were in the previous analysis. The estimated true slopes range from about -1 to 4, which is slightly narrower than large-sample normal theory led us to expect.

The exploratory analysis in Table 5 reveals that gender (but not race or age) may account for a significant amount of variability in the intercepts. The obvious next step would

Table 5. Simple Hierarchical Model for QT Interval as a Function of BMI: Exploratory Analysis

	MALE	WHITE	AGE
INTERCEPT	-12.695	-3.434	-.055
S. E.	3.235	3.660	.139
T VALUE	-3.924	-.938	-.399

	MALE	WHITE	AGE
BMI SLOPE	.384	.257	-.001
S. E.	.263	.266	.010
T VALUE	1.462	.968	-.050

be to add gender to Equation (5) as a predictor of the intercept. The resulting equation is:

$$b_{0j} = g_{00} + g_{01} \text{ MALE}_j + u_{0j} \tag{9}$$

The parameter g_{01} is significantly different from zero, as predicted by the exploratory analysis, and shows that the adjusted QT interval for males is lower than that for females. An additional interesting finding is that g_{10} is now significantly different from zero, and has approximately the same value as in the previous model, so that as BMI decreases, the adjusted QT interval also decreases.

Example 2: Comparison of Weight-Loss Treatments

This example uses data kindly provided by Darlington (1993) from her dissertation work. Subjects were put on one of two treatment regimens for weight loss, and were measured weekly for up to 12 weeks. Not all people attended all 12 sessions, however, so the data are incomplete. Only a small number of variables from Darlington's study will be used here. One of Darlington's hypotheses dealt with a possible interaction between eating style and the effectiveness of different kinds of treatment. Here, the restraint measure from an instrument developed by Stunkard and Messick will be used to demonstrate how to assess such interactions.

For this model, the observation-level equation is exactly like Equation (1), with weight being the outcome variable, and time (here, in weeks) the only predictor. In the example using Allison's data, weight was already adjusted for height by using the body mass index, while here a different technique will be used: height will be entered as a predictor (control) variable in the individual-level equations.

The predictors in the individual-level equations include height (H), a dummy variable for treatment group (G), score on the restraint scale (R), and the product of group and restraint (GR), to represent an interaction. The resulting equations are:

$$b_{0j} = g_{00} + g_{01} G_j + g_{02} R_j + g_{03} (GR)_j + g_{04} H_j + u_{0j} \tag{9}$$
$$b_{1j} = g_{10} + g_{11} G_j + g_{12} R_j + g_{13} (GR)_j + g_{14} H_j + u_{1j} \tag{10}$$

The results of fitting this model are presented in Table 6. The nonsignificance of the effect of group on the intercept (g_{01}) indicates that the groups did not differ in weight (adjusted for height) at the start of the study. The significant interaction (g_{03}) indicates that the relationship between initial weight and restraint was different in the two treatment groups. Because subjects were randomly assigned, this means either that randomization did not work, or that subjects differentially dropped out of the two groups as a function of their level of restraint. While we will not do so here, the matter can be decided on the basis of additional analyses.

Table 6. Hierarchical Model for Darlington Data, with Weight as a Function of Time

FIXED EFFECT ESTIMATES:

	ESTIMATE	STANDARD ERROR	T STATISTIC	p-VALUE
FOR INTERCEPT				
INTERCEPT	172.642957	6.649304	25.964	.000
HEIGHT	2.990012	1.136981	2.630	.009
GROUP	.916020	6.818901	.134	.894
RESTRAIN	-1.786823	1.175330	-1.520	.128
GxR	3.369513	1.600298	2.106	.035
FOR WEEK SLOPE				
INTERCEPT	-.784360	.185655	-4.225	.000
HEIGHT	-.024534	.033001	-.743	.457
GROUP	.267444	.189054	1.415	.157
RESTRAIN	-.019082	.041212	-.463	.643
GxR	.071033	.055960	1.269	.205

RANDOM EFFECT ESTIMATES:

PARAMETER VALUE	ESTIMATED PARAMETER VARIANCE	DEGREES OF FREEDOM	CHI SQUARE	P-
INTERCEPT	1087.96887	62	8090.6	.000
WEEK SLOPE	.24998	62	119.53	.000

RELIABILITY ESTIMATES:

INTERCEPT	.989
WEEK SLOPE	.179

Using strict significance testing, we find that subjects lost weight at a rate of about .78 pounds per week, which did not differ by group or level of restraint. In particular, the hypothesized group by restraint interaction did not occur. However, both the group effect and the group by restraint interaction were substantively large enough to wonder whether a larger sample size (67 people had enough data to be included in the analysis) would have detected an effect.

DISCUSSION

This paper has emphasized the use and interpretation of the hierarchical linear model, and because of space limitations has given less prominence to measurement considerations. For example, different measures of obesity (weight, body mass index, percent body fat) may produce different results in the same statistical analysis. In the data provided by Allison, different adjustments of the QT interval may give different results.

An important consideration for obesity studies is attrition from treatment. If such attrition is related to final status or progress in treatment, then the estimate of treatment impact will be biased. For example, if those who do not lose weight drop out, then the effect of treatment will be overestimated. In a study such as Darlington's, if one treatment is more onerous than another, causing differential attrition, then the estimate of the relative effectiveness of the treatments will be biased.

At each level of the hierarchical model, limitations exist on the number of predictor variables that can be included. If an individual is measured three times, then at most three predictor variables (including an intercept) can be fit in an equation such as (1), and only two predictor variables if an estimate of within-person variation is needed. Therefore, an important design consideration in this type of study is not just the number of subjects to include (which determines the accuracy with which the between-person effects can be estimated), but the number of measurement occasions for each subject. Good information on statistical power is not yet available for these designs.

A related issue is that for analyses such as was done relating QT intervals to obesity, subjects must vary over time on the variables used as predictors in the within-person equation. If not, the parameters of the model (intercept and slopes) cannot be estimated. If variation is small, then one or more parameters cannot be estimated accurately (the standard error will be large).

The exposition presented here has been at an introductory level, with no discussion of many technical issues involved in multilevel modeling. More details on the approach suggested here and related methods can be found in Bryk and Raudenbush (1992), Goldstein (1987), Gornbein, Lazaro, and Little (1992), and Willett (1988). These sources, in turn, contain further references of interest.

The analyses reported here were conducted using the computer program HLM (Bryk, Raudenbush, Seltzer, & Congdon, 1988). In this program, the model is specified as in Equations (1)-(3). Two other programs specifically written for hierarchical linear models are ML2 (or ML3 for three-level data) by Harvey Goldstein, and VARCL by Nick Longford. Some newer programs for mixed linear models, such as BMDP Program 5V and SAS PROC MIXED can be used to fit these models. BMDP 5V and PROC MIXED can also fit a variety of other models, including various patterns of correlated residuals for time-structured data.

The reader may wonder why such complicated computer programs are needed for these analyses when conceptually it would seem possible to use standard packages. For example, one might fit a regression for each person, and use the estimated regression coefficients as dependent variables in the individual-level analysis. This method would ignore sampling variability of the parameter estimates in the equations for individuals; this is especially a problem when (i) there are few measurements on each individual, as was the case in both examples used here, (ii) the number of measurements varies from individual to individual, or (iii) the range of the predictor variables in the within-person equation varies from person to person, resulting in different standard errors for different people. The use of generalized least squares (GLS) instead of ordinary least squares (OLS) can be an effective solution, but this may be more difficult for most people to do than using one of the specialized packages such as HLM.

REFERENCES

Bryk, A. S., Raudenbush, S. W. (1992) Hierarchical linear models: Applications and data analysis methods. Newbury Park, CA: Sage Publications.

Bryk, A. S., Raudenbush, S. W., Seltzer, M., & Congdon, R. (1988) An introduction to HLM: Computer program and user's guide (2nd ed.). Chicago: University of Chicago Department of Education.

Darlington, D. (1992) Weight loss as a funtion of treatment and personality variables. Unpublished dissertation proposal, CUNY Graduate Center.

Goldstein, H. (1987) Multilevel models in educational and social research. New York: Oxford University Press.

Gornbein, J. A., Lazaro, C. G., & Little, R. J. A. (1992) Incomplete data in repeated measures analysis. Statistical methods in medical research, 1, 275-295.

Willett, J. B. (1988). Questions and answers in the measurement of change. In E. Z. Rothkopf (ed.), <u>Review of research in education 15</u> (pp. 345-422). Washington, DC: American Educational Research Association.

CONTRIBUTORS

David B. Allison
N.Y. Obesity Research Center
St. Luke's/Roosevelt Hospital
Columbia University College of Physicians &
  Surgeons

Teis Andersen
Hvidovre Hospital
University of Copenhagen

Per Björntorp
University of Göteborg

Claude Bouchard
Physical Activity Sci. Lab., PEPS
Laval University

George Bray
Pennington Biomedical Research Center
Louisiana State University

L. Arthur Campfield
Hoffman LaRoche, Inc.

Lindon Eaves
Dept. of Human Genetics
Medical College of Virginia

Robert M. Elashoff
UCLA School of Medicine
Dept of Biomathematics

Cheryl N. Engel
N. Y. Obesity Research Center
St. Luke's/Roosevelt Hospital
Columbia University College of Physicians &
  Surgeons

Leonard H. Epstein
Dept. of Psychology
State University of New York at Buffalo

J. P. Flatt
Dept. of Biochemistry
University of Mass. Medical School

John P. Foreyt
Baylor College of Medicine
Nutrition Research Clinic

Gary M. Foster
School of Medicine
Weight and Eating Disorders Program
University of Pennsylvania

David Garner
Department of Psychiatry
Michigan State University

John S. Garrow
Dept. of Human Nutrition
Saint Bartholmew's Hospital Medical
  College

Steven M Haffner
University of Texas Health Science Center
  at San Antonio
Division of Clinical Epidemiology
Department of Medicine

Stanley Heshka
N.Y. Obesity Research Center
St. Luke's/Roosevelt Hospital
Columbia University College of Physicians &
  Surgeons

Steven B. Heymsfield
N.Y. Obesity Research Center
St. Luke's/Roosevelt HospitalColumbia
University College of Physicians & Surgeons

James O. Hill
University of Colorado Health Sciences
    Center
Center for Human Nutrition

Jean M. Jayo
Wake Forest University
The Bowman Gray School of Medicine

Shiriki Kumanyika
Pennsylvania State University
College of Medicine
Center for Biostatistics and Epidemiology

J. J. McArdle
Dept. of Psychology
University of Virginia

Michael C. Neale
Dept. of Human Genetics
Medical College of Virginia

F. Xavier Pi-Sunyer
N.Y. Obesity Research Center
St. Luke's/Roosevelt Hospital
Columbia University College of Physicians &
    Surgeons

Andrew M. Prentice
Dunn Clinical Nutrition Center

R. Arlen Price
Behavioral Genetics Laboratory
University of Pennsylvania

David M. Rindskopf
Education Psychology Program
City University of New York Graduate
    Center

Barbara J. Rolls
Program in Biobehavioral Health
Pennsylvania State University

Joseph S. Rossi
Cancer Prevention Research Center
University of Rhode Island

Lars Sjostrom
University of Goteborg
Department of Medicine I
Sahlgrenska Hospital

Thorkild I. A. Sorensen
MRC Professor, Dr. Med. Sci
Institute of Preventive Medicine
Copenhagen Health Services
Municipal Hospital of Copenhagen

Albert J. Stunkard
University of Pennsylvania

Theodore B. Van Itallie
Prof. Emeritus of Medicine
N.Y. Obesity Research Center
St. Luke's/Roosevelt Hospital
Columbia University College of Physicians &
    Surgeons

Thomas A. Wadden
Dept of Psychology
Syracuse University

G. Terrance Wilson
GSAPP
Rutgers University

Rena R. Wing
University of Pittsburgh School of Medicine
Western Psychiatric Institute and Clinic

Susan C. Wooley
Psychiatry Department
University of Cincinnati Medical College

INDEX

Carbohydrates (*cont.*)
oxidation of, 143, 148
corticosterone-related increase, 155, 156
relationship to carbohydrate availability,
147
relationship to dietary fat intake, 157
relationship to glycogen reserves, 147
two-compartment model of, 147–149
reserves of, 145, 147
Carbohydrate-to-fat ratio, 144, 145, 152
effect of alcohol on, 157
Cardiovascular disease
abdominal body fat distribution as risk predictor
of, 71–74
body mass index as risk predictor of, 4, 6, 9–10,
11, 12, 47–48
Metropolitan Relative Weight and, 5
weight cycling as risk factor for, 49
Carleton, Richard, 76
Catecholamine metabolites, obesity-related cerebrospinal fluid content of, 208
Caucasian-American women, ideal body image of,
79
Celebrities, weight regain by, 36
Cerebrovascular disease (stroke)
age-adjusted decrease, 18
effect of weight loss on, 46, 47
relationship to body mass index, 8–9
relationship to waist-to-hip ratio, 72
Change
motivational readiness for, 97–98
paradigm shifts in, 76–77
Child neglect, as adult obesity risk factor, 123
Children, obesity in
behavioral economics treatment of, 113–119
activity patterns, 116–117
eating behavior changes, 116
theoretical background, 113–115
prevention of, 90
relationship to parental obesity, 219, 220
Chocolate "addicts", 134
Choice, behavioral theories of, *see* Behavioral economics
Cholelithiasis, weight loss-related increase, 25
Cholesterol levels, *see also* Hyperlipidemia; Hypertriglyceridemia
effect of weight loss on, 24
Cloning, positional, 221
Code of Federal Regulations, Title 21, 29
Coenzyme A, in pyruvate oxidation, 149
Computed tomography (CT), for visceral body fat
distribution measurement, 71, 73
Confirmatory factor analysis, 236
Consciousness raising, 99
Cook, R.D., 248–249
Coping strategies, for weight maintenance, 114,
186
problem-solving skills as, 107, 108
Coronary heart disease
age-adjusted decrease, 18
gender differences in, 211

Coronary heart disease (*cont.*)
morbidity increase in, 18
mortality ratio by Metropolitan Relative Weight,
5
relationship to body mass index, 4, 7, 8–10, 11,
12
weight cycling-related risk increase, 49
weight loss-related risk decrease, 46, 47
Corticosterone, effect on macronutrient balance,
155, 156
Corticotropin-releasing hormone, obesity-related
cerebrospinal fluid content of, 208
Counterconditioning, 99–100
Cultural factors
definition, 79
in perception of ideal body shape and weight,
37, 79–82
in weight loss treatment, 76

Daily weighing, as weight maintenance technique,
105
Danish Adoption Study, 123, 125
Demographic factors, as weight loss treatment outcome predictors, 191, 192
Depression
dieting-related, 30
fenfluramine-related, 177
effect on weight loss, 185
Developing countries, obesity-socioeconomic
status relationships in, 80, 122
Developmental process, as weight loss factor, 107,
108
Dexfenfluramine
carbohydrate intake effects of, 167–168
cardiovascular effects of, 169–170
central nervous system effects of, 170–171
clinical trials of, 177
insulin sensitivity effects of, 169
for smoking cessation-related weight gain prevention, 171
Dextroamphetamine, 176
Diabetes
intermittent caloric restriction therapy for,
165
hyperandrogenicity treatment in, 207
effect of modest weight loss on, 37
non-insulin dependent, relationship to body fat
distribution, 65–69
relationship to body mass index, 4, 7–8, 12
Diagnostic and Statistical Manual-IV, binge eating
disorder diagnostic criteria of, 184
Dietary restraint, as weight loss treatment outcome
predictor, 184, 200
Dieters, eating habits of, 108, 109
Diet industry, 27, 77
Dieting
adverse effects of, 27, 29–30, 32
public opinion regarding, 36
by African-American women, 80
alternatives to, 28–29, 31–32